TRANSCULTURAL RESEARCH
IN MENTAL HEALTH

Transcultural Research in Mental Health

Volume II of *Mental Health Research in Asia and the Pacific*

EDITED BY
WILLIAM P. LEBRA

AN EAST-WEST CENTER BOOK
THE UNIVERSITY PRESS OF HAWAII   1972

Contents

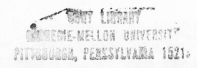

Preface

THE PAPERS in this volume were presented at a conference, Social Change and Cultural Factors in Mental Health, held at the East-West Center, University of Hawaii, during the week of March 17–21, 1969. That conference and this volume are second in a series of four planned in conjunction with the Program on Culture and Mental Health in Asia and the Pacific. The background on the origin of the Program, the commonly-felt need for its creation, and its progress and development have been detailed in the preceding volume (Caudill and Lin, 1969) and in the Program's *Newsletter* (Lebra, Editor). Suffice it to say at this point, the Program is both international—encompassing East Asia and Western Pacific—and interdisciplinary—including the fields of psychiatry, psychology, anthropology, sociology, and linguistics. Funding, provided by the East-West Center, the University of Hawaii, and the National Institute of Mental Health (Grant #MH09243), is gratefully acknowledged.

The conference reported on here was planned by my colleagues, Drs. Robert I. Levy and Thomas W. Maretzki, and myself. It was our intention to maintain the high standards established by Drs. Caudill and Lin in the first conference, to provide broad regional coverage, and to include significant new research. At the same time, we were desirous of developing a more focused program goal which might allow for some degree of coherence in an assemblage so diverse in terms of disciplines and nationalities. Whether we succeeded or not will be left for the reader to judge in the following pages. We are confident from the comments that the participants gained new insights, new breadth, and new colleagues for further research and interchange. It was also our intention that in this conference the number of Asian participants would be equal to or greater than the number of Western. We further hoped that each presentation would stimulate open and free discussion. Although each paper was read in full, copies were provided for all the listeners, thereby obviating translingual communication problems. Approximately equal time was given to formal presentation and informal discussion exchange. Most gratifying to all, I believe, was the fact that this conference did not follow the path frequently taken at similar international meetings where a few monopolize nearly all discussion. This was precluded by the great skill exercised by Dr. Levy as moderator and by, among others, the five discussants—Dr. Howard Blane, Harvard University; Dr. Raymond Firth, London School of Economics; Dr. Alexander Leighton, Harvard University; Dr. Chutikul Saisuree, Chulalongkorn University; and Professor Carmen Santiago, Maryknoll College. In addition, Drs. Richard H. Williams, Ben Locke, and Martin Katz of the National Institute of Mental Health contributed much by their participation. The lively discussions following each presentation, although tape-recorded, unfortunately could not be included here because their length would have entailed a second volume, while severe editing would have done gross injustice to the spontaneity which obtained. Special appreciation should be accorded Dr. Leighton for his Herculean task in presenting a final summation during the last hours of the conference.

Following the conference, most of the participants revised (and often lengthened) their papers, in a few cases almost completely. Some of the papers were edited quite extensively, largely to conform in style and length with the others. Like my predecessors, Caudill and Lin, I have refrained from the temptation of adding comments or interpretation. Two of the participants unfortunately did not submit their papers for inclusion; a third paper was dropped as not research-relevant. Although each of the papers contained in this volume has been read by me several times over, since early March of 1969, it was not until July 1970 that there was opportunity to spend an uninterrupted week solely devoted to the manuscript. This took place at a small hotel in a Japanese resort town. It might have been that the discomfort caused by typing while seated on the floor sharpened my awareness, but in arranging the sequence of papers, I was somewhat overwhelmed by the disparity. At one extreme are the efforts from some of the developing areas where mental health research is still in infancy and where even the prevalence of psychiatric disorders may be unknown in the absence of basic census material. At the opposite extreme are the messages emanating from some representatives of the more developed areas; these form a single theme, that time is running out and if we do not quickly learn to understand and control ourselves, the obvious result will be an early extermination of all mankind. I can only reflect that these seeming disparities accurately depict the present scene and to note that our hope was to bridge a gap, to establish communication, and to understand.

William P. Lebra

Honolulu, Hawaii
December, 1970

PROBLEMS OF DEVELOPMENT

1. Prospects of Psychiatric Research in a Multiracial Developing Community: West Malaysia

ENG-SEONG TAN, M.B.B.S., C.P.M.

Department of Psychological Medicine
University of Malaya
Kuala Lumpur, Malaysia

Ethnic Composition and Cultural Background

West Malaysia has a population of approximately nine million people. About fifty percent of the population are of Malay or Indonesian extraction, thirty-five percent of Chinese extraction, and less than fifteen percent of Indian, Ceylonese, or Pakistani descent. A very small proportion of the people includes a large variety of ethnic groups including Eurasians, Europeans, Arabs, Filipinos, Australians, etc. Until very recently most of the ethnic groups were socially isolated from each other, although they lived contiguously, and even now there is limited social intercourse between the ethnic groups. Intermarriages are few and far between. There is a rather distinct, although by no means exclusive, rural-urban distribution of the main ethnic groups. Before independence in 1957, the Malays were largely a rural people, whereas the Chinese and the majority of the Indians were urban. Thus, there were fairly distinct differences in the economic levels and the social positions achieved by members of the various ethnic groups. Although the royal families in each of the Malay states have been Malays, most Malays before independence were economically depressed and held rather lowly social positions. Most of the wealthy sections of the population were either Europeans or Chinese who also formed the bulk of the commercial community, while many positions in the civil service and the professions were held by people of Indian extraction. Since independence, however, the government has initiated many programs to provide more opportunity for education and social advancement for the economically deprived Malays. This has at times raised outraged protests of discrimination from the non-Malay sections of the population, but on the whole the programs have helped create a more equitable distribution of wealth in the country.

From the linguistic point of view, West Malaysia with its poly-ethnic population is in many respects a veritable Tower of Babel. There are many local variations in the Malay language, and indeed there are not a few dialects among the isolated communities on the east coast of the peninsula. Nor are the Chinese a linguistically homogenous group. Most of the Chinese in the country are immigrants, or descendants of immigrants, from the south coastal provinces of China. Although Hokkien (Fukkienese) and Cantonese are the two chief dialects spoken, there are in fact eight distinct dialects in common use in West Malaysia. In the last two decades or so, a ninth dialect, Mandarin, which became the national language of republican China in the earlier part of this century, took on common usage among the younger generation of the Chinese population because of the rise in the literacy rate of the Chinese who were taught Mandarin in schools. Although Tamil is the most common among the Indian languages, the Indian community in the country is by no means homogenous. The Tamils who come from Madras are the most numerous, but there is also a large group of Malayalams who come from that region in southern India which now forms the state of Kerala. There are also the northern Indians, some of whom are from the states of Bengal and Punjab; most of the Punjabis are Sikhs. The interesting historical note to make at this point is that most of these Indian language or Chinese dialectal groups migrated to West Malaysia, or were taken there by the British colonial government, each to play a very specific role in the early development of the country. The Cantonese and the Hakkas went into the country mainly as tin miners. The Hokkiens arrived as businessmen to run small grocery stores or large rice import agencies. Most of the Tamils were brought as laborers for the rubber estates, the Malayalams as clerks in the rubber estates, and the Sikhs as members of the local police force. Even as late as the years just before World War II, the railroads in Malaya were almost exclusively manned by Ceylon Tamils. In the last two decades the distinctions between these traditional roles of the various ethnic groups in the country have blurred because of increasing educational opportunities which permit greater competition for jobs in the various fields.

Until 1967, ten years after independence, the official language used in administration was English. Notwithstanding this, the government supported, and still supports, schools which are, to use local terminology, in the four language systems, meaning that the medium of instruction in these schools may be in English, Malay, Chinese, or Tamil. Since independence, a national language, the Bahasa Kebangsaan Malaysia (Malay) has been introduced and is now being taught in all the schools. It has become since

1967 the official language of the government, although English is still widely used. There is a program to increase the usage of this language as the medium of instruction in all schools. To my mind, this will obliterate, to some extent, the cultural differences that now exist between one ethnic group and another in the country. A great debate is going on, albeit at an intellectual level, as to whether the process of cultural development should be one of integration of the elements of the four major cultural groups into a common Malaysian culture or assimilation into the Malay culture. Whatever the outcome, and even more essentially, whatever the trend of development itself, the result, although it may be politically desirable, will significantly obscure the distinction between the ethnic and cultural groups. The opportunity for studying the process of cultural change and its implication for mental health should be utilized before it is too late. Though some differences will still persist, as has been demonstrated by Glaser and Moynihan (1963) in New York City, the cultures may no longer exist in relatively pure form as they do now. The cross-cultural dimension of any study will then be somewhat vitiated.

Economic Development

Besides the cultural changes that are taking place, there are programs for far-reaching economic changes. Hitherto, the economy of the country has depended on the production of two commodities, rubber and tin, the prices of which are not at all stable. The government has brought into being programs in education, industrialization, etc., which it hopes will expand the economy rapidly and improve the standard of living in the country. As much as a third of the national budget annually is allocated for education. Foreign investments are very much encouraged in an effort to expand industrial resources and income. However, in spite of all these efforts, unemployment remains a major problem. Moreover, the population is increasing rather rapidly although family planning has been introduced recently. There is an extensive rural development program that allocates land to people who are willing to settle in virgin jungle areas to cultivate cash crops, such as rubber and palm-oil, with the aid of an initial government cash subsidy. The human implication of this program, apart from the promise of wealth in the future, is the transporting of families from their traditional *kampongs* (villages) not to urban areas as in some countries, but to new rural areas, often great distances away from their native villages, to live with neighbors who come from other areas of the country and who therefore speak with slightly different accents and have manners slightly different from themselves. There is, as is to be expected, a slight urban drift of the population, particularly of the Malays. Young people move to the cities in search of jobs in the factories, and many who come are disillusioned by what they find. One distinctive consequence of the urban drift is the establishment of squatter settlements within or on the periphery of cities (McGee, 1967). These illegal settlements have posed difficult problems in such areas as sanitation, housing, employment, and economic planning. Their psychiatric implications are not clear.

All these changes are taking place now and, of course, will continue to take place. If any worthwhile study is to be made of these significant changes in terms of human attitudes, human feelings, and mental health, I feel very strongly that the data must be collected now, particularly if the findings are to be of any value in guiding the direction of the change itself.

Behavioral Science Research

In spite of the note of urgency that I have sounded, I regret to say that apart from a few economic studies, no studies of these changes have been attempted by behavioral scientists for a number of reasons. Malaysia, despite twelve years of independence, is still very British in many ways, and this is reflected in the disciplines established in the local university. Behavioral sciences have a comparatively small place, whereas the humanities are very prominent. It is only in the past few years that the importance of the behavioral sciences has begun to be felt. These remarks are equally applicable in the field of medicine. Most of the practitioners in West Malaysia are graduates of the medical school established in 1905 in Singapore, now the School of Medicine at the University of Singapore. In this medical school, these is no Department of Psychiatry, and a total of about twenty hours of psychiatry is taught in the six-year course. As a result, most of the graduates know very little about psychiatry, and few are interested in making it their life's work. Thus, in Malaya there are currently only eight psychiatrists for nearly nine million people. The establishment of the Department of Psychological Medicine in the new medical school at the University of Malaya in Kuala Lumpur is therefore a very significant development in the field of behavioral sciences in the country. The department has been in existence for just over two years, having been a one-man department for the first six months. Since it became a fully functional clinical department in June 1967, almost all the energy of the department has been expended on services, teaching, and the administrative chores of sorting out the teething problems of such a new venture. The tremendously heavy service and teaching load that staff members in the department have been called upon to carry leaves very little time and energy for research endeavors. Wittkower (1966) stated that this situation occurs in developing countries. Tsung-yi Lin told me that it took him a number of years to get research activities organized in his department in Taipei. On the contrary, E. K. Schmidt, who until lately has been the only psychiatrist working in East Malaysia, which has a population of below one million but covers a more extensive geographical area than West Malaysia, has been able to nearly complete his full-scale research project (Schmidt, 1964). There are many good reasons for this contrast.

Whereas Schmidt has been in Sarawak since 1958, until 1962 in West Malaysia there were no trained psychiatrists resident for any length of time who were interested in psychiatric research. Furthermore, the clinical work load in West Malaysia, because of the greater population pressure, has been heavy enough to prohibit any such endeavors.

Epidemiological Research

The medical school and university hospital of the University of Malaya are located in Petaling Jaya, a major satellite town of the capital city of Kuala Lumpur. The Department of Psychological Medicine is the only psychiatric facility in this huge conurbation of nearly a million people. Although patients are admitted from all over the country, about ninety-five percent of them come from the greater Kuala Lumpur area and about fifty percent of these come from Petaling Jaya itself. The department operates an efficient medical records system from which data about patients are easily retrieved and codified. The data is used for an epidemiological study and for indications of the incidences of psychiatric disorders in a psychiatric facility. Cases have been coded and classified and are currently being processed. When the potential of this project is realized, the feasibility of starting a psychiatric case register for at least Petaling Jaya, if not for the greater Kuala Lumpur area, is high. A nationwide case register such as exists in Denmark would be difficult to set up, but a regional register such as the Camberwell Register in Southeast London (as reported to me by L. Wing) might be feasible. Petaling Jaya has a population of about seventy thousand, a size which should lend itself easily to statistical manipulation. This area would give an inevitable bias to the industrialized and urbanized section of the population, but if the stretches of land just beyond the township of Petaling Jaya were included as well, one could have a fairly ample cross-section of the population of the country, both rural and urban, industrial and agricultural, and including all social classes. A computerized program could be worked out eventually to deal with this information. The project is all the more tempting to undertake if one considers the fact that good demographic data is available for the whole population of West Malaysia and that every adult above the age of twelve is required by law to carry a numbered identity card which can be a very important source of identification in a case register.

The pattern of psychiatric disorders and the incidents of each disorder are unknown in West Malaysia. There are two state mental hospitals in this half of the country. The larger one at Tanjong Rambutan, about 150 miles north of Kuala Lumpur, has about forty-five hundred patients, and in the country the name Tanjong Rambutan has become a household word signifying madness. The other state hospital at Tampoi, on the southern tip of the peninsula, has over twenty-five hundred patients. A number of general hospital psychiatric units in various West Malaysia towns, most of which have been opened in the last few years, include psychiatric units in the general hospitals of Penang, Alor Star, Kota Bharu, and Seremban.

Among the patients admitted to the mental hospitals, there is an overwhelming predominance of severely disturbed schizophrenics. Very few patients carrying other diagnoses have been admitted to these hospitals (Tan, 1964). One sees a different sort of population in the general hospital psychiatric units, particularly in the general hospital psychiatric clinics. Here patients with depression and neuroses are seen more frequently than in the mental hospitals. In the psychiatric world, the name Malaya is traditionally associated with the conditions of *amok* and *latah*, although these two exotic conditions are comparatively rare. In my four years as Consultant Psychiatrist at Tampoi, I saw only five cases who were admitted after having run *amok*. All five turned out to be schizophrenics, according to Bleulerian criteria (Tan, 1965). Cases of *latah* seldom were brought to doctors for treatment. There are a number of comparatively common conditions which have hitherto not received psychiatric attention but are worthy of further scrutiny and detailed study.

Epidemic Hysteria

One such condition is the frequent outbreak of epidemic hysteria, which seems to be confined to Arabic schools in Malaya. These are religious schools in which Islam is taught for half a day, with Arabic the medium of instruction. Students at these schools are exclusively Malay and attend secular schools in the mornings before receiving their religious education in the afternoons. The epidemics of hysteria usually take the form of the students seeing ghosts and having fainting spells. Although most of these schools are coeducational, these attacks usually are confined to girls. The episodes may go on for several weeks, and even months, at a time (Tan, 1963). Qualitatively, this condition is not at all unique. It is in some ways comparable to the condition of *hsieh ping* described by Lin (1953) in his survey of mental disorders among the Chinese in Taiwan. These epidemics in Arabic schools in Malaya also are similar to the epidemic of hysteria occurring in the women of Tristan da Cunha described by Henriksen and Oeding (1940). However, there are a number of differences. The epidemics in Malaya affect a much larger group of people, sometimes forty to fifty girls in any one epidemic, whereas those described by Lin and by Henriksen and Oeding involve fewer people at a time.

Spermatorrhea

A symptom of anxiety neurosis which one sees in the psychiatric clinics in Malaya has not been described in the psychiatric literature. A common complaint of male patients suffering from anxiety neurosis is that of spermatorrhea. Spermatorrhea here is defined as a loss of seminal fluid in the absence of any form of sexual stimulation, physical or psychic, e.g., sexual fantasies, masturbation, or any form of sexual intercourse. Frequently, spermatorrhea is associated with nocturnal emissions, with the patient complaining of two or three emissions each night. Less frequently the patient may complain of losing seminal fluid during micturition. In many instances the patient is impotent as well. In a study of anxiety neurosis patients in the Psychological Medicine Unit of the University of Malaya Medical Center, I found that 44.16 percent of male anxiety neurotics had sexual symptoms. Of these about 25 percent complained of spermatorrhea (Tan, 1969). This complaint will have to be further looked into; possibly, it is largely subjective. I am of the impression that this is very much a culture-bound phenomenon, like the condition of *koro,* which is also seen in Malaya and which has been described by Rin (1965), Yap (1965), and Gwee (1963, 1968). Like *koro,* this idea of seminal loss giving rise to a loss of substance and energy derives from the folklore of Malayan ethnic and cultural groups. Although the condition was seen mostly among the Chinese, there was one Indian case in our series.

Somatic Symptoms in Depression

I have the impression that the manifestations of depressive illness in Malaya are often different from those described in psychiatric textbooks. There is a high frequency of complaints of somatic symptoms by almost all patients diagnosed as suffering from depressive illness. This again, of course, is nothing new. Wittkower (1968) reviewed the literature in this area and suggested a number of reasons why a greater tendency of somatization of psychiatric complaints exists among primitive peoples. My impression is that patients who are educated in the vernacular languages tend to somatize their complaints whereas those who are educated in English, and who are therefore more Western in their orientation, tend to show more of the textbook type of clinical picture. I feel, therefore, that this tendency to somatize depressive complaints correlates negatively with the degree of acculturation in the particular patient. If one could devise a measure of acculturation such as that used by Rin, Chu, and Lin (1966) in their study of psychophysiological complaints in Taiwan, one should be able to test this hypothesis. Western Malaysia is one area in which the opportunity to make a transcultural comparison should be utilized before it is too late.

Selective Mutism

Another problem that is currently being studied in my department is the condition of selective mutism among children. Although we do not have a full-scale psychiatric clinic yet, we are beginning to provide facilities for the evaluation and treatment of children as outpatients. Although few children are brought to our attention, several of them have been received with a selective mutism that tends to occur in situations that are frequent in Malaya. The children would be speaking one language at home and another at school. There could be any combination of the language of schools and dialects spoken at home. A child from a Cantonese-speaking family may attend a Chinese school in which the medium of instruction is Mandarin, or a Malayalam-speaking child may attend a Tamil-speaking school. To my mind the unique contribution of this study will be the cross-cultural dimension that our series will be able to provide.

Other Possible Areas of Study

The few projects that I have briefly outlined above are those in which work is being done currently. The members of my department and I see a large number of other areas in which interesting and fruitful research could be done. Because a large number of cases of attempted suicide are admitted to our university hospital, it would be very interesting to look into the rate of attempted suicide in the country, what social classes they occur in, the modes of suicidal attempts, etc. The population in Malaya may be divided into three main racial groups. Culturally, each of these may be further subdivided into smaller cultural groups and with its own folklore of the causation and treatment of mental illness. "Native concepts of psychiatric disorder" (Murphy and Leighton, 1965) would be an interesting anthropological study in which psychiatrists could collaborate. Indeed, Schmidt (1964) has done much in this subject in Sarawak, East Malaysia. Some work has been done among the Malays in Malaya (Dunn and Colson, 1968). Child-rearing among the different ethnic groups as studied by Djamour (1959) showed that, among the Malays, child-rearing techniques are somewhat different from European techniques. The correlation of data on child-rearing with personality characteristics and psychiatric disease patterns would make an interesting study. I am sure there are many more interesting projects that could be worked on in West Malaysia.

Summary

I referred initially to the rather varied ethnic and cultural groups living in Malaya that would provide suitable clinical material for cross-cultural studies in the field of mental health. I feel there is a sense of urgency in making such studies in view of the cultural and political changes that are taking place in the country which will blur these ethnic and cultural distinctions in the course of time. I briefly described some of the research projects that are being carried out at the Department of Psychological Medicine, University of Malaya, Kuala Lumpur: the tabulating of all the basic data of our patients who are seen at our clinical facility; the peculiar complaint of spermatorrhea as a symptom of anxiety; the tendency of patients to somatize symptoms in depressive illness and its possible relations to acculturation; and the problem of selective mutism among children. I also indicated that there are other interesting possibilities for research, particularly where cross-cultural comparison is important.

ACKNOWLEDGMENTS

I would like to thank Dr. Ronald C. Simons for his helpful comments and Mrs. M. Siew for her help in preparing the transcript.

REFERENCES

Dunn, F. L., and A. Colson. 1968. Medical resources in a Malay kampong. University of California, International Center of Medical Research & Training Annual Report, Spring 1968.

Djamour, J. 1959. Malay kinship and marriage in Singapore. London, Althone Press.

Glaser, N., and P. D. Moynihan. 1963. Beyond the melting pot. Cambridge, Massachusetts Institute of Technology Press.

Gwee, A. L. 1963. Koro—a cultural disease. Singapore Medical Journal 4:119–22.

————. 1968. Koro—its origin and nature as a diesase entity. Singapore Medical Journal 9:3–6.

Henriksen, S. D., and P. Oeding. 1940. Medical survey of Tristan da Cunha. Quoted by J. B. Loudon. *In* Transcultural Psychiatry. A. V. S. de Reuck and R. Porter, eds. London, Churchill.

Lin, T. 1953. A Study of the incidence of mental disorder in Chinese and other cultures. Psychiatry 16:313–36.

McGee, T. G. 1967. The Southeast Asian city. London, G. Bell and Son.

Murphy, J. M., and A. H. Leighton. 1965. Native concepts of psychiatric disorder. *In* Approaches to Cross-Cultural Psychiatry. J. M. Murphy and A. H. Leighton, eds. Ithaca, Cornell University Press.

Rin, H. 1965. A study of the etiology of koro in respect of the Chinese concepts of illness. International Journal of Social Psychiatry 11:7–13.

Rin, H., K. Chu, and T. Lin. 1966. Psychophysiological reactions of a rural and suburban population in Taiwan. Acta Psychiatric Scandanavica 42:410–73.

Schmidt, K. E. 1964. Folk psychiatry in Sarawak: a tentative system of psychiatry of the Ibans. *In* Magic, Faith and Healing. A. Kiev, ed. London, Free Press of Glencoe.

Tan, E. S. 1963. Epidemic hysteria. Medical Journal of Malaya 18:72–76.

————. 1964. Characteristics of patients and illnesses seen at Tampoi Mental Hospital. Medical Journal of Malaya 19:3–7.

————. 1965. Amok—a diagnostic consideration. Proceedings of the Second Malaysian Congress of Medicine 2:22–25.

————. 1969. The symptomatology of anxiety in West Malaysia. Medical Journal of Australia. In press.

Wittkower, E. D. 1966. Perspectives of transcultural psychiatry. Proceedings of the Fourth World Congress of Psychiatry, Excerpta Medica International Congress Series 150:228–34.

Wittkower, E. D., and R. Hugel [1968]. Transcultural aspects of the depressive syndrome. Mimeographed.

Yap, P. M. 1965. Koro—a cultural bound depersonalization syndrome. British Journal of Psychiatry 111:43–50.

2. Psychological Problems and Attitudes of Korean Students

KI-SUK KIM, Ph.D.
Behavioral Science Research Center
Korea University
Seoul, Korea

IN THE YEARS since independence (1945) there has been a rapid increase in number of colleges, universities, and students. Although many youths have received a higher education in Korea in recent years, it can be said that the quantitative expansion of institutions of higher education has not been accompanied by a corresponding rise in their quality. This fact has forced educators and concerned authorities to review higher education seriously and to undertake several measures to remedy the situation. For example, the Ministry of Education has set up a nationwide preliminary college entrance examination to identify unqualified high school graduates before they apply for college. Despite such efforts, however, an important aspect of college education, student guidance, remains largely ignored. The life and problems of Korean students have not yet been given close attention. Although an effort has been made to reorganize and strengthen guidance programs, and guidance centers and counseling services have been established by some colleges and universities, the results of such endeavors are far from satisfactory.

In an effort to prepare the fundamental data necessary for policy-making, and to help improve the existing guidance programs, the Ministry of Education of Korea in 1967 sponsored a research project on student guidance activities in Korean colleges and universities. This study, in which I participated as research director, was a rather extensive one, ranging from a historical survey of student problems to a public opinion poll concerning student guidance. I will report briefly on several findings of the study which illustrate some of the major psychological problems and attitudes of Korean students today.

Survey of the Problems of Students

The problems of students can be approached in two ways. On the one hand, it is possible to analyze what the students themselves consider to be their problems and, on the other hand, to analyze the situations in which students find themselves. Therefore, an attempt was first made to find out what students considered were their problems. A Korean version of the Mooney Problem Check List was administered to 2,876 students, which is approximately 2.2 percent of the total college population in Korea, chosen by stratified random sampling. The check list covers ten problem areas, (1) health and physical, (2) financial, (3) social recreational, (4) sociopsychological, (5) personal psychological, (6) courtship and sex, (7) home and family, (8) morals and values, (9) academic, and (10) future. The problem area with the largest number of responses was that of social recreational. The academic area was second in terms of number of responses, personal psychological was third, morals and values was fourth, future was fifth, sociopsychological was sixth, financial was seventh, family and home was eighth, health and physical was ninth, and courtship and sex was last.

In the social recreational area, the most frequent source of problems, over one-half of the students showed a strong frustration at being unable to satisfy their desire for travel or for a leisurely pursuit of intellectual interests. Lack of opportunity and time to appreciate music and art was another problem pointed out by almost as many students. The academic problem area, the second most frequently cited in students' responses, revealed that over 50 percent of the students complained that they were not having enough contact with their professors and that they needed a good academic advisor. Over one-third of the students were dissatisfied with college facilities, questioned the value of a college degree, and pointed out the indifference of professors towards students.

In the personal psychological area, which drew the third largest number of responses, approximately one-half of the students had too many things they wished to do but could never get done. Also, about 40 percent of them checked frequent daydreaming, regrets, and moodiness as their psychological problems. In the area of morals and values, which ranked fourth in the number of responses, the question of the worth of life was of the greatest concern for many students; 40.3 percent of them said they often wondered what life was really for. Next came indignation at the injustices and corruption in society, and then doubt as to the real value of material wealth. One-third of the students were skeptical about the existence of God or the absolute.

The students' problems about their futures were fifth in rank. Over one-third of the students felt a need for advice on plans for after graduation. They were wondering if they could ever be successful in life or find a suitable spouse. "Frequent feelings of inferiority" was checked by over 40 percent of students in the sociopsychological problem area, which was sixth in ranking. This was followed by lack of leadership (36 percent), and then timidness and shyness (26 percent). Insufficient pocket money and the financial difficulty of their families were reported by over one-third of the students. Most of those who were short of pocket money were reluctant to rely on their parents for it and were seeking part-time jobs. In the family and home area, it was indicated that students feel a heavy psychological responsibility towards their parents. The awareness of their parents' over-expectations of them was painful for many students (42 percent). Also, over one-third of the students had a sense of guilt because of their parents' sacrificing for them to attend college.

In the health and physical area, which was the ninth in the number of responses, over 35 percent of the students said they felt tired most of the time, and about 27 percent reported they lacked enough physical exercise. Of all the areas, the area of courtship and sex was the source of the fewest problems. Among the items checked in this area, the one which appeared most often was the difficulty of finding a good girl or boy friend (38 percent). About 27 percent reported that they could not express their affection to a companion of the opposite sex.

In summary, Korean students seem to feel that they have more problems in the social recreational, academic, and psychological-personal areas than in other areas. The problems of over half the students are (1) unsatisfied desire for travel and leisurely pursuit of intellectual interests, (2) insufficient personal contact with professors, and (3) frustration over not being able to engage in the various activities that appeal to them.

Survey of the Present Situation of Students

I have just described the problems of Korean students as revealed in their response to an adapted version of the Mooney Problem Check List. Since it seems that these student problems can be better understood in the context of the environmental factors in their daily lives, we further attempted a survey of the circumstances of students which may be responsible, to a greater or lesser extent, for these problems. In summarizing the findings, it was shown that about 43 percent of the students were from familes of average income, while 37 percent were from either rich or very rich families. About 20 percent regarded their family as poor or very poor. From these figures, we can judge that about 80 percent of college students are from families that do not face great economic difficulties. However, in the case of male students, the number of students from an upper economic class barely exceeded one quarter (26.9 percent), whereas for female students, the number of students constituted nearly a half (48.7 percent). Students from low-income families constituted one quarter (26 percent) in the case of male students, but only a little over 10 percent (12.5 percent) in the case of female students. This fact seems to suggest that many male students go to college despite difficult economic conditions, while female students do so only if their families are in better than ordinary economic situations.

Turning to the students' sources of meeting school expenses, about 60 percent of the total survey subjects had no particular trouble raising funds for school expenses, while 40 percent had mild or serious difficulties. Comparing male and female students, male students who faced either major or minor difficulties in paying school expenses constitute 45.9 percent within their group, while female students in this category represented 29.5 percent of their group. In terms of the sources of students' funds for school expenses, students who obtained allowances from their families constituted the largest percentage, 75.7 percent. They were followed by those who relied on part-time jobs, scholarships, loans, and help from relatives, in that order. Students of private colleges or universities tended to rely more on their families than the students of national colleges or universities, who depended more on part-time jobs for school expenses. This difference seems to indicate that students of national colleges or universities face more financial difficulties than those of private schools.

The number of students who worked part-time was 25.2 percent of the total questionees. Students were engaged in a total of 36 different kinds of jobs, ranging from tutoring, translation, art design, and surveying to general office work. Of these, tutoring was the most popular with 72 percent of the students engaged in it. As for the time spent by students on their jobs, two hours per day was the most frequent figure; the next largest number of the working students spent three hours a day working, and a considerable number (13 percent of the job holders) worked four hours or more daily. Many difficulties and problems can arise for students who have jobs. When asked to point out the most serious difficulties they encountered when working at their jobs, students gave as their reasons: (1) interference of jobs with their studies, (2) low salary, and (3) health undermined by hard work. Impeded study or impaired health are natural consequences to working students when one considers the amount of time they spend on their jobs. The motive most students gave for having jobs was "to cover living expenses." Additional motives were to raise funds for school expenses and, then, to earn pocket money. A very small number said they took jobs to gain experience and wider personal relations with others. In general, it is obvious that most students took their jobs out of immediate financial necessity.

When students were asked about their motives for entering college, the largest number, representing 30.5 percent, gave a motive of a more or less academic nature, that is, pursuit of advanced studies. This academic reason was followed by the desire for broadening human relations (19.7 percent), for developing potentialities (17.5 percent), and for getting better jobs after college (14.6 percent). From the figures, we can observe that about half the students entered college with the desire of pursuing more advanced studies or developing their specific capacities, and about one-third did so for the more pragmatic reason of having a better future. However, it is to be noted that about 7 percent of the respondents could be considered as having entered college without any sincere or clear purpose. Next, students were asked whether they were in the colleges or the major fields, or both, of their original choices in high school. No less than 37 percent of all the students were in neither the major fields nor in the colleges of their original choices. Only three-quarters of the students polled were in the colleges or major academic fields they originally wanted to be in. Such misplacements illustrate the unfortunate college and university admissions problem in Korea.

The degree of satisfaction with his major field could seriously affect a student's attitude and motivation. About half (45.8 percent) of the students were neutral in their opinion of their major fields. Among the rest, those who were satisfied exceeded in number those who were dissatisfied. However, the fact that dissatisfied students constituted nearly 20 percent of those polled was a matter that could not be overlooked. In general, medicine and pharmacology students were more satisfied with their fields than those in any other area. Also, if the major fields and the colleges agreed with the students' original choices, students showed higher satisfaction with their major fields. If they were dissatisfied with their major fields of study, students were asked to what fields they wished to be transferred. The results showed that the most popular fields to which students wanted to transfer were, in order of preference, social sciences (42.8 percent), natural sciences (18.7 percent), and humanities (16.7 percent). The fields to which students wished to transfer were generally those related to their present fields. The fields to and from which the smallest number of students wanted to transfer were medicine, pharmacology, the arts, and physical education. An interesting fact here is that these findings do not validate the general concept of transfer as a matter reflecting the vocational prospects in a field. In other words, even some of those who are in fields of bright vocational prospect desire to change their major fields, and the fields to which they want to move are not necessarily those with good employment opportunities.

We asked the students whether they had professors who understood them and with whom they felt free to discuss their personal problems. About 80 percent answered in the negative. However, it was clear that personal contact with professors increased in the upper two years to 19.8 percent from the 9.9 percent in the lower two years. Nevertheless, the fact that the majority of students admitted lack of personal relation with their teachers should not be overlooked. As the reason for such a lack of relation, about half of the students gave the fact that they did not seek out their professors. About 30 percent had no intention of making any such contacts. About 9 percent complained of the lack of response from professors. These students expressed their distrust of professors, ascribing their estrangement from professors to the latter's indifference, lack of understanding, self-righteous attitudes, and poor academic achievements. If students are desirous of personal contact with professors, what do they expect from such contact? The answers most frequently checked for this query were consultation on ideas or views of life and academic advice.

Regarding their post-graduate plans, the largest number of students (about 42 percent) said they would seek employment. The next most frequent indication was military service (18 percent). A major exception was, however, for the fields of medicine and pharmacology, in which going abroad to study occupied second rank (25 percent). This exception may be attributed to the better opportunities for study abroad in medicine and pharmacology. The future plans of the students were further examined to determine whether the jobs that students seek are related to their major fields of study. About 70 percent of the jobs cited were related to major fields, but about 20 percent were unrelated, and the rest were undetermined. It is noticeable that about 20 percent of the students polled were definitely planning to get jobs outside their academic fields. In the case of humanities majors, no less than 30 percent were planning to get jobs unrelated to their major fields. Even among the students planning to get jobs related to their major fields, 45 percent were not very confident of finding them. Only 40 percent expressed confidence. The other students (7 percent) had no confidence at all in finding jobs in areas related to their major fields, or they had not considered the matter. The number of students who said they were confident decreased in the upper years, while those with no confidence increased. The reasons given for such a lack of confidence were limited job opportunities and lack of academic abilities. In view of the fact that a great number of students are ready to ignore their academic fields in seeking employment, and that those trying to find jobs related to their fields are not confident of success, there is evident need for a critical evaluation of existing programs of vocational guidance in colleges and universities.

In summary, this portion of the survey reveals that about one-fifth of the Korean students polled were studying under great economic pressure and that about one-fourth of them had part-time jobs. Also, nearly one-fourth of the students were studying in academic fields which they did not originally want to be in. This affects the degree of satisfaction students have with their overall college life. Most of the students misplaced in their academic fields were not enjoying their college life. Furthermore, a majority of students lacked professors with whom they could closely consult concerning personal and academic matters. Among those who planned to find a job upon graduation, about 20 percent wanted to be employed in areas unrelated to their major fields of study. Among those students who planned to seek employment related to their major fields, about half were not confident of success in finding jobs.

Survey of Student Attitudes

In this study, adaptions of Eysenck's Attitude Scale and Chung's Developmental Attitude Scale were used. The fact that both scales were only tentative preliminary forms somewhat limited this study. The subjects for the study were 3,461 students from 41 colleges and universities throughout the country. The Eysenck Attitude Scale, which was developed mainly on the basis of observation of the opinions and convictions of British political parties and groups, was designed to measure attitudes by two subscales: R Scale and 8 Scale. The R Scale attempts to measure the degree of radical and conservative dimension, and the T Scale is designed to measure the degree of tender-minded and tough-minded dimension.

Chung's Developmental Attitude Scale is based on a hypothesis of the possibility of separating attitudes more conducive to national development or moderization from other attitudes. For example, self-confidence falls more under the category of developmental attitude than sense of incompetence. The scale is divided into three subscales: sociocultural, political, and economic which are purported to measure attitudes toward sociocultural, political, and economic issues respectively.

Turning to the results of the Eysenck Scale, our study confirmed the common understanding that male students are more radical than female students. Females are much more conservative and less prone to radical reforms. Also, students in the fields of the social sciences, arts, education, physical education, natural sciences, and engineering proved to be more radical than those in the fields of humanities, medicine, and pharmacology. The prospect of a relatively stable future seems to account for the attitudes of medical and pharmacology students, who were most conservative. It is interesting to note that humanities were found to be in between conservatism and radicalism. Those who professed to be nonreligious showed more radical tendencies than Buddhist students, and Buddhists, in turn, appeared to be more radical than Christians. The location of schools generally did not seem to affect the attitude of students in this regard.

In the T Scale, as a matter of course, females were much more tender-minded than males. In view of the results of both the R and the T Scales, male students were more radical and tough-minded than female students. Students in medicine and pharmacology showed significantly higher tender-minded characteristics than those in any other field. In general, it could be said that students in medicine, pharmacology, and the humanities show more conservative and tender-minded characteristics than the others, and that arts and physical education majors generally show more radical and tough-minded tendencies. In terms of religious affiliation, Christians are significantly tender-minded compared with Buddhist or students with no religion, and Buddhists are more tender-minded than students in the nonreligious group.

When compared with the normal adult group in society, students, in general, had a more radical and yet a more tender-minded attitude. In other words, nonstudent adults were more conservative and yet more tough-minded than students. According to Eysenck, British socialists and conservatives are neither tough nor tender, but they show opposing tendencies in that socialists are radical, while conservatives are inclined to be conservative. Fascists and liberals tend toward conservatism but differ in that Fascists demonstrate a considerably tough attitude, while liberals show a moderate one. Communists are very tough and radical. A comparison of Korean students with those British political groups reveals that Korean students lean somewhat toward radicalism and yet are more tender-minded. We could describe Korean students as tender-minded radicals who believe in social progress through gradual reform.

When we examine the results from the sociocultural subscale of the Developmental Attitude Scale, arts and physical education majors are socioculturally less progressive and more traditional than the other major groups. Social science majors show a more progressive attitude than humanities majors. In terms of the location of schools, students of provincial colleges and universities were more progressive, socioculturally, than students in Seoul. For male students, religion did not seem to have any influence in this respect, but in the case of female students, Christians had more traditional, nonprogressive attitudes than Buddhists or the nonreligious group.

In the political subscale, which attempts to measure attitudes towards political issues, no significant difference was found among the different major groups except between students of arts and physical education and those in the other major groups. Arts and physical education majors show a more traditional and conservative attitude politically. In terms of religious faiths, Buddist students are more development-minded in political matters than Christians. No difference was found between Seoul and the provinces. In the economic subscale that attempted to measure attitudes towards economic development of the nation, male students showed a significantly more progressive attitude than females. In relation to economics, students of natural sciences and engineering are more development-minded than those in other fields, and students of medicine, pharmacology, and social sciences are more development-minded than those in the humanities, arts, education, and physical education. Particularly, the difference between the natural sciences and the humanities is quite significant. In terms of religion, the nonreligious group is more development-minded in relation to economics than are Christians.

Finally, if we survey the overall tendencies of Korean students as reflected in the sociocultural, political, and economic subscales, both male and female students demonstrate the most developmental attitude in the political scale, next in the sociocultural scale, and lastly in the economic scale. In other words, when we attempt to link some attitudes towards national development and modernization, the political attitude is found to be most conducive to development, while the sociocultural attitude and the economic attitude rank second and third respectively.

COMMUNICATION: CULTURAL PATTERNS

3. Tiny Dramas: Vocal Communication between Mother and Infant in Japanese and American Families

WILLIAM CAUDILL, Ph.D.

Laboratory of Socio-environmental Studies
National Institute of Mental Health
Bethesda, Maryland

THE ANALYSIS of a recently published comparison of the everyday behavior of mothers and infants in Japan and America (Caudill and Weinstein, 1969) led Helen Weinstein and me to conclude that, despite areas of similarity, the styles of caretaking shown by the mothers are different in the two cultures and are linked to different patterns of infant behavior. We found that by three to four months of age the infants had already learned (or had been conditioned) to behave in certain distinctive ways in each culture. Abstractly speaking, the infants have learned, at least in nascent form, to be members of their culture, and this has happened out of awareness and well before the development of language. Since the use of his voice is the main way a young infant communicates with his mother (when he is alone, it is virtually the only way), this paper examines the characteristics of vocal communication between mother and infant in Japan and America in order to probe more deeply into the process by which the early learning of cultural expectations for behavior may come about.

Our findings show that when mothers in the two cultures are involved in direct caretaking of their babies, the American mother does more talking to her baby than the Japanese mother while the Japanese mother does more lulling of her baby. At the same time, the American infant has a greater amount of vocalization, and particularly of happy vocalization, than does the Japanese infant. When the babies in each culture are not being cared for, there is no difference in the total amount of vocalization, but the American infant does more happy vocalization than his Japanese counterpart who, on the other hand, does more unhappy vocalization.[1] This paper is primarily concerned with the question of why there should be these differences in the use of the voice by mothers and infants in the two cultures.

In order to answer this question we will review first the general methods and earlier findings of the study as background leading to the present analysis. Secondly, we will look at the pace of life for the mothers and infants across the total observations to see whether a livelier or more leisurely approach to caretaking by the mothers is likely to affect their verbal behavior and whether variation in the awake-asleep cycles of infants is likely to affect the nature of their vocalization. Thirdly, we will turn to a more detailed examination of those times when the infants are awake and inquire as to how quickly, and with what type of verbal behavior, the mothers in each culture respond to various kinds of vocalization by their infants. Finally, we will attempt to draw together and interpret what we have learned.

Background Leading to the Present Analysis

The data for this study come from naturalistic observations made on two consecutive days in the homes of thirty Japanese and thirty American first-born, three-to-four-month-old infants equally divided by sex and living in intact middle-class urban families between 1961 and 1964. Data on the ordinary daily life of the infant were obtained by time-sampling, one observation being made every fifteenth second over a ten-minute period in terms of a predetermined set of categories concerning the behavior of the mother (or other caretaker) and the behavior of the infant, resulting in a sheet containing forty equally spaced observations. There was a five-minute break between observation periods, and ten observation sheets were completed on each of the two days, giving a total of 800 observations for each case. In the analysis already published, these data were analyzed by multivariate analysis of variance using three independent variables: culture (Japanese, American), father's occupation (salaried, independent), and sex of infant (male, female). The effects of each of these independent variables were examined separately while controlling on the other two variables, and culture proved to be overwhelmingly the most important variable. Interactions between the independent variables revealed nothing of importance.

In summary and as background for the further analysis presented here, the general findings by culture in the earlier analysis show a basic similarity in the biologically rooted behavior of the infants in the two countries regarding the total time spent in feeding (sucking on breast or bottle and eating of semi-solid food) and in sleeping, and also show a basic similarity in the behavior of the mothers in the time spent in the feeding, diapering, and dressing of their infants. Beyond these similarities, however, the American infants have greater amounts of gross bodily activity, play (with toys, hands, and other objects), and happy vocalization; in contrast, the Japanese infants seem passive and only display a greater amount of unhappy vocalization. The American mothers do more looking at, positioning the body of, and chatting to their infants; the Japanese mothers do more carrying, rocking, and lulling of their infants.

In interpreting these general findings we feel that, first of all, the mothers in each culture are engaged in different styles of caretaking: the American mother seems to encourage her baby to be active and vocally responsive, while the Japanese mother acts in ways which she believes will soothe and quiet her baby. Secondly, the infants in the two cultures have become habituated to respond appropriately to these differences. We were, moreover, struck by the fact that the responses of the infants are in line with general expectations for behavior in the two cultures. In America, the individual should be physically and verbally assertive, and in Japan, he should be physically and verbally restrained.[2]

We were interested particularly in the greater happy vocalization of the American infant, because it is significantly correlated with the mother's looking at and talking to her baby. In contrast, the lesser amount of the Japanese infant's happy vocalization does not show any clear pattern of relationship with the mother's behavior. This patterning of correlations is intriguing, and it does suggest a different use of vocal communication between mother and infant in the two cultures. However, findings phrased in terms of correlations do not answer the question of how the flow of vocal communication actually proceeds in daily life in each culture. It is possible in this article to enter further into this problem by making use of the sequential property of the data over the 800 observations in each case.

To provide a framework for the sequential analysis of the observations, we will classify observations into what we earlier called states. Each observation may be classified into one of six states which are defined by the infant either being awake or asleep in combination with the mother doing caretaking, being merely present and not doing caretaking, or being absent. Table 1 presents the mean frequency of time in each of these six states over the total 800 observations by culture.[3]

From the point of view of the mother, it is clear in Table 1 that there is no significant difference between the cultures in the amount of time spent in the caretaking of awake babies (state 1). As a minor, but nevertheless interesting, theme, it is true, however, that Japanese mothers spend more time in the caretaking of sleeping babies (state 4). Secondly, Japanese mothers are more passively present in the room with their babies regardless of whether the babies are awake (state 2) or asleep (state 5). Thirdly, there is no difference between the cultures in the amount of time that mothers are absent from awake babies (state 3), but American mothers

Table 1:   Cultural Comparison of Adjusted Mean Frequencies
for Time in Six States

States	Japanese (N=30 cases)	American (N=30 cases)	Correlations*	p <
Infant Awake				
1. Mother present and caretaking	286	321	0.16	n.s.†
2. Mother present but not caretaking	103	53	0.34	0.05
3. Mother absent	106	119	0.08	n.s.
Total infant awake	495	493	0.01	n.s.
Infant Asleep				
4. Mother present and caretaking	52	16	0.37	0.01
5. Mother present but not caretaking	100	32	0.45	0.001
6. Mother absent	153	259	0.42	0.001
Total infant asleep	305	307	0.01	n.s.
Total Observations	800	800		

* Findings are presented in terms of a one-way analysis of variance, in which culture is the independent variable in question, and findings are controlled for the effects of father's occupation (salaried, independent) and sex of infant (male, female). The partial correlation used is the square root of the ratio of (a) the sum of the squared deviations from the mean attributable to culture, to (b) the total sum of the squared deviations minus the sum of the squared deviations attributable to the control variables of father's occupation and sex of infant, and their interactions.

† Not significant

are definitely more absent than Japanese mothers when their babies are asleep (state 6). From the viewpoint of the baby, it is clear that there is no difference between the cultures in amount of time spent awake or asleep.

These findings, from an analysis of the total observations, present, of course, a static picture and say nothing about the sequence in the shifts from one state to another across the observations. Necessarily, the six states do shift, one into another, across the 800 observations, and it is this property of shifts in states that is the first subject of analysis in this paper.

The Pace of Changes in State
for Mother and Infant across the Total Observations

THE PACE OF CHANGES IN STATE FOR THE MOTHER

The point of departure here is the finding in Table 1 that mothers in both cultures spend approximately the same amount of time in caring for awake babies. Nevertheless, it is our strong impression from work with the basic data that American mothers are more in and out of the room during the time their babies are awake and in need of caretaking. Thus, our reasoning is that the pace of caretaking is different in the two cultures despite the fact that the total time spent in caretaking for awake babies is about the same. If true, this difference in the pace of caretaking would help to explain why American babies are more vocal, and particularly why they are more happily vocal. That is, if the American mother is starting and stopping her caretaking more frequently, then she is inadvertently providing more natural opportunities to talk to her baby at the beginning and ending of such periods with the probable effect that her voice will stimulate the baby to respond. (If nothing else, she is providing more times at which she is likely, in essence, to say hello and goodbye to her baby.)

In terms of changes in the six states, the mother can shift her state from active caretaking (states 1 and 4) to no caretaking (states 2, 3, 5, or 6) or vice versa. In addition, because of the way in which the states are defined, it is possible to have a change in state from being merely present but not caretaking (states 2 and 5) to being absent (states 3 and 6) or vice versa. There is some reason to believe that the Japanese mother might be more involved than the American mother in the latter situations because of her more frequent passive presence when the baby is awake and asleep. In any event, the changes of state just described for the mother are logically exhaustive, and Table 2 shows the mean frequency of changes in state and the analysis of the rank-order distribution of the cases by culture.[4]

In Table 2 it can be seen that the American mother, in total, has significantly more changes of state over the 800 observations than does the Japanese mother. It is also clear that the bulk of these changes of state in both cultures occurs in the shift from caretaking to not caretaking or vice versa. The frequency of shifts from being merely present to absent or vice versa is a minor matter, and only one of the four comparisons in this regard is significant: Japanese mothers do seem more to wait until their infants are asleep before shifting from being merely present to absent.

Since we know already from Table 1 that mothers in both cultures spend approximately the same total amount of time in caretaking of awake babies, the most interesting finding in Table 2 is that American mothers have significantly more shifts in state than Japanese mothers from caretaking to no caretaking of awake babies and vice versa. This necessarily means that the American mother is, in fact, doing her caretaking in more frequent and shorter periods and hence is providing more natural opportunities for vocal exchange between mother and infant at the beginning and ending of these periods. In this sense, the American mother may be more attentive to her baby than the Japanese mother, and certainly in her style of care the American mother appears livelier and busier, whereas the style of the Japanese mother is more leisurely.[5]

Table 2: Mean Frequency of Mother's Changes of State and Results of Analysis of Rank-Order Distribution by Culture

| | Mother's Changes of State | | | | | | | | |
| | Caretaking to not Caretaking* Infant is: | | Not Caretaking to Caretaking† Infant is: | | Merely Present to Absent‡ Infant is: | | Absent to Merely Present§ Infant is: | | Total Mean Changes |
Culture	Awake	Asleep	Awake	Asleep	Awake	Asleep	Awake	Asleep	
Japanese (N=30 cases)	16.2	4.5	16.8	3.9	2.4	2.7	2.0	1.9	50.4
American (N=30 cases)	27.1	7.9	26.8	7.9	3.4	1.4	2.5	1.2	78.2
z score	3.37	1.01	2.94	1.76	1.29	2.17	0.83	1.69	3.46
p <	0.001	n.s.||	0.01	n.s.	n.s.	0.05	n.s.	n.s.	0.001

* Includes all changes from state 1(infant awake) or state 4 (infant asleep) to states 2, 3, 5, or 6

† Includes all changes from states 2, 3 (infant awake) or states 5, 6 (infant asleep) to states 1 or 4

‡ Includes all changes from state 2 (infant awake) or state 5 (infant asleep) to states 3 or 6

§ Includes all changes from state 3 (infant awake) or state 6 (infant asleep) to states 2 or 5

|| Not significant

THE PACE OF CHANGES IN STATE FOR THE INFANT

Given the definition of the six states, there are only two ways in which the infant can change his state by himself: he can shift from being awake (states 1, 2, or 3) to being asleep (states 4, 5, or 6) or vice versa. In addition to this, however, the mother either can be involved in the transition of the infant from awake to asleep (from state 1 to states 4, 5, or 6) or not be involved (from states 2 or 3 to states 4, 5, or 6). The same thing, of course, is true for the infant's transition in the opposite direction: the mother either is involved (state 4 to states 1, 2, or 3) or not involved (states 5 or 6 to states 1, 2, or 3).

In general, we already know from Table 1 that infants in both cultures are awake or asleep the same amount of time, but this finding does not tell us whether this behavior is patterned in the same way in the two cultures over the total observations. In approaching the analysis for this paper we did not have an hypothesis about this matter but, as can be seen in Table 3, it does turn out that there is a difference between the cultures.

It is clear from Table 3 that, in total, the Japanese infant is more in and out of sleep across the observations than is the American infant. Closer examination of the findings in the table indicates, however, that when the mothers in the two cultures are not involved in the infants' going to sleep or awakening, there is no difference between the cultures in the number

Table 3: Mean Frequency of Infant's Changes of State and Results of Analysis of Rank-Order Distribution by Culture

Culture	Infant's Changes of State				
	Awake to Asleep* Mother is:		Asleep to Awake† Mother is:		Total Mean Changes
	Involved	Not Involved	Involved	Not Involved	
Japanese (N=30 cases)	4.2	3.5	2.6	5.0	15.3
American (N=30 cases)	1.5	4.2	0.8	4.4	10.9
z score	3.59	1.09	2.44	1.08	2.45
p<	0.001	n.s.‡	0.05	n.s.	0.05

* Includes all changes from state 1 (mother involved) or states 2, 3 (mother not involved) to states 4, 5, or 6
† Includes all changes from state 4 (mother involved) or states 5, 6 (mother not involved) to states 1, 2, or 3
‡ Not significant

of such shifts. Presumably, this lack of difference reflects the similarity in the biological processes of the infants in the two cultures when they are left alone to determine their own behavior in this regard. The greater total number of shifts for the Japanese infants is due obviously to the cultural fact that the Japanese mother is more involved in the active care of her infant, both when he is going to sleep and when he is waking up, than is the American mother.

The next question is: How do we explain the greater involvement of the Japanese mother in the more frequent transitions of her infant? A good starting point in answering this question is to call attention again to the finding in Table 1 that Japanese mothers do more caretaking of sleeping babies. From the earlier analysis (Caudill and Weinstein, 1969:38–39), we know that Japanese mothers proportionately do more feeding, carrying, rocking, and other tasks (wiping face, adjusting bedding, etc.) of sleeping babies than American mothers, whereas proportionately the latter look at their sleeping babies more. The greater feeding of sleeping babies occurs for the Japanese mother largely because she is more content to continue sitting, holding the baby who has fallen asleep with the nipple of the breast or bottle in his mouth; by definition, the mother in this situation is still scored as feeding. The greater looking at sleeping babies for the American mother occurs because she leaves her sleeping baby alone and then returns periodically to the door of his room to check visually upon him, usually without doing any other caretaking.

For the analysis reported in this paper we returned to the basic observational data and examined what the mothers in the two cultures do in all instances in which they are involved in the infant's transition from being awake to being asleep and vice versa. When putting a baby to sleep, the Japanese mother does significantly more carrying, rocking, and lulling than does the American mother who, in contrast, puts her awake baby down in his crib, talks to him briefly, and, after waiting a few moments to be sure he is comfortable, leaves the room. A second but quantitatively less important area of difference is, as noted above, the more leisurely pace of the Japanese mother in terminating feeding after the baby has fallen asleep on the breast or bottle. In either situation in Japan, whether the baby is being carried and lulled to sleep or falls asleep after feeding, the important element is that the Japanese infant by three to four months of age has become accustomed to falling asleep in his mother's arms, at least when he is aware that she is near him. The American infant, on the other hand, by the same age has become used to being put down in his crib to go to sleep by himself.

The different effect upon the infants of these two styles of caretaking is clearly evident in the observations. In Japan, the mother succeeds in putting the baby to sleep while carrying him but when she puts him down, he awakens and cries. She then picks him up, and the process is repeated until finally the baby remains asleep. It is this process that accounts for the greater number of shifts from awake to asleep for the Japanese infant when his mother is involved than for the American infant. It is also this process that provides one of the reasons for the Japanese infant's greater unhappy vocalization. In America, the mother is more likely to leave her awake infant alone to go to sleep by himself, and he is less likely to cry because he has become accustomed to this procedure. When he does cry, the American mother often will briefly pat and talk to the baby but will not pick him up. This bit of extra comforting is usually sufficient to induce sleep.[6]

The greater involvement of the Japanese mother in contrast to the American mother during the infant's shifts from asleep to awake is also related to differences in styles of caretaking in the two cultures. At first, we thought that Japanese mothers were waking their babies more than Americans in order to feed them on schedule in the case of bottle feeding or because of the pressure of milk in the mother's breasts in the case of breast feeding. However, neither of these situations turned out to be so— only two American and four Japanese mothers woke their babies in order to feed them, and in all of these cases feeding was by bottle. The answer to why the Japanese mother is more involved in the infant's waking lies, rather, in what the mothers in the two cultures do to sleeping babies. The American mother, as we indicated, largely restricts her care to checking visually on the baby. The Japanese mother goes beyond this to do significantly more caretaking which involves physical contact with the baby or his bedding. This additional physical care frequently acts as a stimulus sufficient to cause the baby to wake up and often to cry.

The greater involvement of the Japanese mother in her baby's movement in and out of sleep may be interpreted as evidence of a greater concern for the comfort of the baby, but the result of this behavior is that the Japanese infant is more fretful and fussier, specifically in matters concerned with sleep, than is the American infant.[7] At this point a crucial question arises naturally. Why does the Japanese mother persist in a style of care that makes her baby fussier, especially when her goal seems to be that of having a quiet and contented baby? The answer to this question is complex. It would involve us in a comparative cultural and psychological discussion of the self-image and behavior of the mother in relation to her child as infant and adult in Japan and in America. Because of the complexity of this issue, we must defer even a beginning discussion of it until the conclusion of this paper.

For now, however, we believe we have identified one of the reasons for the greater unhappy vocalization of the Japanese infant in the more extensive involvement of his mother in matters related to sleep in contrast to the American mother and infant. Other reasons for the Japanese infant's more prolonged unhappy vocalization will become apparent shortly. We also believe we have identified, at least tentatively, one of the reasons for the greater happy vocalization of the American infant in the more frequent opportunities that the American mother provides for her baby to "talk" to her as she moves in and out of his presence while he is awake.

Since the effects of vocal communication between infant and mother can only really be studied when the infant is awake, we turn now to a closer examination of what happens in the vocalization of infants and mothers in the three states in which the infant is awake.

Mother's Responses to Infant's Vocalization in Various States

In order to explore the effects of vocalization in those states in which the infant is awake, it is necessary first to establish the boundaries of the behavioral episodes to be used in the analysis. From this point on, all data presented in Tables 4–7 are derived from the analysis of what we call bounded episodes which clearly have a beginning and an ending. As explained earlier, the observational data were gathered in ten-minute periods (each containing forty observations made at fifteen-second intervals) with a break of five minutes between periods. Because we want to know what conditions, in terms of differing states, both precede and follow an episode in a given state, the episode itself must be confined within the ten-minute observational period. Moreover, the episode must occur between the second and the thirty-eighth observation because the first and last observations on the sheet are reserved, at the maximum limits of an episode, for the purpose of bounding episodes in terms of the differing preceding and following states. Thus, an episode may vary in length from one to thirty-eight observations or, in actual time, from one-quarter of a minute to nine-and-a-half minutes. By definition, then, a bounded episode is a run of contiguous observations in a given state that is bounded at the beginning and ending by the occurrence of an observation in another state.[8] We call the preceding state the antecedent and the following state the consequent, and whenever possible, an analysis of episodes in a given state is controlled on the antecedent state while looking at the outcome in terms of the consequent state.

Using this definition of a bounded episode, we determined an average score for each case in terms of a particular problem, and then we rank-ordered these scores and analyzed the resulting distribution by culture using a Mann-Whitney U test as the statistic (see note 4). For example, let the general problem be the length of time it takes mothers in the two cultures to respond to the unhappy vocalizations of their infants. One set of data bearing on this problem comes from the following circumstances. The antecedent condition is that the infant is awake and in the presence of his mother (states 1 and 2); the bounded episode occurs when the infant is awake and alone (state 3) and makes one or more unhappy vocalizations (and does not make any happy vocalizations); and the consequent condition is that the mother responds by coming into the awake baby's room (states 1 and 2). The score is the number of observations it takes the mother to respond from the time of the first unhappy vocalization. Suppose that instances of this set of circumstances occur in twenty-nine (twelve Japanese and seventeen American) of the total sixty cases. In each of these twenty-nine cases we obtain the average length of time (that is, the average number of observations) it takes a mother to respond, and then we rank-order the cases on this basis and proceed with the analysis by culture to determine if there is a statistical difference between Japanese and American mothers in the average time of their response to the solely unhappy vocalization of their babies. The logical approach to the ordering and analysis of data that is illustrated by this example was used in all the analyses that will be referred to in the remainder of this paper.

ANALYSIS OF BOUNDED EPISODES IN STATE 3:
INFANT IS AWAKE AND ALONE

The bounded episodes in which the infant is awake and alone can be divided into four types, according to the kind of vocal behavior shown by the infant during the episode: (1) he is silent throughout; (2) he has only unhappy vocalization; (3) he has mixed happy and unhappy vocalizations; and (4) he has only happy vocalization. In addition, when we control on the antecedent state as to whether the infant is awake (states 1 or 2) or asleep (states 4, 5, or 6), and also control on the consequent state as to whether the mother responds to her awake infant (states 1 or 2) or the infant goes to sleep (states 4, 5, or 6), we have a 2 × 4 × 2 design which

Table 4:   Results of Analysis of Rank-Order Distribution by Culture of Time Taken by Mother to Respond to Infant's Vocalization in State Three (infant awake and alone)

Culture	Average Number* of Observations Taken by Mother to Respond from Time of Infant's First Signal When Infant is:				
	Silent: Antecedent Awake	Unhappily Vocal: Antecedent Awake	Unhappily Vocal: Antecedent Asleep	Mixed Vocal: Antecedent Awake	Happily Vocal: Antecedent Awake
Japanese	5.1	5.4	6.2	21.7	8.0
American	2.9	2.7	3.0	11.3	5.0
Number of cases					
Japanese	20	12	10	5	10
American	29	17	4	17	25
z score	2.15	2.04	2.90	2.62	0.93
p<	0.05	0.05	0.01	0.01	n.s.†

* This number is obtained by averaging the averages for the mothers in each culture.
† Not significant

results in sixteen possible logical sequences from antecedent to episode to consequent.

We examined all these logical sequences, but eight of them occurred so infrequently that the data were insufficient for analysis.[9] In the other eight sequences, however, we did have sufficient data. In five of these sequences the consequent is that the mother responds to her infant, and in the remaining three sequences the consequent is that the infant falls asleep by himself. In both classes of sequences the rules of the game were the same for infants and mothers in each culture, and all parties started out alike— the infants were awake and alone, and the mothers were out of the room.

In the first class of sequences, the basic question is: How quickly do mothers in each culture respond to various kinds of vocalization by their babies? The answer is given in Table 4.

As can be seen, in four of the five sequences analyzed in Table 4 the Japanese mother takes significantly longer to respond to her baby. Since two of these four sequences involve solely unhappy vocalization, it seems safe to conclude that the Japanese mother takes longer than the American mother to respond to the unhappy vocalization of her baby when he is awake and alone. This delay is another reason why the Japanese infant is, in general, more unhappily vocal than the American infant.

When the infant is happily vocal, however, there is no significant difference in the time taken to respond by mothers in the two cultures. Note that the average time of response for the American mother is less than that for the Japanese mother in all five sequences (and significantly in four) in Table 4. It seems likely, therefore, that the American mother responds more quickly to her infant regardless of the nature of his vocalization when he is awake and alone.

Using the data presented in Table 4, we can begin to answer another question. Is there a difference in the time taken by mothers in each culture to respond to their infants' unhappy as opposed to happy vocalization? In other words, is the mother making a meaningful discrimination of the kinds of vocalization by her infant? Using the two sequences in which the antecedent is awake, we can compare the responses of the mothers in each culture. It is clear that the American mother responds more quickly to her infant's unhappy than happy vocalization (the average number of observations taken are 2.7 for unhappy and 5.0 for happy, $z = 2.59$, $p < 0.01$); whereas, there is not a significant difference for the Japanese mother (5.4 for unhappy and 8.0 for happy, $z = 0.36$, n.s.). Thus, we may conclude that the American mother is making more discriminating use of the vocal signals of her baby when he is awake and alone. It seems likely that the American baby, as a result, is learning to use his voice in a more refined way than the Japanese baby.

Let us look now at the second class of sequences in which the consequent is that the infant goes to sleep by himself. Our question here is whether there is a difference between the cultures in the amount of time infants take to go to sleep when left to their own devices.

Table 5:   Results of Analysis of Rank-Order Distribution by Culture of Time Taken by Infant to Go to Sleep When Mother Does Not Respond in State Three (infant awake and alone)

Culture	Average Number* of Observations Taken by Infant to Go to Sleep When Infant is:		
	Silent: Antecedent Awake	Silent: Antecedent Asleep	Unhappily Vocal:† Antecedent Asleep
Japanese	5.5	1.7	2.5
American	4.8	1.9	1.8
Number of cases			
Japanese	4	14	7
American	5	20	6
z score	no test used	0.93	0.44
p <	n.s.‡	n.s.	n.s.

* This number is obtained by averaging the averages for the infants in each culture.
† Time taken to go to sleep is measured by the number of observations from the first unhappy vocalization.
‡ Not significant

It is clear from Table 5 that in the three types of sequences for which we have data, there are no meaningful differences between the two cultures in the time taken by infants to go to sleep when the mother does not respond. This finding again argues strongly for the similarity of biological processes in the two cultures when the infants are left to themselves.

ANALYSIS OF BOUNDED EPISODES IN STATE 2:
INFANT AWAKE AND MOTHER PRESENT BUT NOT CARETAKING

As in the preceding section, it is possible to divide the bounded episodes in state 2 into four types of vocalization by the infant—silent, unhappily vocal, mixed vocal, and happily vocal—and to control for the antecedent state as to whether the infant is awake (states 1 or 3) or asleep (states 4, 5, or 6). The consequent state, however, is a bit more complicated and may be divided into three situations: (1) the mother responds by caretaking (state 1); (2) the mother leaves the room (state 3); and (3) the infant goes to sleep in the presence of the mother before there is any action on her part (states 4 and 5). These divisions give us a $2 \times 4 \times 3$ design resulting in twenty-four logical sequences of antecedent, episode, and consequent. In seventeen sequences the data were insufficient for analysis mainly because sequences in which the antecedent or consequent is asleep occurred very infrequently.[10] In the seven sequences for which the data were adequate the antecedent is always awake, and the consequent is either that the mother does caretaking or leaves the room. In the latter situation we know from a content analysis of the data that the mother usually leaves to get something (a bottle, a diaper, etc.) for the baby.

The basic question we are asking of the seven sequences indicated in Table 6 is the same as that asked in the earlier analysis. How quickly do mothers in each culture respond to various kinds of vocalization by their babies? In the present situation, however, the mothers are actually in the room, whereas earlier they were absent, and the rules of the game are much more stringent.

The first finding to note in Table 6 is that once again the American mother is quicker to respond, in general, to her baby, regardless of the nature of his vocalization. In all seven sequences the average time of response is less for the American mother, and this is significantly so in two of the sequences and of borderline significance in two others.[11]

Looking specifically at the response to the unhappy vocalization of the baby, we note that the American mother responds faster than the Japanese mother both by caretaking and by leaving the room to get the things necessary for caretaking. In either case, the longer time taken by the Japanese mother seems likely to increase the amount of the infant's unhappy vocalization, and this reinforces the same reasoning arrived at in the preceding analysis of the situation in which the infant is awake and alone.

The American mother responds more quickly to the happy vocalization of the baby by caretaking than does the Japanese mother. Although it goes beyond the limits of the data presented in Table 6, it is important to know that the response of the American mother more frequently includes chatting to the baby in answer to his happy vocalization, as will be apparent in the next section and has already been indicated at the beginning of this paper from the published results of the more general analysis of the data.

We can use the data presented in Table 6, as we did in the preceding analysis, to test whether the mothers in each culture discriminate between the unhappy and happy vocalizations of their babies by responding more quickly with caretaking to the unhappy vocalization. The results are not significant in either culture in the present situation where the mother is in the same room as her baby, but the pattern of the data is the same as in the preceding analysis. In both cultures the average time of response is less to unhappy vocalization, and the American mother responds more quickly than the Japanese mother (Japanese average time of response: 2.7 to unhappy and 5.4 to happy, $z = 1.63$, n.s.; American average time of response: 1.7 to unhappy and 2.3 to happy, $z = 1.31$, n.s.).

Table 6: Results of Analysis of Rank-Order Distribution by Culture of Time Taken by Mother to Respond to Infant's Vocalization in State Two (infant awake and mother merely present)

| | Average Number* of Observations Taken by Mother to Respond from Time of Infant's First Signal When Infant is:† | | | | | | | |
| | Silent: | | Unhappily Vocal: | | Mixed Vocal: | | Happily Vocal: | |
Culture	Mother Does Caretaking	Mother Leaves Room	Mother Does Caretaking	Mother Leaves Room	Mother Does Caretaking	Mother Leaves Room	Mother Does Caretaking	Mother Leaves Room
Japanese	2.4	2.1	2.7	2.0	9.8	Insufficient Data	5.4	3.5
American	1.8	2.0	1.7	1.0	6.1		2.3	1.8
Number of cases								
Japanese	28	17	19	8	9	0	17	7
American	30	24	16	6	7	1	26	12
z score	1.78	0.81	1.85	2.32	0.85		2.11	0.51
p <	0.08	n.s.‡	0.07	0.05	n.s.		0.05	n.s.

* This number is obtained by averaging the averages for the mothers in each culture.

† Antecedent is awake in all sequences.

‡ Not significant

In those sequences where the infant goes to sleep by himself, the data were not sufficient to control on the antecedent of asleep or awake or to control for the type of vocalization in the episode. If we ignore these controls, however, and deal only with a more grossly defined situation in which the infant is awake in the presence of his mother and then goes to sleep, we do have enough data for a test. The score in this test is the average number of observations, from the beginning of the episode, that it takes the infant to go to sleep by himself. We have data for eleven Japanese and nine American infants, with a Japanese mean of 4.5 and an American mean of 5.8 observations taken to go to sleep. The z score of 1.22 is not significant. This finding again argues for the similarity of basic biological rhythms if the mothers do not interfere.

ANALYSIS OF BOUNDED EPISODES IN STATE 1:
INFANT AWAKE AND MOTHER CARETAKING

In the analysis of bounded episodes in state 1 our basic question cannot be concerned, as it was in the preceding analyses, with how quickly a mother responds to various types of vocalization by her infant, because in state 1 the mother and infant already are in interaction. We can, however, focus on the patterns of vocal behavior between mother and infant and ask how often, on the average, these patterns occur within the bounded episodes of the thirty cases in each culture.

As before, the vocalization of the infant can be divided into four types—silent, unhappy, mixed, and happy. Similarly the vocalization of the mother can be divided into four types—silent, only lulling, mixed lulling and chatting, and only chatting. The combination of these two classifications results in sixteen logical kinds of vocal behavior between infant and mother.

We next examined the data to find out, in fact, which of these sixteen kinds of vocal behavior occurred with sufficient frequency to permit comparative analysis. Our a priori criterion was that a kind of vocal behavior should occur in at least one-third of the cases in each culture. The criterion was met by seven kinds of vocal behavior (these can be seen in Table 7). Nine did not meet it.[12]

Working with the seven kinds of vocal behavior which met the criterion, we looked at the number of cases available when, in addition, we controlled for the infant's being awake (states 2 or 3) or asleep (states 4, 5, or 6) both in the antecedent and consequent states. In this $2 \times 7 \times 2$ design there are twenty-eight possible sequences, but the upshot of our examination was that the great bulk of cases in each culture occurred in the seven sequences in which both the antecedent and consequent are awake.[13] Consequently, there appeared to be little point in controlling for the antecedent and consequent states, and we decided, therefore, simply to examine the average frequency of occurrence of bounded episodes in the seven kinds of vocal behavior over the thirty cases in each culture.[14] Table 7 gives the results of this inquiry.

Table 7: Mean Frequency of Bounded Episodes of Vocal Behavior and Results of Analysis of Rank-Order Distribution by Culture in State One (infant awake and mother caretaking)

Culture	Mother Is Silent:			Mother Chats to Infant:			
	Infant Is Silent	Infant Is Unhappily Vocal	Infant Is Happily Vocal	Infant Is Silent	Infant Is Unhappily Vocal	Infant Is Mixed Vocal	Infant Is Happily Vocal
Japanese (N=30 cases)	5.7	0.8	0.5	3.6	1.6	0.4	1.1
American (N=30 cases)	6.2	0.8	2.5	3.6	1.4	1.4	4.0
z score	0.02	0.30	3.77	0.13	0.24	3.21	4.72
$p <$	n.s.*	n.s.	0.001	n.s.	n.s.	0.01	0.001

* Not significant

It is immediately apparent in Table 7 that the major difference between the cultures is the greater number of episodes in which the American infant, as opposed to the Japanese infant, is happily vocalizing, and this is particularly true when his mother is chatting to him. We believe that this added vocal stimulation and encouragement by the mother carries over to those times when she is silent but the baby is happily vocal, probably in anticipation of a response from his mother. It should also be noted that the American mother chats more to her mixed vocalizing baby who is, of course, making a combination of unhappy and happy sounds. At the beginning of this paper we indicated that there is a positive correlation between the amount of chatting by the mother and the amount of happy vocalization by the baby in the American, but not in the Japanese, cases. From the present analysis we can see that, in fact, there is more of such verbal interaction between mother and baby in the American cases.

Discussion and Conclusion

We began this paper with the question of why should the American infant have a generally higher level of vocalization, and particularly of happy vocalization, while the Japanese infant has more unhappy vocalization. We believe that the evidence we have presented goes a long way towards answering this question.[15]

First of all, the pace of the American mother is livelier than that of the Japanese mother; she is in and out of the room more often and thus provides more naturally occurring opportunities to speak to her baby and for him to respond vocally as she cares for him. The American mother also responds more quickly to her baby's vocalizations than her Japanese counterpart, and, even more important, she differentiates more sharply between kinds of vocalization by responding in a shorter time in answer to his unhappy than to his happy sounds. In this latter regard, the American mother appears to be teaching her infant to make a more discriminating use of his voice. Finally, the American mother has more vocal interaction with her baby than the Japanese mother, especially by chatting to him at the same time that he is happily vocal. All of these findings are part of the American mother's style of caretaking which, we believe, serves to increase her infant's happy vocalization and, more generally, to emphasize the importance of vocal communication.

In contrast, the pace of the Japanese mother is more leisurely and, although she does not spend any more total time in the care of her baby than the American mother, her periods of caretaking are fewer and longer. She is more involved in the process of her baby's going to sleep and waking up. Part of the Japanese mother's style of caretaking is to carry, rock, and lull her baby to sleep with the result that when the sleeping baby is put down, he tends to awaken and cry, and the process begins again. In checking on the sleeping baby, the Japanese mother is more likely to go beyond glancing at him to other care that brings her into physical contact with the baby and that often results in the baby's waking and crying for a brief period. Thus, although the total time spent in sleep is not different for the Japanese baby than for the American baby, the former is in and out of sleep more frequently and is more unhappily vocal during these transitions. The Japanese mother is slower to respond in general to her infant's vocalizations, and she does not discriminate between his unhappy and happy sounds by responding more quickly to one than to the other. Finally, the Japanese mother has less vocal interaction with her baby during caretaking, and this is particularly true for the situation in which the mother is chatting to a happily vocalizing baby. These aspects of the Japanese mother's style of caretaking help to explain why the Japanese infant has a greater amount of unhappy vocalization than the American infant, and also point to a lesser reliance on and refinement of vocal communication between the Japanese mother and infant while, at the same time, emphasizing the importance and communicative value of physical contact.

Earlier we raised, but did not answer, the question of why the Japanese mother should persist in a style of care that led to her baby being fussier. This question is only a part of the even more general question of what lies behind and influences the specific styles of care shown by the mothers in the two cultures. In concluding this paper we can at least outline some of what we believe are the answers to this question.

The mother's perception of her infant and of her relation to him would seem to be different in the two cultures. In America the mother views her baby as a potentially separate and autonomous being who should learn to do and think for himself. For her, the baby is from birth a distinct personality with his own needs and desires which she must learn to recognize and care for. She helps him to learn to express these needs and desires through her emphasis on vocal communication so that he can "tell" her what he wants and she can respond appropriately. She de-emphasizes the importance of physical contact such as carrying and rocking and encourages her infant through the use of her voice to explore and to learn to deal with his environment by himself. In the same way that she thinks of her infant as a separate individual, she thinks of herself as a separate person with needs and desires which include time apart from her baby so that she may pursue her own interests and act as a wife to her husband as well as a mother to her baby. For this reason the pace of her caretaking is quicker than the Japanese mother's, and when she is caretaking, her involvement with the baby is livelier and more intense. This is true partly because she wishes to stimulate the baby to activity and response so that when it is time for him to sleep, he will remain asleep and allow her time to do other things during the day and at night.

In Japan the mother views her baby much more as an extension of herself, and psychologically the boundaries between the two of them are blurred. The mother feels that she knows what is best for the baby, and there is no particular need for him to tell her what he wants because, after all, they are virtually one. Thus, in Japan, there is a greater emphasis on interdependence, rather than independence, of mother and child, and this emphasis extends into adulthood.[16] Given this orientation, the Japanese mother places less importance on vocal communication and more on physical contact; also, for her, there is no need for hurry as the expectation is that she will devote herself to her child without any great concern for time away from him or even for time to be alone with her husband. As we know from other research (Caudill and Plath, 1966), the Japanese child will ordinarily sleep with his parents until he is approximately ten years of age.

Given the differences in these two styles of care, we believe that the infants have learned to respond to each respective style in culturally appropriate ways by three to four months of age. Since the differences that these styles of care elicit in the behavior of infants are in line with the later expectations for behavior in the two cultures, we can say that the infants have learned some of the rudiments of their respective culture by three to four months of age. This learning process takes place well before the development of the ability to use language in the ordinary sense; hence, these infants have acquired before then some aspects of the "implicit culture" (Linton, 1945; Kluckhohn, 1951) of their group—that is, those ways of feeling, thinking, and behaving that go on largely out of awareness and that, in general, characterize the actions of people in a given culture.

We are fortunate in that, by design, we had the opportunity to follow up the behavior of the first twenty of these same children in each culture as they became two-and-a-half and six years of age. We are about to begin analysis of these data. We can, therefore, test at these later ages whether or not the differences in vocal communication which we found in infancy do, in fact, persist over the first six years of life. Our prediction is that this will happen, and that the early differences in behavior which we can already see in infancy will continue to develop along the lines laid down by the two cultures.

ACKNOWLEDGMENT

The preparation and analysis of data was facilitated by the assistance of Mrs. Barbara Schmidt.

NOTES

1. In this article, the terms mother and caretaker are used interchangeably, because in the observations in each culture, it was the mother who did the caretaking more than 90 percent of the time. In the more general study (Caudill and Weinstein, 1969), all of the dependent variables concerning the behavior of mother and infant were precisely defined, and a satisfactory level of interobserver reliability was established for each of them. In this article we use the same definitions for the various kinds of vocal behavior. By infant vocalization we mean any expressively voiced sound, and we did not include hiccups, coughs, etc. Unhappily vocal means any negatively voiced sound, and it has an interobserver reliability of 89 percent in the Japanese cases and 88 percent in the American cases. Happily vocal means any positively voiced sound, and it has a reliability of 70 percent in the Japanese cases and 70 percent in the American cases. The two variables are additive and can be combined into a composite variable called total infant vocalization. The vocalization of the mother is divided into chats and lulls. Lulls is a very delimited variable and means that the mother is softly singing or humming a lullaby or making repetitive comforting noises, with the apparent intent of soothing and quieting the baby or getting him to go to sleep; it has a reliability of 94 percent in the Japanese cases and 100 percent in the American cases. Chats include all other vocalization to the infant, such as talking to him, singing to him in a lively fashion, and playing word games ("boo," "goo," etc.) with him; it has a reliability of 90 percent in the Japanese cases and 83 percent in the American cases. The two variables are additive and can be combined into a composite variable called total talks to infant.

2. Like any broad generalization, this one needs qualification and explanation which is beyond the scope of this paper. Briefly, what is meant is that a child or an adult in America is expected to defend his opinions and rights and to take personal responsibility for his actions, whereas in

Japan a person is expected, much more than in America, to blend in as a member of his important reference groups, and it is the group more than the individual that bears responsibility for actions. (For further discussion along these lines see Caudill, unpublished paper.)

3. The probability values given in Table 1 and in all subsequent tables are two-tailed, meaning that the direction of the outcome of the results has not been predicted.

4. In Table 2 and in all subsequent tables, the more complicated statistical procedure of analysis of variance is not used. Since, in the earlier analysis, we found that culture was overwhelmingly the most important independent variable, culture is used here as the only independent variable in an analysis of the rank-ordered distribution of the cases on a given dependent variable. For example, the sixty mothers represented in Table 2 are first rank-ordered from one to sixty in terms of the number of changes of state shown by each mother, and then this distribution is examined to determine whether there is a significant difference in the ranked positions occupied by American as compared with Japanese mothers. The statistic used in the analysis presented in Table 2 and in all subsequent tables is the Mann-Whitney U test (Siegel, 1956: 116–127). The results of this test can be given as a z score with its appropriate (two-tailed) probability value. Because the test is a nonparametric statistic (that is, the test is made in terms of positions in a rank-order rather than in terms of numerical quantity), the means given in the tables are essentially illustrative and only indicate the direction and an approximation of the magnitude of an effect. The crucial findings are given by the z score and its probability value.

5. Gradually we are coming to believe that activity in and of itself is a value in American culture. It is not too extreme to point to the greater physical activity and play of the American infants and the greater busyness of the American mothers compared to their Japanese counterparts as specific examples of such a value. This line of thought will be developed further as the data collected on the same children at two-and-a-half and six years of age are analyzed.

6. It should be mentioned that these differences in the behavior of the mothers and three-to-four-month-old infants in the two cultures are not influenced by the chance factor of sickness. We did not make observations on days when either mother or infant was ill. In a separate body of research data, the tendency of the Japanese mother to fuss over her sleeping baby is vividly illustrated in several of the cases that Peter Wolff and I observed in Kyoto over the first month of an infant's life during a pilot study carried out in 1963. The results of this study have not been published, as we need to gather more data on the behavior of Japanese mothers and infants during the first month of life. Wolff has already gathered a substantial body of data on American mothers and infants during this very early period.

7. The problem that Japanese have with sleep disturbances is a recurring one in separate studies done by us and others. Iwawaki, Sumida, Okuno, and Cowen (1967) report that nine-year-old Japanese children show significantly less anxiety in general on the Children's Manifest Anxiety Scale than do comparable groups of French and American children ex-

cept on a cluster of three items pertaining to difficulty in going to sleep in which the Japanese children show significantly more anxiety. In a comparative study of Japanese and American schizophrenic patients, we found that the Japanese patients show significantly more symptoms of sleep disturbance (Schooler and Caudill, 1964). (In general, see Caudill and Plath, 1966, on sleeping arrangements in Japan.)

8. The bounded episodes used in this analysis constitute a representative sample of all episodes that are thirty-eight or less observations in length, because it is a random matter over the total observations whether such episodes occur entirely within the ten-minute observation periods or have their beginning or ending during the five-minute breaks. We also examined all longer nonbounded episodes (those of more than thirty-eight observations in length) in the three states in which the infant is awake. These do not occur with sufficient frequency to permit analysis in state 3 when the infant is alone or in state 2 when the infant is in the presence of his mother who is not caretaking. They do occur with greater frequency in state 1 when the mother is caretaking, but a separate analysis of these longer nonbounded episodes reveals the same findings as are discussed in the text for the bounded episodes in state 1.

9. The eight logical sequences in which the data were insufficient for analysis involve three sequences in which the consequent is that the mother responds and five in which the consequent is that the infant goes to sleep. The three sequences in which the consequent is that the mother responds are: (1) antecedent is asleep, episode is silent; (2) antecedent is asleep, episode is mixed vocalization; (3) antecedent is asleep, episode is only happy vocalization. The five sequences in which the consequent is that the infant goes to sleep are: (1) antecedent is awake, episode is only unhappy vocalization; (2) antecedent is awake, episode is mixed vocalization; (3) antecedent is awake, episode is only happy vocalization; (4) antecedent is asleep, episode is mixed vocalization; (5) antecedent is asleep, episode is only happy vocalization.

10. The seventeen sequences in which data were inadequate are: (1) all twelve logical sequences in which the antecedent is asleep; (2) all four sequences in which the infant in the episode is silent, unhappily vocal, mixed vocal, or happily vocal, and the antecedent is awake while the consequent is asleep; and (3) the antecedent is awake, the episode is mixed vocal, and the consequent is that the mother leaves the room. This latter sequence is indicated in Table 6 to maintain the symmetry of the table even though the data were insufficient.

11. As stated earlier, all probability values are given in terms of two-tailed tests meaning that we do not assume that we have predicted the direction of a finding, although by now it would be a fairly safe assumption that the Japanese mother is slower in her response to her infant's vocalization. If we make the latter assumption, then four of the seven tests are significant. What seems remarkable to us, and increases our credence in the findings, is that any of the tests are significant since the mothers start out in this situation by being present in the same room with their babies.

12.   There is, nevertheless, something of interest to be learned from three of the nine kinds of behavior which do not meet the criterion; all three concern the mother's lulling of an awake infant who, respectively, is silent (three Japanese and one American cases), unhappily vocal (six Japanese and one American cases), or happily vocal (two Japanese and no American cases). As indicated, there are more cases of Japanese mothers in all three of these kinds of vocal behavior. The other six kinds of vocal behavior which do not meet the criterion are: (1) a silent mother does caretaking for a mixed vocal baby (two Japanese and five American cases); (2) a mother is mixed vocal to a mixed vocal baby (no Japanese and one American case); and (3) four kinds which never occur in either culture: a mother is mixed vocal, respectively, to a silent, to an unhappily vocal, and to a happily vocal baby, and finally, a mother lulls a mixed vocal baby.

13.   Beyond these seven sequences, there are only two others that contain enough cases to be interesting. In each of these the antecedent and consequent are that the infant is asleep, and both sequences mainly involve Japanese mothers. In one, the mother is silent as she cares for her awake and silent baby (16 Japanese and 2 American cases), and in the other, the mother chats to an awake and silent baby (5 Japanese and 1 American cases). It seems clear that the essence of the meaning of these two sequences has already been covered in the earlier discussion of the greater involvement of Japanese mothers in the waking of infants.

14.   We also did parallel analyses of the average length of episodes, and where appropriate, of the average number of observations per episode of verbal behavior by the mother and by the infant. In general, however, there were no differences between the cultures in the length of episodes or in the amount of verbal behavior within the episodes. Therefore, the best and simplest measure proved to be the one we are using here, that is, the average frequency of occurrence of episodes of a given kind of verbal behavior.

15.   A caution is necessary here. Strictly speaking, our results obtain for first-born infants in middle-class urban families in Japan and America. We feel, however, that our findings have a broader applicability, particularly in the more general form in which they are stated in the concluding section of this paper.

16.   For a discussion of the emphasis on interdependence in its various aspects in Japan see Caudill and Doi, 1963; Caudill and Scarr, 1962; Caudill, 1962, and Caudill, unpublished paper.

REFERENCES

Caudill, W. 1962. Patterns of emotion in modern Japan. *In* Japanese culture: Its development and characteristics. Robert J. Smith and Richard K. Beardsley, eds. Chicago, Aldine.

———. The influence of social structure and culture on human behavior in modern Japan. Paper to appear in Adaptation, adjustment, and culture change (tentative title). G. DeVos, ed.

Caudill, W., and L. T. Doi. 1963. Interrelations of psychiatry, culture, and emotion in Japan. *In* Man's image in medicine and anthropology. I. Galdston, ed. New York, International Universities Press.

Caudill, W., and D. W. Plath. 1966. Who sleeps by whom? Parent-child involvement in urban Japanese families. Psychiatry 29:344–66.

Caudill, W., and H. A. Scarr. 1962. Japanese value orientations and culture change. Ethnology 1:53–91.

Caudill, W., and H. Weinstein, 1969. Maternal care and infant behavior in Japan and America. Psychiatry 32:12–43.

Iwawaki, S., K. Sumida, S. Okuno, and E. L. Cowen. 1967. Manifest anxiety in Japanese, French, and United States children. Child Development 38:713–22.

Kluckhohn, C. 1951. The study of culture. *In* The policy sciences. D. Lerner and H. D. Lasswell, eds. Stanford, Stanford University Press.

Linton, R. 1945. The cultural background of personality. New York, D. Appleton-Century.

Schooler, C., and W. Caudill. 1964. Symptomatology in Japanese and American schizophrenics. Ethnology 3:172–78.

Siegel, S. 1956. Nonparametric statistics for the behavioral sciences. New York, McGraw-Hill.

4. The Use of the Imperative Mood in Postwar Japan

MASANORI HIGA, Ed.D.

Social Science Research Institute
University of Hawaii
Honolulu, Hawaii

TWENTY-THREE YEARS have passed since Japan began democratizing social institutions as a result of defeat in World War II. This sort of drastic social change is bound to have some effect on the language spoken by the Japanese, since social, cultural, and psychological factors are said to be closely related to linguistic changes (Fodor, 1965). When one observes the Japanese language of today, comparing it with usage before 1945, one recognizes certain significant changes, many of which seem to be attributable to the social change. Taking note of such changes can throw some light on the nature of speech as social behavior and on the relationship between language and social structure.[1]

Although languages change continuously, basic structural alterations take place over a long period of time so that one cannot expect to find significant changes at the phonemic, morphemic, and syntactic levels in the Japanese language during the past twenty-three years. Most of the observable changes are at the lexical and usage levels. Some of these have been brought about by artificial means such as governmental decrees and systematic educational programs. As examples, one may cite the limiting of the use of Chinese characters to less than two thousand basic words and the discontinued use of the terms that were used only in reference to the imperial household. However, many of the changes are voluntary or self-imposed in the sense that they are not the products of organized efforts. The increased use of the colloquial style and traditionally Japanese vocabulary in place of the formal or literary style and Chinese loan-words for an effective use of mass media of communication and the increased tendency for both males and females to use a common style of speech in place of the traditional male and female style of speech are some examples. One of the interesting and significant changes in the latter category is the change in the use of the imperative mood, the topic for this paper.

The Japanese people had long been feudalistic and authoritarian, and their use of language clearly reflected this characteristic. For example, there used to be the pronoun *chin* used only by emperors. The use of honorifics was strictly observed, and in referring to oneself, one had to be careful to choose the right pronoun from the set of class- or status-reflecting pronouns. In addressing his equals or inferiors, a Japanese could use pronouns, but if he was speaking to those who were his superiors in status or age, he had to use in place of pronouns their occupational titles, generalized kinship terms, or last names depending upon the setting. The kind of *vous-tu* relation that exists between speaker and addressee in French and other European languages (Brown and Gillman, 1960) and the you-you relation that exists in English did not, and still does not, exist in Japanese. The imperative mood or the command form could be used only by superiors in addressing inferiors or between close friends. From the linguistic point of view, imperial, military, feudal, governmental, parental, and seniority authority in Japan meant the authority to use the imperative mood to command subordinates. Even husbands had the same authority vis-à-vis their wives. This type of authoritarian command used to be convenient and effective in maintaining authority and in getting things done.

The postwar democratization of Japan, however, instilled into her people a sense of human dignity and equal rights for all. As was the case in the United States, words connoting low social status were discarded in favor of new, dignified terms. Thus, maids, janitors, and garbage collectors, for instance, are no longer called as such but as helpers (*otetsudai-san*), custodians (*kanrinin*), and sanitation officers (*eiseifu*). Husbands stopped referring to their wives as stupid wives (*gusai*), and parents stopped referring to their children as piglike children (*tonji*). Government officials and policemen began to assume the role of public servants, at least on the surface, using honorifics or the polite form in talking with citizens. These changes confirm the general notion that the burden of democratizing a language is on superiors. One may say, to emphasize the point, that the Japanese language has become primarily a means of communication, even with the masses, rather than a means of exhibiting authority [2] and an instrument of social control.

As the authoritarian attitude was greatly modified, so was the use of the imperative mood. The defeat in war and the subsequent democratization made it explicitly clear that those who had had the authority to command the nation, students, and children (the political and military leaders, teachers, and parents) had erred in their philosophy and leadership. They had not only lost face, but they had lost the authority to use the imperative mood. The democratization of the Japanese language might have proceeded quickly if those superiors who had lost authority had not regained their superior or leadership positions in postwar Japan. The postwar social change was not accompanied by a drastic leadership change. The situation today is that, on the one hand, there is a socially and psychologically imposed pressure on superiors not to use the imperative mood in giving orders to inferiors, and, on the other hand, there is a habitual urge for them to use it as an effective expression of their requests. This means that they are now linguistically obligated to treat their inferiors as equals, although they still perceive them as socially inferior. The result is a dissonance which must be reduced. At present, it is still too early to tell whether they will modify their perception of the people to whom they speak in accordance with the form of language they feel pressured to use, or vice versa.

The word 'mood' as a grammatical term is somewhat old-fashioned. By this term grammarians refer to the attitude of mind of a speaker with respect to the nature of a statement he makes (Curme, 1925; Jespersen, 1924). If he states a fact or truth, he uses the indicative mood, e.g., 'The earth goes round the sun.' When he makes a statement of supposition, the subjunctive mood is used, e.g., 'If there were no oxygen on the earth, animals would die.' When a command or request is made, he uses the imperative mood, e.g., 'Go round the earth!' These are the three moods that are commonly used, and linguistic utterances are classifiable into these categories. From the linguistic viewpoint, no value or stigma is attached to any of these, and the imperative mood is as good as the others. But from the sociopsychological point of view, a speaker is often, as in Japan, pressured to refrain from using the imperative mood.

Historically speaking, such a sociopsychological pressure is not unique to the Japanese language. Although the imperative mood is commonly used in English today, especially in commercial advertisements, there was some restraint on its use in earlier centuries when either the indicative or the subjunctive mood was frequently used. In addressing superiors or strangers, the following phrases were generally used: 'May it please you . . .', 'I pray you . . .', 'I desire you . . .', 'I beseech you . . .'. Today the word 'please' is regarded as an adverb when it is used with the imperative form, and people are often unaware that it is the abbreviation of the old subjunctive form, 'If it please you'. In addition to these forms, the passive and question forms were popularly used. Many of these are still retained and used in English as indirect or polite request forms. Even a simple indicative form is sometimes used as an indirect method of giving a command. When a husband says to his wife, 'I am hungry', he is not simply referring to his physical state. He is indirectly commanding that his wife prepare a meal for him. It is true that these indirect commands are made by English-speaking peoples even today, but in order to make clear the contrast with the Japanese language, it must be emphatically mentioned that in English the simple imperative form is commonly used in everyday life, and when one wishes to be polite, all one need do is add the word 'please'. This free use of the imperative mood may be due to the fact that the English language does not possess an honorific style of speech as Japanese does, and also the English-speaking peoples have come through the social process of democratization.

At present, Japanese-speaking people may be said to be one step behind English-speaking peoples in the use of the imperative mood. The indirect and polite forms in English are the forms most commonly used by the Japanese, especially in conjunction with the use of their honorifics. Those Japanese who have had a taste of using the straight imperative mood seem to feel that the indicative or the subjunctive mood is irritatingly slow and inefficient in expressing commands. Instead of saying to his class, 'Turn in your reports' (*'Repōto o teishutsu-seyo'*), a teacher nowadays makes such statements as the following:

> 'You are to turn in your reports.' (*'Repōto o teishutsu-surukoto.'*)
> 'I beg you to turn in your reports.' (*'Repōto o teishutsu-shitekudasai.'*)
> 'I would appreciate if you would turn in your reports.' (*'Repōto o teishutsu-shitekudasattara iindesuga.'*)
> 'Won't you turn in your reports?' (*'Repōto o teishutsu-shitekudasaimasenka.'*)

It is linguistically interesting to watch a meeting between so-called radical students, on the one hand, and administrators and professors, on the other. Radical students make it a rule to attack the traditional usage of the Japanese language as part of the Establishment, and in addressing administrators and professors, they deliberately use the lowest form of pronoun (*omae*) and the straight imperative form, e.g., *'damare'* ('shut up'). To them, the use of honorific language signifies a linguistically imposed submission to the existing Establishment, and thus they avoid using it. In contrast to these students, administrators and professors typically keep using honorifics and the indicative or subjunctive mood to express their requests. In such a linguistic situation, a sensible dialogue is difficult, and a meeting often becomes unproductive. A Japanese-speaking person is well aware that when a subordinate or inferior person stops using honorific language and starts using the imperative form and the familiar style of address in talking with a superior person, he is declaring hostilities; and this act often creates an irreversible hostile relation between the two. Inferiors are never expected to talk to superiors in the way in which superiors used to talk to them.

Japanese commercial concerns find it inconvenient not to be able to use the imperative mood in addressing consumers. From the semantic point of view, their basic concern is to say to consumers imperatively, 'Buy our products!' In the prewar years, advertisements and slogans often used the direct imperative form in the literary style such as *'miyo'* ('see'), *'kike'* ('listen'), *'kitare'* ('come'), *'yome'* ('read'), *'kaubeshi'* ('buy'), *'mochiubeshi'* ('use'), *'kōdokuseyo'* ('subscribe'), as this style was considered somewhat neutral in terms of superior-inferior relations. Today these imperative words are no longer used, because the literary style is rarely used in everyday life. Most advertisements are phrased in the indicative mood using colloquial Japanese, and occasionally requests are made in indirect and somewhat ingenious ways that will be described below. I randomly selected several issues of magazines and newspapers of Japan and the United States and compared their advertisements in terms of the use of the imperative mood.[3] The statistics showed that whereas 62 percent of the American advertisements used the imperative mood and 38 percent used the indicative mood, none of the Japanese advertisements used the imperative mood, 30 percent used various indirect forms, and 70 percent used the indicative mood. Most of the American advertisements using the indicative mood were in the nature of public relations statements. It should be pointed out that when Japanese products are advertised in American magazines using English, there is no significant difference in the use of the imperative mood between the advertisements of American products and those of Japanese products.[4] Most frequently used imperative words are: 'try', 'see', 'compare', 'be', 'get', 'take', and 'come'. The reverse of this is also true. When American products are advertised in Japan using the Japanese language, those imperative words disappear, and the indicative mood becomes the predominant mode of expression. The ubiquitous advertisement of Coca Cola in many parts of the world is that imperative sentence, 'Drink Coca Cola'. In Japan, it is not directly translated as *'Coca Cola o nome'*, but indirectly as *'Coca Cola o nomimashō'*, which means: 'We will drink Coca Cola'.[5]

The various techniques of making commands or requests by Japanese commercial concerns may be regarded as euphemistic. One technique is to state only the object and omit the imperative verb as in *'Okurimononi X o'* ('X for a gift') and *'X o dōzo'* ('Please X'). The imperative verb 'buy' or 'give' is implicit. The question forms like *'Tameshite mimasenka'* ('Won't you try?') and *'Otameshi kudasai'* ('Will you have the favor to try?') are commonly use. Apparently, these euphemistic expressions do not satisfy advertisers, and they have now begun to use the imperative mood directly by having comedians, coquettish women, and children utter imperative sentences. It is surprisingly true that comical expressions, coquettish appeals, and feminine and baby talk reduce the offensiveness of the imperative mood to a great extent. Thus, comedians, coquettish actresses, babyish singers, and verbally facile children are in demand for producing radio and television advertisements. This phenomenon indicates that as long as the speaker somehow clearly manifests his inferiority to the listener, even in an artificial way, he can use the imperative mood, although its commanding effect may be reduced. The use of baby talk, for example, evokes a nurturant-baby situation (Ferguson, 1964) in which the listener-consumer is placed in the superior position of nurturant and is asked to patronize the advertiser who assumes the inferior role of baby.

Another technique, which is likely to gain at least transitory popularity, is to use English where imperative sentences are needed. 'Stay white' is an English sentence used by one shirt manufacturer, and 'Open bonnet [sic]' [6] is a sentence used by an automobile oil producer. The reason why this technique may spread widely is that since English is a required part of the school curriculum, simple English imperative sentences are understandable to every postwar educated Japanese.

This use of English as a euphemistic technique reminds one of a linguistically interesting phenomenon that took place in Japan immediately after the war. It was the use of the English pronouns 'you' and 'me' in Japanese sentences by those who came in contact with English-speaking people. This was the time when the Japanese did not use Japanese pronouns as often as they do now. In Okinawa and in the Japanese-speaking community in Hawaii, the same phenomenon can still be observed. One even hears the Japanized pronouns 'you-ra' and 'me-ra' as the plural forms of 'you' and 'me'; ra being a Japanese suffix to indicate plural.[7] The instances cited here seem to indicate that a foreign language, both in grammar and vocabulary, can act as a kind of catalyst for a language which is in a transitional or transformational stage.

In many Japanese organizations, superiors plan various programs for the purpose of creating a feeling of togetherness between superiors and inferiors and among inferiors. After taking subordinates to drinking parties or on recreational tours while keeping a seniority rule and practicing paternalism toward them, superiors quietly but surely win an acquiescence from their inferiors to use the imperative mood in giving them orders. Thus, in Japan, drinking and group touring are considered to be the most effective means of cultivating close human relations and breaking the language barriers described so far.[8]

A question of significant interest for linguistically oriented social scientists is: What will be the future of the Japanese imperative mood after the present ambivalence? Several possibilities are conceivable. One is that with the increased use of the polite form by all as the standard style of speech, the imperative mood may be replaced by the indicative and subjunctive moods in colloquial Japanese. In this case, vocal factors, i.e., volume and intonation, may become the characteristic attributes of command or request forms rather than the traditional grammatical form (Hockett, 1958). This is perhaps the most desirable. Another possibility is that the kind of commercialism mentioned above will create a neutral and inoffensive way of uttering an imperative sentence. Comical, feminine, and baby talk may become standard ways of saying an imperative sentence. An undesirable possibility is that authoritarianism may rise once again in Japan and with it, the use of the imperative mood only by superiors as in the prewar years. If this takes place, it may mean that the postwar democratization of Japan has failed. In reaction to the current violent students movements, Japan is witnessing the beginning of some reactionary movements. From the linguistic point of view, radicals and progressives are struggling for the use of the imperative mood by all or, if that is impossible, for its total disuse; reactionaries and conservatives are trying to regain control over its use for superiors. The former are also trying to establish a linguistic usage whereby inferiors can address superiors by pronouns.

Japanese linguists agree that the Japanese language is in a state of confusion and that there is a need for specifications of what may be accepted as standard Japanese (Kindaichi, H., 1966; Kindaichi, K., 1959; Ono, 1968; Yazaki, 1960). If language is to be related to cognition and if language usage is to reflect the structure of society (Hoijer, 1954), it seems to be much more important for the entire nation to create and sustain a democratic and humanitarian society than for linguists and governmental commissions to prescribe an ideal standard speech. Martin (1964), who studied speech levels in both Japan and Korea, predicted that the use of different speech levels, including honorifics, will not die out, even if feudalism is replaced by democracy in these countries. However, the critical factor in the use or disuse of different speech levels, including honorifics, does not seem to be a simple replacement of feudalism by democracy, but the extent of the loss of authority in such a change on the part of superiors such as political leaders, teachers, and parents. Viewed from this point, Martin's prediction may be upheld in Korea, where it was the Japanese who lost authority. As the Japanese colonial rule ended in Korea in 1945, the superior-inferior relations were broken between the Japanese and the Koreans, but such relations among the Koreans remained almost intact. As was mentioned earlier in this paper, the superior-inferior relations are somewhat ambivalent among Japanese today because the loss of authority on the part of the prewar superiors has been incomplete. This ambivalence is clearly reflected in the use of the speech levels by Japanese. In this sense, one may say that the future of the Japanese imperative mood depends upon how the present superior-inferior relations change in the future.

NOTES

1. Stalin (1951) felt that the Russian Revolution had not affected the Russian language and wrote papers to the effect that language was not a superstructure and, therefore, remained unaffected by changes in the base or the economic structure of society.

2. Prewar pupils were forced to memorize the so-called Imperial Edict on Education (*Kyōiku Chokugo*), but the language used was so difficult that they recited it by rote without understanding it.

3. These were Asahi Shimbun, Shūkan Yomiuri, Bungei Shunjū, Honolulu Star-Bulletin, Newsweek, and Life.

4. These were the Asian editions of Time and Life.

5. This Japanese sentence is often translated into an imperative English sentence as "Let us drink Coca Cola," but the original Japanese is only connotatively imperative and not grammatically imperative.

6. In American English this may be phrased as 'Open the hood!'

7. The Japanese suffixes *wa*, *ga*, *no*, *o*, and *ni* were also used to indicate the case of these pronouns: subjective, possessive, or objective.

8. In American occupational settings, too, superiors seem somewhat restrained from using the imperative mood. According to one survey (Ervin-Tripp, 1964, 91), "the imperative form is most often used to inferiors, and more often for easy than difficult or unusual services.... The yes-no question is the most typical request form to superiors."

REFERENCES

Brown, R., and A. Gilman. 1960. The pronouns of power and solidarity. *In* Style in Language. T. A. Sebeok, ed. New York, John Wiley and Sons.

Curme, G. O. 1925. College english grammar. Richmond, Virginia, Johnson.

Ervin-Tripp, S. 1964. An analysis of the interaction of language, topic, and listener. American Anthropologist 66, no. 6, part 2:86–102.

Ferguson, C. A. 1964. Baby talk in six languages. American Anthropologist 66, no. 6, part 2:103–14.

Fodor, I. 1965. The rate of linguistic change. The Hague, Mouton.

Hockett, C. F. 1958. A course in modern linguistics. New York, Macmillan.

Hoijer, H. 1964. Language in culture. Chicago, University of Chicago Press.

Jespersen, O. 1924. The philosophy of grammar. London, Allen and Unwin.

Kindaichi, H. 1966. A new treatise on the Japanese language. Tokyo, Chikuma. [In Japanese]

Kindaichi, K. 1966. Japanese honorific. Tokyo, Kadokawa. [In Japanese]

Martin, S. E. 1964. Speech levels in Japan and Korea. *In* Language in Culture and Society. D. Hymes, ed. New York, Harper & Row. 407–15.

Ono, S., ed. 1968. Reviewing the Japanese language. Tokyo, Yomiuru Shimbun. [In Japanese]

Stalin, J., 1951. Marxism and linguistics. New York, International Publishers.

Yazaki, G. 1960. The Japanese language of the future. Tokyo, Mikasa. [In Japanese]

FAMILY DYNAMICS, SOCIALIZATION,
AND PERSONALITY DEVELOPMENT

5.   Family Life and Delinquency:
       Some Perspectives from Japanese Research

GEORGE DeVOS, Ph.D.

Department of Anthropology
University of California
Berkeley, California

HIROSHI WAGATSUMA, Ph.D.

Department of Sociology
University of Pittsburgh
Pittsburgh, Pennsylvania

IN AMERICAN SOCIAL SCIENCE one finds general acceptance of the notion that the family serves as the principal agency of socialization. There is less consensus on the question of how personality development takes place in the matrix of the family. Generally speaking, there are today relatively few adherents to hereditary, constitutional explanations of socially conforming or socially deviant behavior. One must note, nevertheless, that early studies of family lines, such as those of the Jukes and the Kalakaks, which were assumed to confirm heredity as the cause of deviance, had considerable influence on research in the relationship of family lines and delinquency. Such influences are found in prewar Japanese writings on delinquency, whereas in postwar research the environmental approach is in almost total ascendancy. Sociological theorists in Japan and in the United States have long opposed biological interpretations and have sought instead to demonstrate that economic conditions and the oppression of impoverished segments of society were the main sources of family disintegration and degeneration. The early literature therefore focuses on poverty, rather than heredity, as the chief source of delinquency and crime within society.

          Neither of these earlier approaches examines the internal dynamics of family life itself. Rather, the determinants of delinquency were sought in the genes or in the nature of the external situations within which families functioned. To some extent the situational approach still characterizes many sociological explanations. The determinative nature of family life or cultural traditions affecting socialization are considered secondary to the economic and social pressures that have been statistically correlated with the selective occurrence of delinquency in particular class and ethnic segments of the society. A psychocultural approach, on the other hand, while not denying the determining influence of socioeconomic considerations, emphasizes instead that an understanding of socially deviant behavior lies in the particular mechanisms of socialization that occur within the family. Psychoanalytically oriented psychotherapy has provided us with insights into the mechanisms of socialization, but the direct application of the psychonanalytic approach tends to emphasize the vicissitudes of the individual while neglecting to perceive the family as an interacting unit functioning within a particular culture or subculture. An approach emphasizing the family as an interacting subcultural system allows for greater attention to the sociological variables as they interact with the psychological processes of socialization that occur within the family.

In viewing the recent research literature on family studies in Japan as well as in the United States, we note that a number of authors have attempted to categorize highly complex family relations as a determinant in delinquency formation. We have classified these studies of the family into categories in which the principal foci of attention are: (1) the family as a social environment, (2) types of discipline and expression of affection in relation to personality development, (3) problems of separation and deprivation, and (4) what we term induction theories of intrafamilial processes. Induction theories are those mainly concerned with direct social learning and those based upon the relation of conscious and unconscious motives in the parental generation as they relate to delinquency formation in children. In our own intensive research with 50 families in Arakawa Ward, Tokyo, we have examined our results in the context of these previous studies, but we have paid more attention to the parents of the delinquents than to the delinquents per se. From this standpoint, we have gained additional insight into previously published conclusions and interpretations. We shall now briefly report some of our results in the context of Japanese research generally.

Influence of Poverty and Broken Homes
on the Appearance of Delinquency

We shall not consider here the various overall statistical analyses of the relation of depression and prosperity to the incidence of crime and delinquency;[1] there have been detailed studies more directly related to family conditions as they affect the incidence of delinquency in children. The assumption of many of these earlier studies was that the impoverished condition of the family itself was a principal cause of crime and delinquency.

One can quote from the Japanese research literature studies that parallel those done in the United States. A number of these studies suffer from inadequate methods of control, however. For example, Takemura (1953:221) attempted to demonstrate that after World War II, the middle-income groups were more stable and had a generally lower incidence of delinquency than either high-income groups or poor families. He sought to demonstrate this differential by obtaining from a number of prisons the relative incidence of individuals within certain stated family incomes. He found that 3 percent of delinquents came from what could be considered wealthy families, whereas 21 percent came from families that were characterized by day-by-day work income or government welfare support. In contrast, in a particular high school, he found that only 0.7 percent represented the wealthier group, and only 3.2 percent represented students from very poor families. He, therefore, came to the conclusion that in prison both the very wealthy and the very poor are over-represented. It must quickly be pointed out that such a study does not take into account the lack of representativeness of one high school (which is compounded by the fact that students select high schools on the basis of their perceived social status) or the various factors that lead to differences in institutionalization versus probation in Japanese adjudication of juvenile cases.

In more recent and more carefully controlled studies that are concerned with other factors besides poverty in the family, no such remarkable differences were obtained. Tatezawa (1954:17–19) reported that poor families were somewhat over-represented when compared with nondelinquent controls. Ushikubo (1956) found that there were more boys from impoverished families in delinquent groups than in nondelinquent control samples, although the differences were not very great.[2] Today, in Japanese studies poverty is regarded as an indirect rather than a direct influence or also a consequence of family instability as well as being directly causative of delinquency per se. Poverty, for example, may induce the mother to leave the home to work which results in the neglect of her children. Poverty may force families to seek residence in neighborhoods where the social inducement to delinquent activity is high. Poverty may also be a source of conflict between family members. Conditions in Japan today are such, however, that the juvenile delinquency rate is increasing, as we have indicated before, in spite of the total increase in the national average income and in spite of the fact that radical unemployment does not exist. Shortly after the war, the impoverished condition of the country probably contributed to the very high rate of stealing and other offenses against property by juveniles and adults. The Research Institute of the Ministry of Justice (1960) suggested that recent juvenile delinquency has notably increased among individuals from middle-income families. We may raise the question whether this demonstrates an increase in juvenile crime among those families previously classified as middle income, or whether with increasing prosperity, a number of families that were previously classified in a lower-income bracket have moved up into the middle-income classification in the Japanese statistics without improving their relative economic status. The statistics, therefore, may not show a radical increase in middle-income delinquency per se but rather a general shift in the prosperity of the country at large.[3]

Another aspect of family living that is often compared with incidence of delinquency is the living conditions of the household. Resident space does show some correlation with delinquency, although interpretations of the facts differ. Although the ratio of Japanese residents to space available per individual is radically less than that of the United States, still some comparability occurs. Tatezawa (1954:16) reported that there is some slight inverse correlation between residence size and delinquency. In a recent study, Ono (1958:103) pointed out that in his statistical comparisons he found less *tatami* (floor mat) area of living space for boys involved in delinquent groups than for his control sample. Institutionalized delinquents, he found, are apt to have less space at home than noninstitutionalized delinquents on probation. He suggested the possible selectivity of court adjudication. The judges may take such factors as the presence of an intact home or living condition into account when they decide whether to put the individual on probation or to send him away to an institution. Studies, therefore, based only on comparison of institutionalized delinquents with nonmatched normal controls are apt to be spurious in regard to such features. Furthermore, the study in no way demonstrates that living space is correlated with delinquency independent of family income. Using matched samples in the same area, we found in a comparison of fifty familes that there is actually slightly less space per person in the families without delinquents than in those with delinquents.[4]

The Effects of Broken or Disrupted Homes on Delinquency Formation

Perhaps of all the factors in family life, that of broken homes has received the most detailed statistical examination in attempts to understand the genesis of delinquency. Historically, we find numerous studies that see the broken home itself as a condition causing delinquency, disregarding other explanations or psychodynamic interpretations. More recent studies see the broken home as symptomatic of the type of relation within the family, and they indicate that only when certain patterns of interpersonal relations also exist in the family will a broken home lead to delinquency.

One of the earlier studies on the question of broken homes was done in Japan by Yoshimasu (1952) between 1927–29. Although Yoshimasu's theoretical orientation was that of a psychiatrist interested in heredity, he nevertheless attempted careful empirical studies of delinquents' environmental differences. He found that 62 percent of the delinquents in institutions were from broken homes. He later replicated the study over a two-year period, 1931–33, with a study of 100 juvenile prisoners and obtained similar results; 65 percent of the cases were from broken homes. Higuchi (1953) in a follow-up study compared his results with those of Yoshimasu and Tani (1929) and found that 48 percent were from broken homes, a rate considerably lower than reported by either Tani or Yoshimasu but higher than that of a secondary school control sample in which only 24 percent of the individuals came from broken homes. Higuchi, also using a noninstitutionalized delinquent sample as a control, found that 37 percent were from broken homes, a figure between that for institutionalized delinquents and to the secondary school sample. One might anticipate that a high rate of broken homes would exist in Japan owing to the large-scale dislocation and the many casualties of the war. That these studies show an overall lower rate of broken homes than prewar studies may bring into some question the accuracy of the earlier statistics or may attest to a higher incidence of broken families in the past than one would expect from the generally held belief that Japanese family ties are weakening. Higuchi did not relate the differences between institutionalized and noninstitutionalized delinquents to questions of administrative policy as Ono (1958) did. Rather, he sees the differences as related to degrees of severity of disturbances of both an emotional and a delinquent nature.

Mizushima (1955), in a similar study, did not find as great a difference between recidivists and nonrecidivists with regard to the incidence of broken homes as reported by Higuchi. Ōura (1957) carefully pointed out that the question of broken homes versus unbroken homes is not simply a question of intact families, but that delinquents actually have more cases of step-parents or parent-surrogates in the so-called intact families than is true for the nondelinquent controls he used. Therefore, it must also be considered that nondelinquent youths are more apt to have their natural parents than are delinquent youths. Ono (1958) pointed out that there is only a slight difference between boys on probation and normal controls in respect to the incidence of broken homes, while the institutionalized delinquents differ significantly from those on probation and those in normal samples. The overall results, therefore, would indicate some selectivity in adjudication among delinquents which results in higher rates of commitment to institutions for those coming from broken homes. It may also indicate, however, greater frequency of occurrence, severity, or visibility among those coming from broken homes.

Some Western studies concerned with broken homes have attempted to test whether there is any differential effect according to the sex of the young delinquent. Studies in Japan, however, show no differential between young male and female delinquents (Takemura, 1953:95).

Studies concerned with the age of the delinquents have revealed in a number of cases that, among individuals who start their delinquent activities earlier, the rate of broken homes is greater than among those who start later. Similar results were obtained in several Japanese studies explicitly concerned with age. Takemura (1953) compared the rate of broken homes of delinquents in a children's training school, juvenile reform training schools, and a juvenile prison. The average age of the inmates was lowest in the children's training school, medium in juvenile reform training schools, and highest in the juvenile prison. The rate of broken homes was 76 percent in the children's training school, 58 percent in the juvenile reformatory, and 48 percent in the juvenile prison. This study did not discuss whether the adjudication that led to placement at early ages was influenced by the absence of the one or both parents. Therefore, one may question the yet unsupported conclusion that the effect of the broken home shows up in earlier delinquency.

Other studies of broken homes have attempted to ascertain whether the absence of a father or of a mother is more consequential in delinquency formation. In Japan, there have been several studies related to this problem. Yoshimasu (1952:145–46) cited statistical research from which he concludes that homes broken when the child is less than five years old produce a higher incidence of delinquency when the mother is not present, whereas homes broken when the child is more than five years old show a higher incidence of delinquency when the father is not present. Similar results to those of Yoshimasu are reported by Higuchi (1953).

We have no statistics in Arakawa Ward of the relation of delinquency to broken and intact families, since by design our sample consisted only of presently intact families. We could make no direct comparison, therefore, of the immediate effects of a broken home versus an intact home. Nevertheless, among our subjects, we were able to obtain some previous evidence of the differential occurrrence of family disruption in the families considered. Of the parents of our delinquents, 58 percent had a previous marriage in contrast to 26 percent among the parents of nondelinquents, over twice the rate. Many of the disruptions were caused by war deaths in both groups; however, there were considerably more disruptions due to divorce or separation in the delinquent sample (Table 1).

This finding is related to that of Ōura (1957). Ōura found that in comparing delinquents who had good prognosis with delinquents who had bad prognosis, the latter came more often from families in which the parental home was broken by divorce or separation. There was no difference between delinquents and nondelinquents in broken homes owing to death. Other studies indicate that step-parents are found more frequently in delinquent homes than in those of nondelinquents (Suzuki, 1957; Tsubota, 1955). Some authors unfortunately are prone to relate such results to stereotypes of wicked or unfeeling step-parents rather than to more complex factors arising from attitudes held by the child in situations of parental loss at given periods of psychosexual development.

The influence of family disruption is not limited to the immediate parental generation. The personality and attitudes of parents are shaped by their own experiences as children and are passed on indirectly to their children. According to the restrospective reports of the parents, there were

Table 1: Marital Disruptions and Irregularities over Two Generations in Arakawa Delinquent and Nondelinquent Sample Families

	Nondelinquent (19)						Delinquent (31)					
	Parents		Grandparents				Parents		Grandparents			
			Paternal		Maternal				Paternal		Maternal	
	Fa	Mo	FaFa	FaMo	MoFa	MoMo	Fa	Mo	FaFa	FaMo	MoFa	MoMo
Intact families (one marriage)												
One generation*	14 (74%)		15 (79%)		16 (84%)		13 (42%)		13 (42%)		15 (48%)	
Two generations†	8 (44%)						2 (6.5%)					
Broken first marriage‡												
Death	3	2	0	0	0	0	8	5	6	3	3	1
Divorce or Separation	2	3	3	3	3	3	8	11	11	14	10	12
No legal marriage	0	0	1	1	0	0	2	2	1	1	3	3

* Delinquent versus nondelinquent: $p < .05$

† Delinquent versus nondelinquent: $p < .01$

‡ Death versus divorce and no marriage: Chi² not significant

many more disruptions reported in the grandparent generation of the delinquent subjects of our Arakawa Ward families than for the grandparents of the nondelinquent controls. Only 2, or 6.5 percent, of the families of delinquents were intact for two generations. This contrasted with 44 percent of the nondelinquent families whose grandparents on both sides remained together until the given parent interviewed was at least 12 years of age. There were 6 common-law liaisons in 5 different families of the 31 families in the delinquent sample as opposed to a single common-law liaison in the nondelinquent sample. Our small-scale data would, therefore, support the contention that a history of family disruption is related to the appearance of delinquency in children even when the present family circumstance is intact.

From a cross-cultural perspective of the studies presented, many studies both in the United States and Japan consist of a rather mechanical juxtaposition of events, limited to simplistic surface interpretations. At this point it is well to issue a caveat at direct statistical comparisons between cultures or, for that matter, between present results and those obtained more than 20 or 25 years ago in either the United States or Japan. For example, studies of the effects of divorce on delinquency in Japan seem to be more conclusive than similar studies in the United States which do not seem to differentiate between the effects of broken homes owing to separation and those owing to death. In comparing results between Japan and the United States, one must note cultural differences in the divorce rate. Divorce is much more common in the United States than in Japan and, hence, is, in effect, possibly much less indicative of extreme difficulties between parents. In any comparative cultural context, the meaning of a statistical correlation between one form of social behavior and another must be interpreted in relation to the overall frequency or social expectancy of either pattern.

Similarly, one must guard against the supposition that more recent studies can be interpreted as disproving previous ones when results are different. It may well be that the recent American studies are more careful and critical and therefore have found less correlation than those of the past; or it may be that the social situation is gradually shifting and that at the turn of the century questions of poverty and broken homes both in the United States and Japan may have shown some mechanically higher intercorrelation than today. Moreover, we cannot rule out the possibility that the nature of delinquency is gradually changing so that such factors play less important roles among the delinquents today than in the past. The generalization we would wish to make from the foregoing material, however, is that a simple correlational juxtaposition does not lead to understanding causative factors in delinquency but merely indicates the direction in which one must look. Evidence of poverty or overt family disruption may be secondary to the effects of parents' personalities and basic attitudes on children who become delinquent. To resolve such issues, more intensive studies are necessary. Finding statistical relationships is only a first step in scientific inquiry.

Parental Relationships: Love, Discipline, and Family Cohesion

Among those authors concerned with the relation of parental attitudes to delinquency formation, there is general unanimity that the two key factors to be considered are the expression of love and the manner of maintaining discipline and supervision in socializing the child. Family disruptions owing to parental discord as well as overt separation are denied by none as causative factors. However, researchers differ in assessing the relative importance of maternal and paternal care and family cohesiveness and in their concept of how delinquent attitudes are shaped by family patterns. Do they derive from direct conscious experiences or from unconscious, less accessible layers of personality?

In surveying the considerable literature on delinquency in both Japan and the United States, one finds studies which have focused attention on one or another set of variables. The realities of parental interaction with children are very complex, and it is difficult to order the variables in any unilinear fashion for presentation. We have found it expedient in the following discussion to begin with the Gluecks' (1950) relatively successful construction of a prediction scale with five variables. These five factors showed the greatest ability to differentiate between predelinquent and nondelinquent groups at the time of first school entry. Subsequent studies in New York and elsewhere have attested to high predictability using this system of relatively simple forced ratings.

In Japan, Tatezawa (1954) has replicated the Gluecks' study on a far smaller scale with amazing similarity of results. According to Tatezawa, 77.3 percent of nondelinquent families manifested adequate supervision on the part of the mothers in contrast to 13.2 percent of the families of delinquents. Similarly, the discipline of the fathers was considered adequate in 51 percent of the families with no delinquents but in only 2 percent of the delinquent subjects. The affection of mothers toward sons was considered adequate for 77.3 percent of nondelinquents. This contrasted with only 32.1 percent for the delinquents. Affection expressed by fathers toward sons was adequate in 64 percent of the nondelinquent cases but in only 20 percent of delinquents. Cohesiveness of family was positive in 85 percent of families of nondelinquents but equally adequate in only 38 percent of the delinquent sample.

Hiroshi Ushikobo (1956) also used the Gluecks' method in a study matching 121 delinquents and 120 controls. The same factors were used in obtaining matched controls in samples. Comparing delinquents and controls, he found that the rate of broken homes, educational level of the family, and the occupation of parents did not differ between normals and delinquents. On the other hand, disciplinary attitudes and behavior indicative of lack of family cohesiveness were most important. He found general punitive attitudes of both parents toward delinquent children. Frequent changes of residence, economic instability, emotional conflict, tension within the family, and lack of joint family activities of a pleasant sort were significantly more frequent in the families of delinquents than in the nondelinquent group.

Our intensive study of 50 Japanese families produced very apparent differences between delinquent and nondelinquent samples when we rated our cases in accord with the Glueck criteria.[5] In respect to fathers' discipline, we concluded that 58 percent of the fathers in our nondelinquent sample showed adequate, consistent discipline compared with none of the fathers of delinquents. Conversely, 18 out of 31 fathers of delinquents evidenced withdrawal or laxity or both in their discipline. Only 1 father of nondelinquents was so categorized. In respect to the supervision of the mother, only 2 mothers of delinquents obtained an optimal rating; 15 out of 31 showed unsuitable maternal supervision. Of the mothers of nondelinquents, 18 out of 19 were rated favorably in this respect.

On the ratings of affection or love, the nondelinquent fathers in only 2 instances were rated unsatisfactory compared with 16, or over half, of the delinquent fathers. No mothers of delinquents were rated unsatisfactory compared with 19, or 63 percent, of the mothers of delinquents who displayed insufficient maternal affection in one way or another.

In respect to family cohesion, no nondelinquent families were rated as unintegrated or totally lacking in cohesion, whereas 11, or 35 percent, of the families of delinquents were rated as totally unsatisfactory. Conversely, 12 families of nondelinquents, or 63 percent, were considered to show sufficient cohesiveness compared with only 1 family among those with delinquent children (Table 2).

There is no question in our minds that in spite of the obvious rigidities entailed in rating families either in a trichotomous or dichotomous classification in respect to these criteria, the results do point up significant differences between the families of our delinquent and nondelinquent subjects.

Sasaki (1962) investigated the family patterns of 81 delinquent boys encountered in the Kobe family court. Families were classified into either basically "rejecting" or "neglecting" or "other." Those from rejecting families tended to act in lone offenses, while those who had neglecting families tended toward group or cooperative offenses. Kobayashi, Mizushima et al. (1963) found evidence suggesting the same three types of problem children by observing cases referred to a child guidance center in Tokyo. Although the family background material available was sometimes limited, they found definite tendencies for socialized delinquents to have neglecting and/or rejecting parents, while more aggressive children tended

Table 2: Glueck Scores of Arakawa Families

	Normals	Delinquents	Fisher's Exact Test
Discipline by father			
a) Suitable	11	0	A–B p < .001
b) Lax	1	18	A–C p < .001
c) Overly strict or erratic	7	13	B–C p < .05
Supervision by mother			
a) Suitable	18	2	
b) Fair	1	14	A–BC p < .001
c) Unsuitable	0	15	
Affection of father			
a) Positive	17	15	A–B p < .005
b) Basically negative	2	16	
Affection of mother			
a) Positive	19	12	A–B p < .001
b) Basically negative	0	19	
Cohesion of family			
a) Good	12	1	
b) Some	7	19	A–BC p < .001
c) None	0	11	

Table 3: Sib Position of Normal and Delinquent Children in Arakawa Sample*

Sib Position	Normals (19)	Delinquents (31)
Only child	2	2
Only child, only son	3	2
Youngest child, only son	1	2
Oldest child	3	5
Oldest son with older sisters and younger brothers	4	6
Youngest child with older sibs	5	3
Middle son	1	11

* Not middle son versus middle son: p < .025

to have rejecting parents. Overinhibited neurotic children were found, in many instances, to have strict or overanxious parents.

Sib Position and Manifestation of Delinquency

In our Arakawa study, we were interested in the relevance of family size and sib positions to delinquency, since we considered these factors as sources of relative neglect of some growing children. In Japan, it is a common observation that the eldest son has been treated differently from other children in the family. It has also often been said that in the patterns of urban in-migration, it is more often the second sons of rural families who go into the city. We were interested in the relation of sibling position to possible manifestation of delinquency, since one would presume the possibility of relative degrees of neglect or rejection related to sibling position in Japanese families. We, therefore, explored both the sibling position of the parents and of the children in our sample. We found some differences that were significant even for our small sample. Our normal controls showed a lower average number of children (2.95) compared either with the isolate (3.45) or social (3.75) delinquent groups. In the sib position of delinquent controls, we found the middle or second son overrepresented. Eleven out of 31 of our delinquent subjects were in this sib position, compared with 1 out of 19 of our normal subjects. Of the normals, the subjects tended to be either the oldest child, the oldest son, or the youngest child, in contrast to the social and isolate delinquent subjects (Table 3).

Going back one generation and examining the sub positions of the parents, we found that although it was less important to examine sub positions of the children regardless of sex, it was highly relevant to examine the sib position of the parents with sibs of the same sex. Nine out of 19 of the fathers of our normal subjects were first sons compared with 8 out of 31 of the fathers of delinquents. Three out of 19 fathers of normals were second sons compared with 18 out of 31 fathers, or 58 percent, of delinquents. This would appear to be a highly signficant difference. Among the fathers of normal children, fathers who were fourth sons or sons of even larger families occurred in 5 out of 19 cases, or 26 percent, compared with only 2 out of 31 fathers of delinquents, approximately 7 percent (Table 4).

Turning to the mothers, we also find some significant differences. The first and second sib positions are slightly less represented among mothers of delinquents than among fathers, whereas 11 out of 31 of the mothers of delinquents in our sample are third or later-born daughters in their own families. This is over 35 percent of the mothers or stepmothers of delinquents compared with 2, or about 10 percent, of the mothers of the nondelinquent sample. What these figures suggest is a position of relative neglect of the parents of delinquent subjects which may contribute to the relative neglect of one or more of their own children and, in a sense, to the

Table 4: Sib Position of Parents of Normal and Delinquent Children in Arakawa Families

| | Normals | | | | Delinquents | | | |
| | Husband | | Wife | | Husband | | Wife | |
	Child	Son	Child	Daughter	Child	Son	Child	Daughter
First	6	9	7	10	6	8	9	12
Second	5	3	4	7	10	18	8	8
Third	1	2	0	1	8	3	4	7
Fourth or more	7	5	8	1	7	2	10	4
Total	19	19	19	19	31	31	31	31

Fisher's Exact Test

	Not 2nd son	2nd son*
Fathers of nondelinquents	16	3
Fathers of delinquents	13	18

$p < .005$

* This category includes most middle sons as defined for Table 3, Test 1, but includes some youngest sons (2nd of 2 sons) and excludes some middle sons (3rd of 4, etc.). The correlation is therefore all the more striking.

continuation of a pattern of experience which contributes to delinquency along with other convergences of experience.

Patterns of Mothering and Developmental Disturbances

While one can make some general assessments of the attitudes of parents toward children derived from case history material, relatively few of the features on which these interpretations are based are quantifiable. In our study of the Arakawa families, we gathered materials from each of the parents concerning the problems they encountered in bringing up their children. We also asked them to describe what they remembered of their early mothering, including the use of breast and bottle, food habits, and toilet training, without direct questioning concerning the appearance of specific symptoms. From this material two very clear patterns appear that differentiate statistically the delinquent children from the nondelinquent controls (Table 5). The one pattern related to feeding shows that 17 out of 19 of the normal controls were breast-fed. In the 27 cases where the material seems reliable for the delinquents, 9 were solely bottle-fed and 3 were fed by a combination of breast and bottle. We tabulated all reports of thumb-sucking or nail-biting and found that no such symptoms were reported by the mothers or fathers of the normal controls, whereas 9 out of 31 mothers or fathers of delinquents reported such problems specifically for those children who became delinquents. This finding agrees with the case findings of the intensive comparative study of Ivy Lee Bennett (1960:176–78)[6] in England and also with previous findings which she reports for Australia.

It is not necessary here to recapitulate psychoanalytic theories about the possibilities of problems arising from the early mother-child relation. One must note, however, that findings relating breast-feeding and delinquency would not, in all probability, be applicable to the United States where the cultural mode in recent years has been bottle-feeding. Therefore, one cannot assume the same degree of motivational and attitudinal differences for bottle-feeding American mothers as for bottle-feeding Japanese mothers since the mode in Japan is still breast-feeding, especially in lower-class and traditional segments of the population.

Although our material on feeding problems per se was less clear-cut, showing relatively few such problems and, seemingly, no relation to delinquent behavior, there was a striking difference in our sample in the reporting of enuresis. Only 2 out of the 19 normal families, or 10 percent of the cases, reported bed-wetting into the school period in contrast with such reports in 13 of 31 families of delinquents, or 42 percent of the cases. This finding of the relation between enuresis and delinquency has been reported previously in psychiatric literature. Michaels and Goodman (1939) and Michaels (1938) report that the highest percentage of enuresis in their studies was found in rejected or neglected children including delinquents and the lowest number in so-called overprotected children. There are numerous

Table 5: Feeding Patterns and Childhood Symptoms of Nervousness in Arakawa Samples

Feeding	Normals				Social Delinquents				Isolate Delinquents			
	Total	No Symptoms	Suck Bite	Enuresis	Total	No Symptoms	Suck Bite	Enuresis	Total	No Symptoms	Suck Bite	Enuresis
Breast	17	16	0	1	8	4	1	3	7	3	2	4
Breast/bottle	0	0	0	0	2	1	1	0	1	1	0	0
Bottle	2	1	0	1	7	3	4	2	2	0	1	2
Unknown	0	0	0	0	3	1	0	2	1	1	0	0
Total	19	17	0	2	20	9	6	7	11	5	3	6

	Normals (19)	Delinquents (31)	Significance*
Breast feeding	17	15	A versus B+C
Bottle feeding	2	9	p < .025
Breast/bottle feeding	0	3	
Unknown	0	4	
Enuresis	2	13	
Oral symptoms	0	19	G versus H
No symptoms	17	12	p < .001
Oral and/or enuresis	2	19	

* Using Fisher's exact test, one-tailed

interpretations given for the continuance of enuresis in children, but the generally accepted cause is lack of appropriate gratification for certain emotional needs. It is sometimes interpreted as a substitutive form of gratification or passive sexuality of a repressed nature. It often seems to be a masked form of masturbation allied with a high degree of covert aggression. It is sometimes related to sibling rivalry or to deep-seated fears or anxieties and very often seen as a disguised expression of repressed hostility toward the parents. Karpman (1948) presents a configuration which suggests that enuresis in delinquents is part of a general syndrome of immaturity and insecurity. It is highly correlated with other symptoms, such as poor sleeping habits, thumb-sucking, nail-biting, and temper tantrums. These all suggest some common fundamental disorder of personality.

The fact that in our cases 19 out of 31 delinquent children, or 61 percent, manifested one or more of the specific symptoms of enuresis, nail-biting, or finger-sucking is a startling cross-cultural affirmation of the findings in the United States of psychoanalytically oriented theories in regard to personality syndromes of predelinquents. Only 2 out of 19 nondelinquent controls, according to the retrospection of the parents, manifested any such problems. It must be noted that, in our nondelinquent group, out of the 2 bottle-fed children, 1 was enuretic. However, no correspondence between breast and bottle-feeding and enuresis was found in the delinquent children since 7 enuretics were breast-fed and 4 enuretics were bottle-fed. Oral symptoms were found in 3 breast-fed delinquents and 6 bottle-fed, indicating some slight correspondence between bottle-feeding and finger-sucking but no correspondence between bottle-feeding and enuresis.

Other Aspects of Parental Personality and Behavior Including Delinquency in Children

The Gluecks' large-scale study concerned itself with the many other variables, not selected for the final prediction scale, which may be considered under the rubric of general family atmosphere and organization. They found the following differences significantly present in delinquent in contrast to nondelinquent families: less planning of household routines, less concern with cultural matters, less self-respect, and less ambition to improve their status and that of their children. Standards of conduct were poorer in homes of delinquents generally than in homes of nondelinquents, and the quality of family life was less positive and less concerned with welfare of the children. The Gluecks also found that although parents of delinquents and nondelinquents stemmed from similar backgrounds as far as the size of family and other economic considerations were concerned, there was a larger number of cases of serious ailments, mental retardation, emotional disturbance, drunkenness, forced marriages, and criminality in previous family members among delinquents. In our small Arakawa samples, the higher tendency for drunkenness in the parents and grandparents did not reach significance. Regardless of whether these attributes were hereditary or environmental in origin, they must have had some adverse influence upon the parents of the boys, who, in their turn, had to assume the responsibilities of marriage and children. There was no difference in the Gluecks' sample of age of marriage or disparity of ages between parents; nor were there age differentials in our Arakawa samples. However, there were other differences indicative of significant discrimination between parents of delinquents and parents of nondelinquents. More of the parents of delinquents made what could be termed forced marriages, and they were more burdened with serious ailments, mental retardation, emotional disturbances, drunkenness, and previous criminality. No such tendencies except for drunkenness showed up in our Arakawa material.

In Tatezawa's replication of the Gluecks' study, he found no significant difference in the use of income, but he found greater significance related to a more systematic family routine in the nondelinquent families than that in the delinquent. The nature of the marital relation of father and mother showed significant differences in Japan as well as in the United States. Although the nature of recreational activities within families was important as a discriminator in the Gluecks' study, it did not appear in the Japanese family as might be expected because of the different nature of the customs of togetherness in Japan and the United States. It is very unusual for Japanese fathers to spend much time in recreation with their families. The work habits of the father in Japan had less importance, although there was some tendency noted in the expected direction. Considering the difference in cultures, the degree to which similar patterns were found in Tatezawa's material is rather striking to that demonstrated in the Gluecks' study, in terms of qualities of family atmosphere. Our Arakawa study also concurred in the finding that the fathers of delinquents were less positive in relating to their children than those of nondelinquents. (This evidence was included in our general scoring of discipline and affection.)

There were a number of early studies concerning the influence of so-called immoral homes, immoral atmospheres, or immoral individuals in the family on juvenile delinquency. In a postwar study by Higuchi (1953) which examined the mental condition of the families of 73 reformatory inmates, it was shown that 17 percent of the families had criminal members and 7 percent had alcoholic members. Of another 214 delinquents in a medical reformatory, 14 had criminal fathers, 2 had 2 criminal parents, 20 had criminal siblings, 39 had alcoholic fathers, 2 had alcoholic mothers, 11 had an alcoholic father and an alcoholic mother. In addition, 50 individuals had family members whose conduct was considered in some way reprehensible. It is probable that the parents did not actively encourage their children to follow their way of life, but in an atmosphere where parents have trouble with the law, there are bound to be other types of conflict among other family members. Higuchi's interpretation of his data was based somewhat upon his belief in hereditary influences on delinquency.

In our examination of the Arakawa family background, no evidence other than the number of broken families in the delinquent groups was significant. There was proportionately greater evidence of a drinking problem and of black market activity among the delinquent sample in the immediate postwar period, but these trends were not significant. Therefore, we do not interpret the influence of so-called immoral parents by simple imitation directly as inducive of delinquency. What may be necessary in the interpretation is a further consideration of the nature of the actual relation between parent and child. It seems that the induction of a son by his father into a professional criminal career is a very rare phenomenon; even when the father is a criminal, identification or imitation on the part of the son occurs only through some father-son conflict so that it is the negative aspects of the identification that may cause the continuity in criminal careers from one generation to the next.

Latent negative attitudes toward authority may be as important as manifest behavior. Adelaide Johnson (1949) in her work with Szurek (Johnson and Szurek 1952) and Robinson (Johnson and Robinson 1957), has produced very striking material suggesting how the mechanism of "induction" for delinquency operates within certain families at both a conscious and an unconscious level.[7] Johnson's work points out that parents may project various forms of gratification for their own poorly integrated forbidden impulses in the acting-out behavior of one or more of their children by some form of unconscious permissiveness or inconsistency toward the child when these behaviors appear. She points out how the parents of the delinquent child unconsciously encourage the child's immoral or antisocial behavior. The neurotic needs of the parents, whether of excessive dominating, dependent, or erotic character, are vicariously gratified by the behavior of the child or in their relations with the child. Because the parents' needs are unintegrated, unconscious, and unacceptable to the parents themselves, the child's behavior is not consciously condoned but is punished. But discipline is often administered with guilt and ambivalence. The child sometimes learns to exploit and subsequently to emotionally blackmail the parents. Especially illuminating is the case history material reflecting parent-child emotional and behavioral involvements.

Japanese studies related to any form of unconscious parental induction theory are lacking. We could not qualify any of our Arakawa material to support the induction theory of delinquency, but we did find interview material in several of our cases from Arakawa, and from the Sapporo Family Court and clinics in Tokyo, that supported the presence of such features in some delinquent families. In presenting some of our case history material elsewhere, we shall illustrate instances of what we consider to be induced delinquent behavior. It is useful to have an awareness of the presence of such mechanisms in understanding family interaction patterns. It is doubtful, however, that such patterns can be qualified in such a way as to lead one to see them as a necessary occurrence in the appearance of delinquency; rather, we must consider induction as part of socially inherited patterns that manifest themselves over generations in the same families.

Role Behavior and Marital Dissatisfaction in the Arakawa Ward

A necessary but sometimes neglected consideration in studies of parental interaction and parental behavior toward children is the effect of social status and internalized attitudes on how one should fulfill one's social role. American social scientists are less sensitive to the effect of internalized role definitions than are students of Japanese culture. In examining the Japanese tradition in family relations, one is made aware of the fact that the father is very often respected for his social role position rather than for himself as an individual. In the past, the father's position was considered unassailable within the family, even if he were, from a personality standpoint, unlikeable or inadequate in his role fulfillment. Formal behavior in the family was defined by roles, and the growing male child would witness the fact that upon reaching maturity he would be afforded similar recognition no matter what he felt subjectively about his own insufficiencies.

In the Arakawa sample, we judged that in a number of cases one could discover a tradition of disparagement toward paternal figures in the grandparent generation. In the perception of the mothers of delinquents, their own fathers often seemed equated with their present husbands as inadequate. Some stated directly that in their family lives males tended to be weak, and husbands were pictured as isolate, spending much time away from the family, in a number of instances manifesting patterns of problem drinking. In some of the cases there were reports of periodic outbursts on the part of the man, sometimes resulting in physical violence directed against the wife or child. This pattern is not infrequently reported for certain American ethnic groups, especially in lower-class settings where drinking is part of a tradition brought from Europe. Characteristically, in lower-class ethnic groups the social status of the father, in terms of the mother, manifests antagonism or disparagement or both.

We must note that the Japanese lower class, as a whole and on the surface at least, upholds the traditional dominant status of the father. The degree to which the status was not maintained by women is not documented, but we may surmise that the ideal of the dominant father was often advocated in the past as it is in the present. The breakdown of status and role maintenance with some of our Arakawa families may not be simply a new phenomenon. However, with social mobility the tradition that a bride support the traditional occupational role of the husband, be it ever so low, may find less social support than in the past. Where occupational role is considered hereditary, there tends to be little conflict in respect to social status. In contrast, in the current ideology of mobility in American families, there is no comparable position protecting male status. The only guides for perception of male adequacy available to women are the highly visible success patterns of middle-class achievement.

CIRCUMSTANCES OF MARRIAGE IN ARAKAWA FAMILIES

One of the considerations specific to Japanese marriage is whether the marriage was based on a degree of free choice or whether it was arranged by family, employers, or other mentors for what was judged to be the benefit of the married couple. It is possible to contend that this factor may influence the nature of cohesiveness experienced by the spouses. Blood (1967) found only slight indications of greater cohesiveness in a sample of middle-class love marriages as compared with arranged marriages. In our own Arakawa sample, we classified marriages as either basically love marriages or basically arranged marriages. We found (Table 6) no really significant difference between our normal and delinquent samples, although there was a very slight trend for a larger proportion of love marriages among the parents of delinquents (9 out of 31), especially in the instance of the parents of isolate delinquents (4 out of 11). There were 5 out of 19 love marriages among the normals, or approximately 1 out of 4, as was true for the social delinquents. Among the isolates there was a 1 to 3 ratio. This does not seem to be a very meaningful consideration among factors influencing delinquency formation in children.

RATINGS OF SOCIAL STATUS

In examining our Arakawa sample, we were interested in finding some measures relating status and role considerations to marital satisfaction and compatability. We sought, therefore, to gain some overall estimates of the present social status of our families as well as some estimates of the social status of both the parental and maternal grandparent generation, and we attempted to set up some indices of status characteristics by which we could make comparisons. Previously in research in Nagoya and elsewhere

Table 6: The Number of Arranged and Love Marriages in Arakawa Families

	Normals	Delinquents	Isolates
Arranged marriages	14	15	7
Love marriages	5	5*	4*
Total†	19	20	11

* Including one case of common law marriage
† No significant statistical differences

(Muramatsu et al., 1962), we adapted and modified the Index of Status Characteristics developed by Warner (1963) and his associates in their intensive study of American social class.

Our criteria were education, occupation, income level, and living conditions. We rated present families and attempted to rate the grandparental families as accurately as possible on the information gained about them through our interviews. We were able to gain some estimates, admittedly subjective, of possible upward or downward mobility as it was retrospectively perceived by our subjects, which allowed us to compare how individual spouses placed themselves in respect to their own parents.

Our results indicated that although we had sought, in our criteria for selecting families through school teachers, to use only lower-class individuals, there was some variation in social background, even in our fairly homogenous sample. Thirty of our sample were what could be termed upper lower class, and 8 were lower lower class. However, 10 families were rated to belong to the lower middle class, and one had to be rated middle middle class. (In one family we could attempt no ratings due to a lack of crucial information.)

The results indicated greater status consistency in the normal groups. Most of the families of the normal controls belonged to what could be termed upper lower social status (15 out of 19), whereas the families of the delinquents varied; 7 were categorized as lower lower, 15 as upper lower, and 7 as lower middle. We also found that the status ratings of the normal group were more consistent; that is to say, education, occupation, and living conditions tended to be approximately on the same level, whereas the delinquent groups were more apt to show inconsistencies in this regard. One can therefore state that in our sample, as measured by the particular indices used, there was evidence of greater status stability in the families of nondelinquents.

RATINGS OF DISSATISFACTION

Aware of the strong emphasis on role behavior in the traditional Japanese family, we were somewhat surprised by the readiness of the Japanese women in our sample to express, rather directly, dissatisfaction with their marriage. Such expressions of dissatisfaction were not limited to the mothers of delinquent subjects, although the degree and strength of the dissatisfaction were much more severe in these women. We believe that some of this dissatisfaction is related to the fact that all of these women find themselves in a relatively low status within Japanese society, married to husbands who, in many instances are relative occupational failures.

While interviewing each of our 50 husbands and wives, we asked them a hypothetical question: "Would you or would you not again marry your present spouse, if you were to repeat your life over?" We probed further into the reasons, either positive or negative, for attitudes expressed about the marital partner. We obtained fairly detailed descriptions of marital

Table 7:   Marital Satisfaction in Arakawa Families

Degree of Satisfaction	Normals		Social Delinquents		Isolate Delinquents	
	Husband*	Wife†	Husband*	Wife†	Husband*	Wife†
	19	19	20	20	11	11
A (satisfied)	16	10	6	2	4	3
B (ordinary)	3	2	8	3	4	0
C (dissatisfied)	0	5	6	3	2	3
D (very dissatisfied)	0	2	0	12	1	5

* Husbands: Normal versus delinquents: $p < .005$
† Wives: Normal versus delinquents: $p < .01$

Table 7a: Marital Satisfaction in First Marriage and Remarriage in Arakawa Families

Degree of Satisfaction		Normals		Social Delinquents		Isolate Delinquents	
		Husband*	Wife†	Husband*	Wife†	Husband*	Wife†
		19	19	20	20	11	11
First	A(satisfied)	13	9	6	2	2	2
Marriage	B(ordinary)	1	1	3	2	1	0
	C(dissatisfied)	0	4	2	3	1	1
	D(very dissatisfied)	0	0	0	4	1	2
Remar-	A(satisfied)	3	1	0	0	3	1
riage	B(ordinary)	2	1	5	1	3	0
	C(dissatisfied)	0	1	4	1	0	2
	D(very dissatisfied)	0	2	0	7	0	3

* Husbands: Normal versus Delinquents: not significant
† Normal versus Delinquents: $p < .01$

life by seeking out illustrative material from our subjects. As a result of these interviews, we attempted classification of each husband and wife according to the overall estimated degree of marital satisfaction or dissatisfaction. In general, in all our groups, husbands were either guarded or tended to express mild satisfaction with their spouses, whereas wives tended to be frank and open. The parents of nondelinquents were generally far more positive in tone than those of delinquents. Of those we could rate as basically satisfied or dissatisfied, we found 10 satisfied as opposed to 7 dissatisfied women among mothers of nondelinquents. This was contrasted with only 5 satisfied as opposed to 23 dissatisfied in the delinquent samples (Table 7).

We examined the differences between spouses married only once compared with those with remarriages. Twenty out of our 50 couples were remarried. There were 5 remarriages among the parents of normals and 15 remarriages among the parents of delinquents. Table 7a reveals a general tendency to less satisfaction on the part of both spouses in remarriages; it is particularly apparent in the wives. Therefore, one is struck with the fact that although we have officially intact families, the manifest attitudinal evidence directly suggests the relative lack of cohesiveness in the families of delinquent subjects.

Table 8 would indicate that almost all women, whether in the normal or the delinquent sample, find little satisfaction in their remarriage. Only 2 out of the total of 20 remarriages were satisfactory. In the normal sample, the one satisfactory remarriage was by a woman who perceived her second marriage as upward in status, whereas the remaining 4 saw the remarriage as downward. In the social delinquents, the one woman whose remarriage was upward gave a somewhat neutral rating of satisfaction, whereas 7 out of 8 rated their marriage downward and were very dissatisfied. The result with the mothers of isolate delinquents is inconsistent, in that 4 out of 6 saw either upward mobility or no difference and only 2 saw downward mobility, yet 5 out of 6 rated their marriages as unsatisfactory. In the first marriages, the normal group in 7 out of 14 cases seemed to perceive no mobility in comparing husbands with fathers, again indicating a greater degree of status stability than in the delinquent subjects. Five out of the 7 rated their marriages satisfactory. An additional 3, who rated their marriages satisfactory, saw the marriages as upward-moving in status so that 9 out of the 10 women in the normal sample who rated their marriages positively perceived their marriages as resulting in no less social status than they experienced in their own families. We must again state that we have no objective evidence of the actual status of people in the grandparent generation. It may well be that the retrospective description of the social status of the grandparents vis-à-vis the status of the present husband is colored by present attitudes of satisfaction or dissatisfaction, and we cannot determine the status from our available material.

Table 8: Status Discrepencies in Remarriage and Wife's Marital Satisfaction or Dissatisfaction in Arakawa Families

Wife's Mobility	Normals Degree of Satisfaction			Delinquents Degree of Satisfaction			Isolates Degree of Satisfaction		
	A	BC	D	A	BC	D	A	BC	D
First marriage									
One or two steps up	3	0	0	1	0	1	0	0	1
No mobility	5	0	2	0	1	2	0	0	0
One or more steps down	1	1	2	1	1	4	2	0	2
Total	9	1	4	2	2	7	2	0	3
Remarriage									
One or two steps up	1	0	0	0	1	0	1	0	2
No mobility	0	0	0	0	0	0	0	0	1
One or more steps down	0	1	3	0	0	8	0	0	2
Total	1	1	3	0	1	8	1	0	5
Total present marriage									
One or two steps up	4	0	0	1	1	1	1	0	3
No mobility	5	0	2	0	1	2	0	0	1
One or more steps down	1	2	5	1	1	12	2	0	4
Total	10	2	7	2	3	15	3	0	8

Satisfaction related to perceived mobility up or no change versus perceived mobility down: $p < .01$
Mobility versus remarriage not significant
Mobility versus delinquency not significant

Attitudes of the Parents of Delinquents toward Their Own Parents

In an effort to gain a two-generational picture, we not only used status assessments but also attempted to rate as accurately as possible the attitudes held by each spouse toward his own parents. This evidence was comparatively fragmentary in many respects, and we recognize that some of our ratings are of questionable validity. We present our findings, therefore, with considerable caution.

The attitudes of the normal control families toward their own parents were generally more positive than those of the families of delinquents. The husbands in the normal control families in 10 out of 19 instances gave generally positive descriptions of their own fathers compared with 3 who were generally negative. In the remaining cases, the statements were either so bland or so ambiguous that one could make no determination. The mothers in these families rated their own fathers positively in 10 cases and negatively in 2. The mothers were rated positively in 13 out of 19 instances and negatively in 5. Altogether, the ratings were approximately 3 times as many in a positive direction as in a negative direction (Table 9).

In the social delinquents, one gains a contrasting picture. The husbands rated their own fathers positively in 6 instances and negatively in 7, their own mothers positively in 7 and negatively in 5. The mothers were even more negative in their ratings of their own parents. Only 5 rated their fathers positively compared with 9 basically negative ratings, and only 7 mothers were rated positively compared with 11 who received a negative rating.

The parents of isolate delinquents were even more extreme in their negative ratings. Four husbands rated their own fathers positively compared with 7 negatively, and 6 rated their mothers positively compared with 4 negatively. The most extreme negative ratings were by the mothers of isolate delinquent children. Only 1 mother rated her own father positively compared with 6 basically negative ratings. Only 2 rated their mothers positively compared with 6 negative ratings.

Grouping together all the mothers of delinquent subjects, we find that only 6 out of the 31 saw their own fathers in a positive light compared with half who gave their fathers a definitely negative rating. Only 9, or less than a third, rated their mothers positively, whereas 17 out of 31 gave their mothers a negative rating. These findings of basic attitudes of parents toward grandparents of juvenile delinquents are very striking. Although we must warn that the evidence in a number of instances is quite fragmentary, the findings are sufficiently notable to indicate the continuance of negative interpersonal attitudes from one generation into the next.

As far as we were able to determine, ratings of satisfaction and dissatisfaction were not related to whether the marriage was seen as a love marriage or an arranged marriage. As we have indicated, the proportion of

Table 9: Overall Ratings of Attitudes Held toward Their Parents by Husbands and Wives in Arakawa Families

Attitudes	Normals — Degree of Satisfaction			Delinquents — Degree of Satisfaction			Isolate Delinquents — Degree of Satisfaction		
	A	BC	D	A	BC	D	A	BC	D
Husband's attitude towards his father	10	6	3	6	7	7	4	0	7
Husband's attitude towards his mother	11	5	3	7	8	5	6	1	4
Wife's attitude towards her father	10	7	2	5	6	9	1	4	6
Wife's attitude towards her mother	13	1	5	7	2	11	2	3	6
Total	44	19	13	25	23	32	13	8	23

Total Ratings in Each Group

Rate	Normals	Delinquents	Isolate Delinquents
A	44	25	13
BC	19	23	8
D	13	32	23
Total	76	80	44

Significance: Husband's father: $p < .05$ Wife's father: $p < .005$
  Husband's mother: not significant   Wife's mother: $p < .025$
  Husband's father and mother: $p < .05$ Wife's father + mother: $p < .001$

arranged marriages to love marriages was slightly higher for the normal group in comparison with the delinquent group.

Conclusions

In brief, our research on delinquency tends to confirm a number of previous conclusions about the influences of family life and delinquency. According to research, in Japan similar social and psychological factors are at work as in the United States. In both cultures, social deviancy in youth is apt to occur among those suffering neglect or deprivation in their formative years. In our specific research with Arakawa families, we are able to find indirect indices supporting these conclusions. We are also able to find, by use of indirect indices, a relation between the interpersonal attitudes of parents toward one another and the appearance of delinquent behavior in at least one child.

Our study has little new to offer in respect to psychodynamic theory as applied to delinquency. Its chief virtue is its examination of generational continuities in familial patterns. The karma of delinquency does not start *de novo* within one generation. It results from a number of factors influencing the grandparents as well as the parents of delinquents. That the grandparent generation in our sample provides such striking evidence of interpersonal disruptions is indicative of this fact.

We were also able to find evidence relating delinquency to specific features of the family, notably sibling position. This finding relates to the illness in the eldest son and youngest daughter within Japanese families. Our results, therefore, further the contention that the relation of the total psychocultural environment of the family to the psychosocial problems of the individual requires more intensive investigation than is presently being undertaken.

ACKNOWLEDGMENTS

This paper will appear in modified form as part of a volume now in preparation. Delinquency in Japan, by G. DeVos, K. Mizushima, and E. Hunn. Research work was funded by the National Institute of Mental Health, Grant MHD 4087. Additional support has been given by the Center for Japanese and Korean Studies, University of California, Berkeley and the Social Science Research Institute, University of Hawaii.

NOTES

1. They are to be reviewed in another context in Delinquency in Japan by G. DeVos, K. Mizushima, and E. Hunn, in preparation.

2.   It is also possible that actually the importance of poverty for delinquency is decreasing with time. After World War II there were many boys who stole as a means of survival in a very difficult economic situation, but such cases are now very rare.

3.   There is some tendency among Japanese, as well as American, statisticians to define class affiliation simply by income classification.

4.   In all our families the space problem would be considered intolerable by most American standards. It is not unusual in our samples to have from five to seven individuals living in a room approximately 9' × 12'.

5.   It must be noted our ratings were done with prior knowledge of which families were delinquent. However, we rated the families independently and found very few differences in our overall ratings.

6.   See also Bennett, Tables 34, 35, and 36, pp. 505–506.

7.   See also M. E. Giffin, A. M. Johnson, and E. M. Litin, "Specific Factors Determining Anti-Social Acting Out," in American Journal of Orthopsychiatry 24, 1954:668–84; E. N. Rexford and S. T. van Amerongen, "The Influence of Unresolved Maternal Oral Conflict Upon Impulsive Acting Out in Young Children," in American Journal of Orthopsychiatry 27, 1957:78–87; E. Jacobson, "Denial and Repression," in Journal of the American Psychoanalytic Association 5, 1957:61–92.

REFERENCES

Bennett, I. 1960. Delinquent and neurotic children. New York, Basic Books, Inc.

Blood, R. O., Jr. 1967. Love marriage and arranged marriage. New York, The Free Press.

Glueck, S., and E. Glueck. 1950. Unravelling juvenile delinquency. Cambridge, Harvard University Press.

Higuchi, K. 1953. Psychiatric study of juvenile delinquency after the war. Judicial Report 41. Tokyo, Ministry of Justice. [In Japanese]

Johnson, A. M. 1949. Sanctions of superego lacunae of adolescents. *In* Searchlights on delinquency, K. R. Eissler, ed. New York, International University Press.

Johnson, A.M., and S. A. Szurek. 1952. The genesis of antisocial acting out in children and adults. Psychoanalytic Quarterly 21:323–43.

Karpman, B. 1948. Milestones in the advancement of knowledge of the psychopathology of delinquency and crime. *In* Orthopsychiatry, 1923–1948: Retrospect and Prospect. Lowrey and Sloane, eds. Menasha, Wisconsin, George Banta.

Kobayashi, S., et al. 1963. Background of problem children. Reports on Annual Meeting of Japan Psychological Association, 404.

Michaels, J. C. 1938. The incidence of enuresis and age of cessation in 100 delinquents and 100 sibling controls. American Journal of Orthopsychiatry 7:460–65.

Michaels, J. C., and S. E. Goodman. 1939. The incidence of enuresis and age of cessation in 1,000 neuropsychiatric patients: with a discussion on the relation between enuresis and delinquency. American Journal of Orthopsychiatry 9:59–71.

Mizushima, K. 1955. A study on the prognosis of social adjustment of delinquents. Japanese Journal of Educational Psychology 2, 4:45–54. [In Japanese]

Muramatsu, T., et al. 1962. The Japanese: culture and personality. Tokyo Reimei Shobō. [In Japanese]

Ono, Z. 1958. An empirical study of the causes of delinquency. Family Court Investigator's Report 3. Tokyo, Secretariat of the Supreme Court of Japan.

Ōura, K. 1957. Delinquent juveniles and family. Family Court Monthly 9:59–101. Tokyo, Secretariat of the Supreme Court of Japan. [In Japanese]

Research Institute of the Ministry of Justice. 1960. Crime and its prevention in Japan. Tokyo, Ministry of Justice. [In Japanese]

Sasaki, Y. 1962. Relations between family, neighborhood and behavior traits in delinquency. Family Court Probation Bulletin 1:83–93. [In Japanese]

Suzuki, T. 1957. Delinquents and the family. Family Court Report 50:105–88. Tokyo, Family Court Probation Officers Training Institute. [In Japanese]

Takemura, H. 1953. Sociological study of juvenile delinquency. Judicial Report 6, no. 4. Tokyo, Judicial Research and Training Institute. [In Japanese]

Tani, T. 1929. Psychiatric study of juvenile offense. Psychiatria et Neurologia 31:38–50. [In Japanese]

Tatezawa, T. 1953. The function of family court probation officer and prediction of juvenile delinquency. Case Studies no. 2. Tokyo Family Court, Family Case Studies Group. [In Japanese]

———. 1954. Prediction of juvenile delinquency. Family Court Reports 35:271–334. Tokyo, Family Court Probation Officers Training Institute. [In Japanese]

Tsubota, M. 1955. Stepmothers and the problem adolescents. Case Studies 32:36–41. Tokyo Family Courts, Family Case Studies Group. [In Japanese]

Ushikobo, H. 1956. Family background of juvenile delinquents. Penal Administration 67, no. 11:21–31. [In Japanese]

Warner, L. 1963. Yankee city. New Haven, Yale University Press.

Yoshimasu, S. 1952. Criminal psychology. Tokyo, Tōyō Shokan. [In Japanese]

6. Suicidal Attempts among Children in Japan

RYURO TAKAGI, M.D.

Department of Neuropsychiatry
Kyoto University
Kyoto, Japan

IT IS GENERALLY FELT that a psychological study of the causes of suicide among children is very difficult—first, because suicide rarely occurs and second, because of the impulse and unexpected nature of the act when it does occur. According to Bender and Schilder (1937), reviewed by Kanner (1957), deprivation or lack of parental love is a major cause of childhood suicide. Ohara et al. (1963) note the following common factors: (1) Suicide often occurs in a defective family; (2) environmental factors such as family, school, and residential area play an important part; (3) enuresis, tic, myopia, cerebral palsy, and stuttering, which may lead to an inferiority complex, are often found in the medical history; (4) many who have attempted suicide have been delinquent at one time or another; and (5) while rare, there are some cases of psychoses. In England, Connell (1965) reviewed causal themes as well as presenting his intensive clinical investigations of suicidal attempts in childhood and adolescence. He stressed that severe disturbances exist in the child's relationships with members of his family and that the relationship between the child's depression and suicidal threats and attempts should not be neglected.

These studies suggest the possibility of a psychological analysis of suicide among children. Therefore, we collected as much data as possible (including interviews with the children themselves) on four unsuccessful cases in the Hiroshima Child Education and Training Home, one unsuccessful case in the Kyoto Juvenile Detection and Classification Home, and one successful case in the Shūtoku Child Education and Training Home in Osaka. We studied the life histories of these cases, and, in addition, we carried out a psychiatric study of two children under fifteen years of age (chosen from patients of outpatient clinics in the child psychiatric division, Department of Neuropsychiatry, Kyoto University Hospital) who at one time had attempted or expressed a desire to die by their own hands. I shall first review these eight cases, commencing with the case of an eleven-year-old boy who committed suicide, and then proceed to a summation and analysis.

A Successful Suicide Attempt

Case No. 3, Y. K.   Sex: male; age at death: 11 years 10 months. Y. K. was born in Okayama in October 1951 as the eldest legitimate son of S. K., the father, and K. K., the mother. Both parents were brought up in a complicated family relationship. The father, a short stumpy man, labored as a longshoreman. He had fallen into alcohol addiction before marriage, and after marriage continued to indulge in drinking and gave little money to his family. He was extremely introverted when sober; but for the most part he was intoxicated and very emotional, talkative, self-centered, and aggressive.

Born as an illegitimate child, the mother was a woman with a relatively firm personality fostered by hardship. Neighbors said that she was too good for her husband. She tried to earn a living by making dresses at home but often lost patience with sewing. It was not uncommon for her to run away to her mother's home and to speak of killing herself. However, no particular information has been found to indicate her incapable of raising children. She committed suicide by drowning on July 26, 1955, at the age of 27, when her son, Y. K., was 3 years and 9 months old. One month before this she had undergone artificial abortion in the fifth month of pregnancy, because she would not have been able to support another child. Thereafter, she exhibited so-called hysterical traits and often had hypochondriacal complaints such as headaches. According to the police report, she was in ill humor on the day of her suicide after having been reproved by her landlady who was also her aunt. Around seven o'clock in the evening she quarrelled with her husband, who had just returned from work, and she left home about eight. The husband was not concerned since it was common for her to go to her mother's home after a quarrel, but the next day her body was found on the seashore. Because no note was left to confirm the evidence of her intent and no external wound was found, the postmortem examination report designated her death as suicide by drowning.

As a result of the mother's death, the younger brother was adopted by a friend of the father, and Y. K., 3 years and 9 months old at the time, was committed to the care of his paternal grandmother who lived thirty minutes' walk from the family's house and with whom they had maintained rapport. The father went to Osaka to work as a day-labor longshoreman. As his alcohol addiction worsened, he scarcely maintained any contact with his mother and son, and his working days became very few.

The boy seems to have been well loved by his grandmother. His kindergarten teacher remembers him as a pale, meek, and gloomy boy with few friends, somewhat lacking in independence. His intelligence level was ordinary or a little below average.

In March 1958, the boy, now 5 years and 5 months old, was sent to his father in Osaka because the grandmother, suffering from neuralgia, was unable to care for him. Right after this, the boy ran away from home and subsequently was committed to the care of the Suita Child Guidance Center on the grounds that his father was incapable of bringing him up. Each time he was placed in the Center, however, he ran away to his father; thus, the protective care of the Center was alternately suspended and resumed. While intoxicated, the father would go to the Center to reclaim his son, arguing insistently that his right to raise his son was being violated. Two or three hours later, however, having sobered, he would tearfully plead with the case worker to care for his son. When the boy ran away from the Center, the Center officials would leave him with his father. Under the father's care, he would run away as well, and he began to commit acts of delinquency. Such was the changing relationship of the father, the son, and the Child Guidance Center.

The commital paper of the Suita Child Guidance Center, which finally decided to send him to Shūtoku Gakuin (Child Education and Training Home) in November 1959, reads as follows.

> The father and son live under a bridge in Suita City.
> The father, who is a day-labor longshoreman, leads a loose life
> addicted to drinking and does not send his son to school. He
> orders his son to buy liquor at night. He was so unqualified
> for his son's upbringing that the boy wanders around the
> neighborhood and steals when hungry or wanting a little
> money. Gradually, the boy has progressed to offenses such as
> stealing from a locked house. Frequently, he steals his father's
> money and gets scolded, which results in his avoiding home.
> The area of his vagrancy has extended to another prefecture.
> For example, immediately before being sent to the Home, he
> ran away to Tsuruga with a year older boy (Y.M.), who lived
> under the same bridge.

In accordance with the decision for committal, the boy was taken to Shūtoku Gakuin where, howling, he refused to be separated from his father. On the afternoon of the first day, he ran away (which constituted escape) and never returned to the Home.

He returned to his previous way of life in Osaka for about one year. In February 1960, at 8 years and 4 months of age, he ran away to his grandmother's in Okayama, and the Okayama Child Guidance Center took him under its protection. This time the boy, accompanied by his grandmother, looked entirely different and showed a very cheerful expression. The following is an extract from the record in Okayama Child Guidance Center: "I.Q.: 96. (Speech and behavior during the test are normal.) Diagnosis: Ordinary intellectual faculties. Mental mechanism of neglected children." Finally, he was placed in Okayama Minori Gakuen (Child Education and Training Home), where he detested learning and often went out without the knowledge of the Home's administrators.

In May 1960, he was taken back to Osaka by his father and admitted to Suita-daiichi Elementary School. There he continued to commit delinquency and run away so that local police notified the Child Guidance Center seven times from March to June of 1960. In April, at 9 years and 5 months of age he ran away again to Okayama as a stow away on a train. In July, he entered Shutoku Gakuin and was put into solitary confinement. He was moved to an ordinary room in October because of his good behavior. In January 1962, at 10 years and 2 months of age, he was forcibly reclaimed by his father. To the teachers' surprise, he reappeared one month later on February 2, 1962, with his friend and volunteered to be admitted to the Home; this had never happened in the history of the Home.

Here is a quote from the Home's diary written by teachers.

> Y. K. and Y. M. visited the Home past four o'clock
> in the afternoon. Y. K., who left the Home after his New
> Year's Day leave, said that they had left home leaving a note
> because Y. M., his friend (a sixth grader in elementary
> school), had been ill-treated by his parents and that they
> wanted to become good children in Shūtoku Gakuin.

The next day, Y. K.'s father went to the Home to take him back. The boy ran in a vain attempt to escape. Thereafter, since he continued being truant, joining delinquents, running away, and wandering, he was placed in solitary confinement in the Home in November 1962. At this time, he was 11 years old. On April 3, 1963, he was removed to an ordinary room, and, showed evidence of regained stability. On April 30, the Home was obliged to release him since the father threatened to take him back by force.

Admitted once again to Suita-daiichi Elementary School, he attended classes for only three days and resumed former ways—keeping bad company, running away, being vagrant, and stealing—until he was caught with C. M. stealing 500,000 yen ($1,400) from a car. He was sent to Shūtoku Gakuin to be confined for the third time. He was placed in the Home a total of five times, by referral in four cases and by voluntary admittance once.

As time went by, Y. K. regained his cheerfulness, though he frequently violated regulations by, for example, such as talking with a child in the next room. On August 30, 1963, nothing strange was observed in his behavior during the day. He had supper as usual, and at half-past seven a child came to give him a glass of water and a can of insecticide to be sprayed in his room. Then teachers and staff started their supper, and the children were expected to study. At twenty to nine, when a child was sent to bring him a mosquito net, Y. K. was found hanging by his undershirt from a low iron bar of the corridor window of the room.

The following observations of his mentality, recorded by Suita Child Guidance Center, seem pertinent to his suicide. They were written before his last entrance to the Home on August 14, 1963, sixteen days before the suicide.

> I.Q.: 91 (by Shin-Tanaka B, Japanese version of the Stanford-Binet Intelligence Test)
> Uchida-Kraepelin's Accumulation Test: very poor (under 10 per minute). Partly owing to absence from school, intellectual faculties remain undeveloped. Poor in discretion, withdrawn, restless, easily flattered, and extremely unstable in actions. A boy of the kind who acts as he wishes without judging the circumstances.

During the boy's stay in Shūtoku Gakuin, the father visited him a few times each month. These visits were always striking. He never appeared at the home sober. He would tearfully caress his son, pressing his cheek against the boy's, and give him a box lunch, caramels, or some sweets. When he recovered from his intoxication, he would become very serious, or more often, would leave the Home before entirely sober. During their meeting the boy would remain extremely tense, silent to whatever the father said, and refuse to eat whatever had been brought for him, despite the father's encouragement. The father evidently loved him in his own way. He would repeat to the teachers: "My son is not to blame"; "It's other people that make him do so"; or "This is a good boy." While he stubbornly refused to listen to the teachers, they had, on occasion, heard him telling his son not to do wrong. At the news of his son's suicide, he came to the Home the next day and cried over the body in an almost maternal manner, saying, "Why did you leave me alone? Take me with you." It was also noted that his working days were fewer when the boy was released from Shūtoku Gakuin into his custody than when the boy was not with him.

The teachers generally felt that the boy was somewhat different from other children in the Home. He looked pale, in rather poor health, and did not try to make friends. He usually kept silent and never boasted about his offenses, as is often the case with children in a home of this kind. Lacking any striking talent, he preferred odd jobs, such as cooking and cleaning, to heavy labor and physical exercises. He was obedient to his teachers. He liked to stay in his room, reading comic books, and occasionally, in excitement, he fought with others but seldom played cheerfully.

In the Home's diary, dated from fall to winter of 1961, during his second sojourn, teachers made the following observations. The day after an excursion, during which he grew closer to a woman teacher, he told her that he loved his father best of anyone in Japan, yet his need for love from her and dependence on her were strong. For example, he never let his demands be ignored, and however busy she might be, he would call loudly, "Teacher!" Equally important for our understanding of his personality is the fact that, driven by a childlike appetite for knowledge, he asked many questions such as; "How was the earth made?"; "What is a cloud made of?"; and "What kind of stars are those?"

I had an opportunity to interview Y. K.'s friend, Y. M., who spoke as follows. "It was fun to read books together at night at Y. K.'s place or to eat sweets which uncle (Y. K.'s father) gave us. We also enjoyed playing cards. Uncle was very nice sometimes, but when he drank, he beat Y. K., who was afraid of him."

The foregoing is an outline of the history and suicide of case no. 3, Y. K. Unfortunately, we have only a part of the picture. The police report is the only source of information on his mother's suicide. Also, his delinquent acts and running away have not been followed up minutely enough to illuminate his relationship with his father. Concerning his stealing of 500,000 yen, the investigation ended with no details about the use of the money. It is not clear to what extent the father might have been involved in this theft. According to neighbors, he came to approve of his son's stealing in such indirect ways as sending him for liquor, knowing he had no money. All this, however, is only guesswork. We can obtain little information from the father who is usually under the influence of liquor. What should be noted here, more than the above-mentioned findings, is the largely hidden part of the father's relations with his son which appeared to involve a kind of secret promise or a rather emotionally entangled tie inviolable from the outside.

In order to provide a psychological explanation of the formation of the boy's personality and his unhappy ending, the following factors are noted: deprivation after mother's death, upbringing by grandmother, problem of poverty and hunger (which explains his delinquency in an earlier stage since he would have had a very practical reason for stealing a lunch box), his companions, and so forth. These factors, however, are common to juvenile delinquents. A biological study might explain his suicide, in connection with his mother's, as hereditary depressive psychoses. All we know about her, however, is that she had felt emotionally unsettled, that she was a woman with a so-called hysterical personality, and that this tendency worsened after an artificial abortion, all of which is not enough to confirm that she was in a pathologically defined depressive state.

The most striking factor in this case is the abnormal relation between the boy and his father. The father was a typical alcoholic—very shy, with a strong inferiority complex—who tried to escape from reality by means of liquor. After the death of his wife, the boy became the only one in the world whom he could dominate and thereby love. Because of this, his desire to possess his son and to keep him under his care became all the stronger. The boy, therefore, became indispensable to the father's maintainance of his life. The boy, who was entirely dependent on his father, gradually grew away from his influence and began to feel hostility towards the always drunken man who was inconsistent in his attitude to the boy and who did not always accept the boy's love. As the means of escape from his father, he began to run away from home. The father began to feel uneasy about his love for the son who tried to turn away from him and who grew to criticize him. Thus, ambivalent feelings toward each other became stronger on both sides as the boy grew older. This compulsive and symbiotic relation was almost done away with when the boy voluntarily reentered the detention home and succeeded in following a stable way of life there. The father, on the contrary, felt all the more uneasy and tried to keep a tie between them, even by indirectly accepting his son's delinquency. With all his attempts at running away, his delinquency, and his futile life in the Home, the boy was repeatedly taken back to his father. His act of suicide can be regarded as a final attempt to rid himself of this relation with the father. Whether the act of suicide was impulsive or premeditated to the extent of tearing his shirt into a rope, we can interpret the essential psychodynamics which drove the boy to death as mentioned above. This interpretation would also allow us to understand his mother's death in terms of a similar mechanism. The father was dependent upon, as well as dominant over, his wife and son, and they finally succeeded in cutting this inescapable tie of ambivalent feelings toward him.

A Case of Childhood Schizophrenia

Case No. 2, U. Y.   Sex: female; age at suicidal attempt: 11 years U. Y. was born when her father was 55 years of age and her mother 31. The father, second husband of her mother, died a little after her birth. Her stepfather, a Korean peddler, third husband of her mother, began to cohabit with the mother when U. Y. was 3 years of age, but they have had no children. There is also a daughter by the first husband who is U. Y.'s half sister (four years older) and who works as a dressmaker. The family is very poor.

The girl was average in physical development, but her mental development was retarded. She was far behind the average in speech development. At the age of 2 she could only cry or make strange sounds instead of speaking. By 4 years of age she could speak a little, but she acted in a contrary manner by striking others when only slightly touched or throwing things about and crying. Soliloquy was often noticed, when she seemed to be in a calm mood. In the first grade of elementary school, this tendency toward contrariness became more noticeable. Whenever wrong answers in her notebook were pointed out, she slapped those who had shown the errors. Later, she secretly made the corrections. She showed her dislike for school by not getting up until ten o'clock in the morning and by not always going to school after leaving home. Instead, she played in the street, soliloquized, and disrupted traffic by throwing stones or pieces of wood. This often brought her to the attention of the police. At school, too, she always acted contrary to other pupils and sometimes attended only for lunch.

The stepfather punished her for her actions by swinging her around by the hair or by hitting her against a pillar. When the child enjoyed handicrafts, he scolded her for making the room untidy. When she played outdoors in the mud, she was scolded for getting dirty. Thus, she cried every day. As she grew older, by the third or fourth grade of school, she learned to run away from her stepfather, to curse him, and to hide from him in a closet. She came to soliloquize more frequently, never studied, rejected any words by others, uttered words of profanity which shocked even adults, and played with much younger children in the neighborhood. In the fifth grade at 11 years of age, her antagonism toward her stepfather deepened, and she would display an edged tool and say, "I'll kill Dad." She also took to playing with matches. Almost every night she would run away from home with her belongings and be brought back by a policeman or a member of the fire department. In addition, she began to steal money from home to spend for food. The stepfather, who was very cruel to U. Y., passed as an agreeable and sincere person among his neighbors. The mother, being a complaining woman as well as timid, seems to have obeyed all of her husband's orders.

One day, during the fifth year of elementary school the stepfather's scolding made her defiant as usual. She cried, "I'll kill myself" and threw herself into a river, but she was soon rescued. Because of the defective family environment and her delinquent acts—neglecting school, staying out, stealing money, and attempting suicide—it was decided to refer her to H. Child Education and Training Home. The psychological test given at that time reads as follows: "C.A.: 11 years 0 months, M.A.: 6 years 10 months, and I.Q.: 62 (by Tanaka-Binet)." At the Home, too, she never listened to teachers, troubled them, and continued to be as aggressive as ever. She was very quick to hide whenever she was in a bad mood. Soliloquy was also remarkably noticed here. The teachers at the Home were at a loss to treat her. When the author visited the Home to investigate this case, she was 11 years and 10 months old. At that time, she was able to maintain relations with other people and was rather dependent and even friendly, although she could suddenly become aggressive and would cry out without provocation. Left alone, she would soliloquize. The soliloquy evidently constituted a dialogue with a certain object and could be called an auditory hallucination or daydreaming. Self-centered and stubborn, U. Y. had no self-control and was emotionally unstable.

In accordance with my recommendation, she was transferred to K. Mental Hospital, where again I had the opportunity to examine her. She held a favorite doll all the time, talked to it, washed its hair, or washed its shorts as if the doll had wet the bed. (In fact, she had enuresis herself.) Her letter to the superintendent of the Home shocked us. It read: "I'll be married. Will you agree, teacher? As I have no friends in the hospital, I can find no other way than marriage. Help me with this, please."

When she walked, she would soliloquize: "You fool, Mr. Takeda [the teacher in charge of her at the Home]. You fool, Mr. Takagi [the author]. You shall soon see! To put me in a place like this! I'll make you cry. I'll strike you to death with this bar." After drinking a mouthful of water, however, she would change her mood and cry, "That's not true. No, no. Mr. Takeda, Mr. Takagi, come and take me with you!" When one of the nursing staff did not accede to her demands or urged her to do something that did not please her, she would either run away into a closet or a bathroom, bite at the nurse, or curse.

Because of her extreme deprivation in personal relations, she developed a dual personality which alternated reliance with aggression and trust with mistrust. From time to time, she lived in a world of illusion, divorcing herself from reality in such ways as projecting her need for love on her doll or talking with an hallucinatory object. The suicidal attempt itself may have been nothing more than an episode to call attention to her distorted life or morbid experiences. This case is worthy of notice by those interested in the circumstances of suicide because of the impulsiveness of the patient's action.

Unsuccessful Cases Connected with Pleasure-seeking in Sleeping Drugs

Case No. 1, C. S. Sex: female; age at suicidal attempt: 9 years, 6 months. The girl in question was separated from her father by divorce soon after birth and heard nothing of him until the news of his death reached her one year before her attempted suicide. She has a sister by the same parents who is three years older. The mother remarried five years after the divorce. Since then C. S. has been brought up by her grandparents and has lacked parental love. The family is poor (her grandfather is a peddler) and receives financial assistance from the government. Since C. S. has been in elementary school, she has been rough and restless, has interfered with others in class, and done poorly in school work. Since she is self-centered, she frequently quarrels with her friends, although she is, on the other hand, dependent upon them. She had enuresis until she was 8 years of age.

From 8 years and 9 months of age, she would steal her grandfather's money to buy small articles of food and gradually began to keep company with delinquents. Whenever she had money, she visited movie theaters one after another but would see only fragments of the films. She was frequently truant from school. Meanwhile, she learned to seek pleasure in sleeping drugs.

It is reported that at the age of 9 years and 6 months, she stole 500 yen and attempted suicide with sleeping pills. This attempt was unsuccessful, but the details are not clear. Her explanation of this experience is quite ambiguous, but she insists that she really wanted to die. After this occurrence, she continued to cause trouble by stealing money from her sister, coming home late at night (explaining that she had gone to her father's grave, because she had dreamt of him), and stealing money from her teacher at school. The Child Guidance Center, therefore, decided to refer her to the Child Education and Training Home.

The psychological test given at that time reports as follows: "C.A.: 9 years 11 months, M.A.: 9 years 4 months, I.Q.: 94 (Tanaka-Binet). Poor in abstract words and in synthetic reasoning. Persistent." The Rosenzweig-Picture-Frustration Study indicated the patient's self-centeredness, aggressiveness, lack of self-reflection or self-reproach, and lack of cooperation—in short the undeveloped state of her mentality was observed. In the Rorschach test, no sign of intellectual disturbances was shown. She gave a response strongly suggesting her frustration which might explain her incapability of controlling her own actions in spite of her seeming adaptability to society. Without any evidence to prove her intent to commit suicide, it would be hard to prove that pleasure-seeking in sleeping drugs was not her only goal. We might conclude that in her desire for family love, she tried to seek her father in an illusive world.

Case No. 6, M. K.   Sex: Female; age at suicidal attempt: 13 years, 10 months. The girl was born when her father was 37 years of age and her mother 26. She has a sister 4 years older. The father, a shrewd type of man and fond of society, was a hard worker and seems to have been engaged in a brokerage or related business. He was sentenced to imprisonment at hard labor on charges of taking a bribe and swindling when the girl was 2 years and 4 months of age. Somewhat later, when he fathered a child by another woman, her parents divorced by mutual consent. After the divorce, the mother left M. K., then 4 years old, with the maternal grandparents and went off to cohabit with another man. The girl was reared, for the most part, by her maternal grandparents so that she loved them best of anyone during her early years, but she came to dislike her ill-tempered grandfather. Being hard-of-hearing, he spoke loudly and became markedly nagging. The grandmother, though given to grumbling, brought up the girl with affection. The mother, after parting from the man, came back to her parents and worked in an office. The girl was then 8 years of age. Her father visited her once in a while. Her older sister, still attached to the father, would ask him for pocket money, but M. K. disliked this. In the fifth grade of elementary school at 10 years old of age she learned of the relationship between her father and mother.

In spite of an unhappy childhood, she performed well in elementary school. She was very shy and quiet and had only one friend. In the second term of the first year of junior high school, she joined a group of delinquents (mainly third-year students) and went out with them at night. In October of that year at 13 years and 2 months of age, she first experienced sexual intercourse. As she cut classes more frequently, her class ranking showed a downward trend. Her delinquent tendencies were accelerated from December of that year through January of the next year to the extent that she began to work as a live-in waitress at a coffee shop without the knowledge of her family and ran away to Kyushu where she had sexual relations with several men. In May, during the second year of junior high, she stole clothing and other items from a next-door apartment. Her promiscuous conduct utterly perplexed the school authorities who finally gave up all efforts on her behalf. She established a close relationship with the leader (K.) of a delinquent gang and believed that she had fallen in love with him. About the same time, Y., a disreputable character (25 years old), began to run after her. He pursued her to school and insisted that she become his wife. Presumably dismayed at being followed continually by him, the girl, who had never taken sleeping drugs, attempted suicide with ten tablets of hyminal. She left a note saying that she was in love with K. This attempt failed.

The psychological tests given to her at middle school, the Juvenile Detention and Classification Home, and the family court report as follows: "I.Q.: 102 (by Shin-Tanaka B). No particular difficulties suggested by Uchida-Kraepelin's Accumulation Test. Vanity-minded. Bold and sociable, though lacking seriousness. Regarded as so-called hysterical character." The latter trait was confirmed by my interview with her. It was also noted that immediately prior to menstruation, she would become unstable in mood, uncontrollably excited, and interested in going out for pleasure. It seems, however, that this was not always the case in the Child Education and Training Home. Incidentally, the suicide was attempted eleven days before her expected menstruation, not immediately before it.

The suicidal attempt of this girl may be regarded like the former case, as one type of reaction by a delinquent girl who has at one time or another experienced sleeping drugs. This case, however, is marked by the sexual relationships involved. We can find motives of suicidal attempt, as seen in adolescence or adulthood, though in a very early stage in such facts as her attempt to escape the man whom she hated and the note left for the one whom she loved.

The two cases cited above are not only typical examples of unsuccessful suicidal attempts in puberty but are also typical in that they follow a formula course: defective family—running away—delinquency—sleeping pills—suicidal attempt.

E. N., the next case, followed the same formula course. However, she is distinguished from the others in that the depressive state in manic-depressive psychosis has more to do with the occurrence than the former two cases (especially that of M. K., Case No. 6). As I did not have an opportunity to interview her, instead of her life history and course of delinquency and suicidal attempt, I shall only quote the reasons for the decision by the Hiroshima Family Court referring the girl to the Child Education and Training Home.

Case No. 7, E. N.   Sex: female; age at suicidal attempt: 14 years, 7 months. The girl had been raised by her grandmother since the death of her father when she was 3 years of age. She attended elementary school and junior high school; in August 1961, when she was in the first year of junior high school, she was taken back by her mother. Except for being solitary, without any close friends, she did not seem to have any problems during that period. According to her own explanation, she was violated by delinquent boys in October 1961 and again in October 1962; since that time, delinquent boys in her neighborhood had pursued her.

On January 15, 1962, her elder brother (19 years old at that time) was arrested on a charge of murder. This was a turning point, since her delinquent acts rapidly multiplied in such ways as going out for pleasure at night, staying out without asking permission, and keeping an unhealthy companionship with boys. In the third year of junior high school (1963), she attended school for only two days and ran away on April 17 to an inn where she had sexual relations with a delinquent boy. She was located by the police and sent home. Though she moved, on this occasion, to the home of her aunt (her mother's sister) of her own accord, she ran away on April 20 to join a delinquent group. When she quarrelled with them, she took sleeping pills, was found nearly unconscious by the police, and was sent back to her mother. Around May 7, she ran away again, and she began working and living in a coffee shop under a false name. Again, she was found and taken into police custody. In spite of her mother's and teacher's urging that she attend school, she never gave up her delinquent acts of truancy, running away, and sexual promiscuity. Given her inclination to disobey her guardians and to avoid their supervision, it was considered likely that she would commit an offense in the future.

Although the mother of the girl has lived with a common-law husband since February 1953, no conflicts in particular so far have occurred between the mother, the common-law husband, and the girl. It is understood that her rapid degradation resulted from her feelings of isolation which suddenly expanded and were driven to the surface by the arrest of her brother. This, together with her unhealthy relationship with boys, increased her inherent tendency toward vanity and so-called hysterical character. As it did not seem likely that she would receive guidance toward normal development at home, it seemed better to refer her to the Child Education and Training Home and place her under special guidance. In accordance with the Juvenile Law, I committed her to the Child Education and Training Home.

In the referral papers cited above, she is described as a so-called hysterical character. Manic-depressive psychoses were also noticed in the teaching records of the home where she was committed on June 14, 1963. She remained in a depressive phase from her entrance to the home in June through late September when improvement was shown. She entered a manic phase in October and November when her interest in the opposite sex increased. During December, minor changes in mood, provoked by physical illness, were observed. At New Year's, she pledged to seek hope and to work cooperatively to make a good home and school record. An appendectomy in February brought a brief recurrence of low spirits, but she recovered to graduate on March 5. She found employment shortly thereafter. This case should be attributed to manic-depressive alternation of mood or cyclothymic temperament.

Cases of Periodic Psychoses in Puberty

Case No. 5, M. H.   Sex: female; age at suicidal attempt: 13 years, 7 months. The girl, M. H., was illegitimate. Her mother was a maid, and her father was unnamed. She was adopted by her mother's employers, the H.'s, who had no children. When she was 9 months old, her mother went off to live with her husband. After that, she visited the girl once a year and wrote letters frequently. When the girl entered elementary school, her mother paid her a visit which turned out to be the last. M. H.'s real mother was a cheerful, sociable woman though rather frivolous; her real father was apparently a normal man. We have no information, from such details as are available, concerning a predisposition of manic-depressive psychosis from either side.

The girl grew up normally and never suffered from any serious illness except tonsillitis in childhood. When she was in the sixth grade of elementary school at 11 years and 3 months of age, she had her first menses. For about half a year after, she seemed disturbed about it and said, "Why should I have this? I wish I were a boy."

The adoptive family was fairly well-off. The adoptive father, an office worker, was cheerful, sociable, and tidy. He loved the girl very much and had slept with her for two or three months before she attempted suicide.* The adoptive mother, who was an easygoing, casual woman at home,

---

* Note to the reader: Co-sleeping heterosexually within the nuclear family, especially mother-son and father-daughter, is common in Japan. As W. Caudill and D. Plath have shown ("Who Sleeps by Whom?" *Psychiatry* 29, 1966:344–66), such arrangements tend to blur the distinctions between the generations and between the sexes. EDITOR

was introverted and nervous with others outside the home. Like her husband, she loved the girl, rather overprotectively, and according to her account, she had spoiled her.

When she was in the sixth year of elementary school (after her first menses), she asked her foster mother if she were an adopted child and was given a vague answer. Someone heard her say, "I won't die while I am in junior high school. When I enter high school, I'll commit suicide." It is hard to tell whether this suicidal desire was caused by a slight depressive phase which had already existed or was merely an emotion peculiar to puberty.

In the second year of junior high school at 13 years and 1 month of age, she was in love with a boyfriend. On July 23 of the same year at 13 years and 4 months of age, "wishing to die," she ran away to another prefecture and was taken into protective custody. This happened a day before the onset of her menstrual cycle. She embarrassed her father on the train by asking, "You are not my real father, are you, Dad?"

The girl came to believe that the I.s, a brother of her adoptive mother and his wife, who often visited her home, were her real parents, because the couple treated her with affection. Towards the end of August, she asked her adoptive parents why she was not permitted to go to live with her real parents. At a loss to explain their relationship, the adoptive parents falsely acknowledged that the aunt and uncle (the I.s) were the real parents and then asked the I.s to consent to this deception.

On September 15 at 13 years and 6 months of age, after having left a suicide note with a classmate, she ran away from school. A teacher found her shopping for a cutting instrument at a cutlery store. On that day she was entirely stupefied and quiet. Her upset adoptive parents tried to make her believe that she was the daughter of the uncle and aunt. To meet M. H.'s demands, they took her to the I.s' home. The girl, who had been depressed for a few days, soon had menses and thereafter remained at the I.s without any problems during October.

In November, she began to shut herself in again and became mutistic. Many notes to her parents were written during those days. On November 23, the second day of menstruation, she went on a picnic with her friends. When she returned home, she went out and purchased a train ticket, but she was detected on the train and returned to her home. At this time she was heard to remark, "I don't want to be a grown-up. Their world is so filthy."

The next day, her adoptive parents brought her to the neuropsychiatry department at my hospital where I had an opportunity to examine her. Though cheerful, she was unable to accurately verbalize her experience. All she could say was that her running away was motivated by a desire to die and that although she partly felt like admitting that desire, she also found it ridiculous. No amnesia was detected during the three occurrences. While she was usually rather talkative, she tired of speaking or became mutistic in these depressed phases.

I gave her thyroxine and watched her prognosis. As no periodic depressive state appeared for the successive six months, I stopped the medical treatment. In a five-year follow-up I have found her healthy, mentally and physically, and she has not resorted to further attempts at suicide. Her I.Q. is 125 by WISC; V: 130, P: 113, and she is usually talkative, cheerful, active, unyielding, and industrious.

This case belongs to a group which exhibits periodic psychoses in puberty and is noteworthy as one in which biological factors and the long-cherished negative idea of life, or anxiety, were combined. This is also a good example of how we can successfully shut out the periodically repeated idea of suicide—a short phase of depression—by consistent reinforcement of her belief that her aunt and uncle were her real parents and by the administration of thyroxine.

Case No. 4, N. D.   Sex: female; age at suicidal attempt: 12 years. The father is a manic-depressive psychotic, with an especially noticeable manic phase. The father's elder sister suffered from depressive psychosis at around age 20 but has now recovered. His elder brother, by a different mother, was schizophrenic and died of tuberculosis; and his elder sister, by another mother, and a paternal cousin have both committed suicide. Thus, numerous instances of psychoses, especially affective psychoses, are dominant on the paternal side. Five years ago, the father was taken to the Department of Neuropsychiatry, Kyoto University Hospital, because of extreme manic excitement. Since then he has had no severe phases except for periodic sullen states. He belongs to an acromegaloid rather than to a pyknic type. He owns a printing company, and the family is fairly well-off. The girl has a brother four years her junior. The mother, nervous and unyielding, devotes herself to the education of the girl, though with too much expectation. No one can deny that she is rich in parental love.

Since 11 years and 11 months of age, she has had periodic depressive states which have appeared monthly. Her depression was accompanied by autonomous nervous disturbances such as vomiting and anoretia and with insomnia which would improve in a week or so. Before the onset of a depressive period, she was cheerful for a few days—manic phase. She showed psychic symptoms of the depressive phase such as suddenly becoming mutistic and motionless as if she had lost all strength or feeling gloomy and pessimistic. She also became susceptible to tears and worried about trifles. Since her first menses at the age of 13 years and 11 months, her manic-depressive manifestations had become shorter and milder, and she seemed to have become almost stabilized. For medical treatment, I gave her 15 mg. of Levopromazine before the arrival of each phase which could be predicted with relative accuracy, and when the phase worsened, the amount of medication was increased as necessary. Thyroxine was found ineffective in this case. In the five-year follow-up her manic-depressive phases, lasting seven to twelve days, are still recurring, and she has not yet reached complete recovery.

Though the girl told her mother of a wish to die during her depressive phases in June 1963 at 12 years of age and in September of the same year at 12 years and 3 months of age, she has not taken any action to this end. As the girl was intellectually above average, like M. H. in the former case, I sought to elicit some introspection on her desire for death, but my efforts were in vain, and no further explanation was obtained other than "I want to die" or "I wanted to die." This may suggest that in suicide or suicidal attempt among children, the idea of death itself is not concretely established but remains very obscure and vague. Yet, bound up with the vague idea of death, desire for death is provoked by a certain mental condition (especially in the last three cases, a periodic depressive state of emotion).

According to our study of depressive states in childhood, suppression of will or impulse is generally dominant, while experiencing emotions such as sorrow—unlike in adulthood—finds expression only in a feeling of melancholy or is at least rarely expressed as a subjective experience of children. Also pertinent is that a desire for death or a sense of guilt is very unusual in childhood. It can be seen, therefore, that very rare cases do exist where children have a pessimistic view of life or a desire for death. This is true especially when emphasized by a prolonged latent sense of anxiety toward life.

Summary

The above eight cases of suicide, successful and unsuccessful, concern children under 15 years of age. Table 1 depicts the major factors of each case. Although it is risky to draw any general conclusions about suicide among children under 15 years of age solely on the basis of this data, we may point out the following as striking: (1) Except for the one successful case, all (the seven unsuccessful cases) are girls. (2) The three incidents of running away or staying out without permission, delinquency, and pleasure-seeking in sleeping drugs are closely related to suicide. Especially noteworthy is the fact that all except case no. 4 have run away from home. (3) All except case no. 4 were either brought up by someone other than their own parents or lacked one of the parents. In short, they grew up in broken homes. (4) Their I.Q.s are not at all low except in case no 2. Also, in case no. 2 where a low I.Q. was shown, a Rorschach test revealed considerable intellectual attributes rather than mental retardation. (5) Four cases, that is half the total, are obviously psychotics. In three of them, suicide was attempted in the depressive phases of either periodic psychoses in puberty or manic-depressive psychoses, with experience of auditory hallucination beginning at the age of 4 or 5 (Takagi, 1959).

In light of the preceding points, these cases might be sorted into two groups. The first is a group of children from defective families who underwent deprivation in their early ages and followed the formula course

Table 1:   Eight Child Suicide Attempts: A Summary

| | | | | | History of Delinquency | |
| | | | | | --- | --- |
Case	Age at Time of Attempt	Method	Result	Run Away	Age at Time of First Act	Form
1. C.S.	9 yrs. 6 mos.	Sleeping drugs	Unsuccessful	+	8 yrs.	Stealing
2. U.Y.	11 yrs.	Drowning	Unsuccessful	+		Running away
3. Y.K.	11 yrs. 10 mos.	Hanging	Successful	+	6 yrs.	Stealing
4. N.D.	12 yrs.	Suicidal desire only		–		None
5. M.H.	13 yrs. 7 mos.	Shopping for cutlery	Unsuccessful	+		None
6. M.K.	13 yrs. 10 mos.	Sleeping drugs	Unsuccessful	+	13 yrs.	Sexual offense
7. E.N.	14 yrs. 7 mos.	Sleeping drugs	Unsuccessful	+	13 yrs.	Sexual offense
8. Y.G.	15 yrs.	Sleeping drugs	Unsuccessful	+	10 yrs.	Stealing

Table 1: (Continued)

	Condition of Family					
Real Father	Real Mother	Fosterage	Remarks	I.Q.	Psychiatric Diagnosis	Remarks
Deceased	Separated from child	Grand-parents		94		Details unknown
Deceased	Lived with child	Sister	Stepfather: violent	62	Childhood schizo-phrenia	Fell ill probably at four or five years of age; hospitalized
Separated from child	Deceased	Grand-parents	Real father: alcoholic	91		In order to cut off symbiotic relationship with father; placed in a solitary cell of child edu-cation home
Separated from child	Lived with child		Father: manic-depressive psychosis	120	Periodic psychosis in puberty	Under remis-sion; res-ponding to treatment
Deceased	Deceased	Step-parents	Stepparents: rather well-off	125	Periodic psychosis in puberty	Psychiatric treatment progressing favorably
Deceased	Separated from child	Grand-parents		102	Hysterical character	
Deceased	Separated from child	Grand-parents	Brother: co-offender	98	Manic-depressive psychosis	Remission; secured employment
Deceased	Deceased	Step-parents, baby sitter	Rejected by stepparents	105		

of delinquency from running away to suicide. They were driven to death, having lost their place in this world and being unable to find anyone on whom to rely. The second is a group of children exhibiting manic-depressive psychoses or periodic psychoses in puberty who attempted suicide with a desire for death arising in a depressive phase. Case numbers 1, 3, and 8 belong to the first group, and case no. 4 belongs to the second group. The other cases, however, appear to be borderline cases. We must understand that any actual case has both psychosociological and biological causes as well as both normal-psychological and psychopathological causes.

All the cases reported here concern children in prepuberty or puberty—a transition period between a parent-controlled environment and the wider society which involves complex problems of adjustment. In this paper, however, only factual material of the cases were reported in the expectation that there would be further discussion of mental health in puberty on another occasion.

REFERENCES

Bender, L., and P. Schilder. 1937. Suicidal preoccupation and attempts in children. American Journal of Orthopsychiatry 7:225–34.

Connell, P. H. 1965. Suicidal attempts in childhood and adolescence. In Modern perspectives in child psychiatry. I. J. G. Howells, ed. London, Oliver & Boyd.

Kanner, L. 1957. Child psychiatry. 3rd ed. Springfield, Charles C Thomas.

Ohara, K., et. al. 1963. Suicide in children: a viewpoint from family pathology. Clinical Psychiatry 5:375–79.

Takagi, R. 1959. Periodic psychoses in preadolescence. Psychiatrica et Neurologia Japonica 61:1194–1208.

7. The Family and the Management of Mental Health Problems in Vietnam

TRAN-MINH TUNG, Lt. Col., M.D.

Military Medical School
Saigon, South Vietnam

TO SAY THAT the family is an ubiquitous factor in life in Vietnam is a truism hardly worthy of mention except for the practical applications that one may possibly draw from it. Corruption among civil servants has been explained by familial contamination, as have softness or compassion in Communist soldiers and desertions among government troops. Therefore, practical measures for the prevention of the noxious influences of familial ties have been devised in civilian and military services.

In medical practice, the patient's mental health is greatly affected by his family's attitudes. If Dr. Michael Balint had written his book in Vietnam, I imagine he would have named it "The Physician, the Patient, His Family, and His Illness." Indeed, the physician, be he a general practitioner or a specialist, always seems to have to cope with one relative or another when he treats his patient. Almost invariably, someone from the family has escorted the patient to the doctor's office. Someone will stay with him through his hospitalization to feed him, to nurse him, and to give him his medication. In most cases, the relatives more than the patients are the ones to be convinced before the patient can start or continue a therapeutic program.

By the same token, the daily practice of psychiatry in Vietnam clearly shows the impact of the same factor in every detail of its conduct.

The family stands incessantly between the patient and the psychiatrist, filtering the communication, buffering the physician's action, altering his relationship with the patient, helping or sabotaging, but always transforming the course of his efforts for diagnosis, treatment, or rehabilitation. The family is so much in the forefront that it must be taken into account in the same manner that one makes allowances for the patient's idiosyncratic response to a drug. Moreover, as a student of human behavior, the psychiatrist cannot help but wonder about the pressures coming from the same source and bearing on the personality of his patient. The Vietnamese individual is so deeply immersed in his social environment, so strictly bound by familial ties, and dependent in so many ways upon his kinship group, that there is hardly a doubt that part of his mental pathology must stem from these factors.

The influence of the patient's family in the practical aspects of his mental health problems is a concrete thing that can be analyzed and determined. With some imagination, useful conclusions may be drawn in the management of mental health programs. One comes to more uncertain ground when he seeks to estimate the participation of the family in the incidence, form, and outcome of mental illnesses. The problem is formidable if only because of the difficulties of research methodology and the elaborate technical organization implied by any probing efforts into these areas. The difficulties arise mostly in the field of theory and doctrine, when one has to analyze, appreciate, and interpret the data so obtained. Certainly one cannot expect any clear-cut and simple answer to the questions asked.

Taking these difficulties into account, I will deal only with the practical problem of the family as a factor in the management of mental illness in Vietnam, and in doing so, I shall present my views as impressions gained from experience and observation rather than as rigorous scientific demonstrations supported by proof and research. The merit of the analysis, should it have any, lies in the opportunity to formulate hypotheses, raise issues, ask questions, and possibly point out areas that need to be further and more systematically explored.

Conditions that explain the intervention of the Vietnamese family, in the course of medical treatment to one of its members, are as follows. (1) The Vietnamese family, as a self-sufficient social unit, is accustomed to looking after the health of its members, as it provides them with food and education. Physicians, hospitals, and medicine in general are but instruments to that end, whereas the initiative and the responsibility of treatment remain with the family. (2) Out of true affection and sincere preoccupation for a loved one, the family expresses a serious concern for a sick member, especially when he is helpless and seemingly in need of compassion. (3) The third reason resides in the situation of medicine in Vietnam, the resources of which are so limited that physicians are happy and grateful for any help, however small or clumsy it may be.

The factors just stated become much more evident if the illness is a mental one. Because of its special nature, mental disease either renders the patient completely helpless and dependent upon his relatives or makes him troublesome and dangerous and in need of his family as a safeguard and for protection. In some cases, the family's interests as well as social and moral obligations entail its keeping charge of the mentally ill member throughout the course of his disease.

To begin with, most often it is the relatives, annoyed or alarmed by the early symptoms of abnormality, who initiate the entire medical program by taking the patient to the doctor. This fact is most readily seen in the case of psychoses. Out of 100 psychiatric patients admitted to government hospitals, about five are brought in by the police as emergency cases suffering from symptoms such as alcoholic delirium or acute excitement. Not more than ten are voluntary admissions, and the rest are hospitalized at the request of a next of kin. Patients of the last two categories are invariably accompanied to the hospital by one or many relatives, and this holds true even for some who are committed as a measure of public safety. The fact is striking even for less disturbed mental patients, such as neurotics treated in outpatient clinics and private practice. My impression is that not more than 20 percent of such patients receive consultation unaccompanied by relatives, and perhaps only 10 percent of the female patients do so. These figures are only the visible consequences of a complex process that involves various factors which can act to the advantage or disadvantage of the patients.

Mental disease is accepted by the average Vietnamese as a fact of life, somewhat mysterious, but not extremely awful or shameful, bearing no special stigma, and bringing to the family only as much embarrassment as would the improper behavior of one of its members in a public place. Of course, discretion is preferred, but the group is not overly anxious to hide the patient or his illness. Besides, as illnesses go, and with rare exceptions, mental disease does not appear very dramatic, that is, not as appalling or life-threatening as the more familiar pathological conditions such as fever, diarrhea, etc. Therefore, to those who live closely with the patient, minor changes may go undetected. Even gross modifications of behavior sometimes seem to be only normal reactions explainable by plausible reasons. Thus, recognition of a mental pathological state often is delayed, even though one might think that close observation by family members should have helped to raise an early warning.

By the same bias, most families believe that a member's abnormal behavior, when it is finally noticed, is just some minor ailment that requires no more than casual attention and the use of some nostrum or family remedy. They seldom think a visit to the doctor, much less to a psychiatrist, is warranted.

Optimism or ignorance, or both, makes it difficult for the physician to convince the family of the necessity to hospitalize the patient. In fact, the main obstacle and the major objection usually posed to such a measure is a practical one and, paradoxically, springs from a real concern for the patient. In regard to comfort, hospitals, especially Vietnamese state hospitals, have never been very attractive, and it seems cruel to leave the patient in the hands of strangers who will never care for him as his own family would. Therefore, if one is compelled to hospitalize a kin, someone, often a female member of the family, escorts the patient and nurses him during his stay at the hospital. Entire Montagnard families in the central Vietnamese highlands camp out week after week in hospital courtyards while waiting on their ill members. In the rest of the country, only one or two relatives will remain in the hospital, but even that is a great inconvenience for the family.

Conditions are slightly different in mental hospitals that do not authorize such living-in practices by patients' families except in very special cases. Still, the families feel an obligation not to desert the patients, and they will try to visit their relatives as frequently as permitted by hospital regulations —every day perhaps, if the hospital is not too far away from home. Families always bring some food, "to nurse him," as the saying goes. Obviously, this family practice could quickly become the source of much family hardship and the cause of much anxiety and guilt among those members who feel that they are obligated to visit the patient.

Thus, the family will react to the slightest sign of the patient's improvement by asking for his discharge notwithstanding the psychiatrists' objections. Partly for this reason, the average stay in Choquan and Hué Psychiatric Hospitals, which are located in downtown sections of the two capitals, is not more than thirty days. On the contrary, for Bienhoa Hospital, thirty miles away from Saigon, there is a different and very distinct pattern in the length of stay. About 30 percent of the cases are discharged after the three or four months spent in the intensive care unit where family visits are frequent—weekly or biweekly. If not discharged, the patients are transferred to the chronic section where they stay for an average of three years. Visits of the family then become less and less frequent, and the hospital administration often cannot even locate the next of kin when the patient finally is discharged. It is my impression that the stronger the sense of obligation on the family's part, the stronger its guilt feelings will be. One of its defenses against this particular anxiety is the rationalization about the incurability of the patient's condition, almost to the point of his rejection into oblivion. One thing is certain—after a while, the family reorganizes itself in the absence of the patient, and it is never easy to make room for him should he return home.

Needless to say, the atmosphere in hospital wards is greatly influenced by the existence or the absence of family visits, and visits tend to become an extrinsic factor that can change the symptomatology or disturb the results of the therapeutic program. This influence greatly complicates the task of the psychiatrist, even though it may help him eventually and imperceptibly. For the implementation of any treatment or rehabilitation program planned for the patient outside the hospital, the physician must rely more heavily on the family than he cares to, and in many instances he must do so entirely aware that it is the only way he will obtain positive responses from the patient.

For example, shortage of auxiliary personnel does not permit the psychiatrist to use qualified help to follow up his patients. Consequently, even to administer medication, he must depend upon the patient's relatives, who are particularly prone to alter or discontinue the prescribed tranquilizers if the patient experiences any alarming side effects or if the psychiatrist is not available to reassure them.

In a subtle but often decisive way, the general attitude of members of the family reflects the course of the patient's illness and helps or hinders the hospital's therapeutic action. The problem is universal, and the tactics of any psychiatric treatment certainly calls for some manipulation of the patient's immediate environment, at least as an accessory to the main course of therapy. In Vietnam, given the especially close-knit organization of the patriarchal family, very often the family is not an accessory to treatment but the crux of the matter. Except for its importance in treatment of its members' mental health, many aspects of the problem still remain unknown. Deeper and more ingenuous research must be undertaken before one can offer more than broad generalities.

In the same line of thought, one point is worthy of note: the problem of the family has its impact also upon the psychiatrist's personality which in turn affects the therapeutic program. The psychiatrist's view of the case and his approach to the patient's problem are certainly determined by his own background, education, and training. Very often the psychiatrist himself has many unresolved conflicts on the subject of family, between the inherited traditional standards and the modern concepts and ideas taught by his Western teachers. If the problem presented by his patients duplicates his own, it will be a hard task for the doctor to remain objective. How much this will hamper his efforts to help them, and how the problem can practically be solved, are subjects of general interest which have special importance in societies witnessing rapid and radical changes such as Asia and Africa.

The subject of this paper is remarkably untreated in medical literature, which is often irrelevant to the particular problems of medical practice in Vietnam; only recently has medical psychology, psychiatry, and sociology been introduced in the curricula of Vietnamese medical schools. Most of the time, physicians play it by ear each time they have to deal with a patient's family. The most sophisticated physicians facetiously name the process "public relations." The majority look on it as a nuisance, either to be ignored or disposed of in the authoritarian manner; i.e., by giving orders or browbeating people instead of trying to understand or to help them.

The psychiatrist, because of his training, is more prudent and more people conscious, if not more family conscious, than other medical specialists. He senses and sees how much his efforts depend upon other people, at least key persons such as the members of his patient's family. Therefore, he will try to manipulate the family in the hope of enlisting their cooperation for the patient's benefit. In most cases, the family is approached when the opportunity arises without any forethought or systematic intention to utilize the family as a therapeutic agent.

Simultaneous treatment of family members has been undertaken on occasion often out of sheer scarcity of psychiatrists. My experience is not large enough to permit a definite impression of the usefulness of simultaneous treatment. The main objection is that the psychiatrist has many difficulties handling the transference, particularly when he is struggling with some problem very similar to those among his various patients. Joint treatment of family members has not been attempted, to my knowledge, perhaps because at first sight it does not seem acceptable to a Vietnamese mind for the following reasons: the natural seclusiveness of the average Vietnamese, his fear of losing face if he is to bare his soul before those who know him, and the strict etiquette that asks the ascendants to preserve their prestige at any cost and the descendants to continue their respect to their elders regardless of their intimate feelings.

Many practical approaches have been suggested to capitalize on the support available from the family to the patient during his illness. Among them, I advanced in 1963 the idea of a day hospital as the most practicable and immediately usable project to take advantage of the desire of the family to wait on the patient and to make the maximum utilization of the meager resources of public hospitals. Various reasons, primarily perhaps the novelty of the idea, have prevented its realization, but I still think that it is worthwhile and that the project should be given a fair trial.

The extension and improvement of outpatient psychiatric facilities in different hospitals have been undertaken primarily to decongest overcrowded public hospitals. Outpatient facilities are completely successful, as the number of patients treated and the positive medical results indicate. The success of the outpatient program can be shown by patients' dramatic improvement, often obtained as a result of tranquilizing drugs and also by the enthusiasm demonstrated by families that are spared the burden, material and moral, of having to nurse their patients away from home.

Conversely, the negative aspect of the problem of the family has been taken into consideration. In 1964, the efforts of the Mental Health Bureau in the Vietnamese Ministry of Health resulted in the creation of a rehabilitation village that harbored seventy patients selected from among the convalescents who were about to leave Bienhoa Mental Hospital after three or four years of treatment. In half-way houses situated at the hospital's periphery and completely independent of treatment facilities, the patients are virtually left to themselves; they even earn their pocket money by cultivating the plot of land belonging to their community, or they hire themselves out to the farmers in the neighborhood. The objective is to help the patient prepare himself for reintegration into normal life, especially for returning home and regaining his place as a responsible member of the family, no longer a burden or an object of pity. The results are not easy to assess in relation to individual cases, but the hospital staff has applauded the community plan to the extent that it is considered to have obtained sufficient credit to double the village's capacity in fiscal year 1970.

In summary, the participation of the family in the care of the patient, including actual medical procedures, is a reality that confronts any physician practicing in Vietnam; family participation in treatment is so commonly seen that it is taken for granted. Yet, many questions must be raised and answered about the nature of family intervention, the extent of pressures exerted upon the family members, the direction of their action, the possible responses of the patient, the effects on the diagnostic and therapeutic program, and their impact on the patient-physician relation, especially in a psychotherapeutic setting. In a broader perspective and with less utilitarian approach, many problems remain to be solved in order to determine the influences of the family group on the individual's personality and his mental health. These questions and others in the same vein will have to be answered for the sake of knowledge, if not for the sake of action, for they are problems especially pertinent to the preoccupations of developing countries such as ours, where cultural changes and historical events may be the source of many conflicts between the individual and social institutions and the cause of political turmoil, social unrest, and personal unhappiness.

8. Psychodynamic Structures in Vietnamese Personality

WALTER H. SLOTE Ph.D.

Columbia University
New York, New York

FOR SOME TIME NOW, my extended research interest has been the study of the psychodynamics, within the cultural-historical sequence, which go into the making up of the personality structure of the rebel and the revolutionary. It was within the context of this interest that I went to South Vietnam during the summers of 1966 and 1967. The original study was devoted to an intensive, psychoanalytic exploration into the lives of four Vietnamese, leaders within their sphere of dissent and chosen because they constituted an elite among the forces opposed to both present and past regimes. As the analysis of the data proceeded, my attention became focused on certain broader dimensions of Vietnamese cultural character structure. This led to my return to South Vietnam in 1967 to gather additional data and to test the hypotheses developed from the original limited sample on a more extensive population in which the element of dissent was disregarded. The results of this second study are presented in this paper.

The assumption upon which this research is based is that, within the subterranean world of the unconscious, man is more alike than not. The deeper the dynamics and motivational patternings in terms of layering of consciousness, the more likely they are to represent universals which can be extrapolated. There is wide differentiation in behavioral and ideational style from one person to another, and there may be significant variation in individual motivation for a particular act; but the deeper one probes into the unconscious, the more apt one is to find patterns which are broadly applicable. Within personality, it is the qualitative—not the quantitative, the patterning, the structural integration, and the inter- and intra-group interaction—that differentiates one culture or subculture from another. Thus, although each of us as individuals shares most, if not all, of the personality dimensions to be described in this paper, we do not share the specific contextual format. I trust that this statement will suffice to establish the qualification of universality as we examine the dynamics that emerge.

This research, and all behavioral research presently being conducted in South Vietnam, labors under one crucial limitation—we have, at present, very little basic anthropological data on the area. The anthropological research that has been done is of excellent calibre, but there is far too little of it. The essential cultural foundations, upon which all behavioral research must, of necessity, be based, are for the most part unknown. The result is that each researcher is forced to study not only his particular area but also the cultural conditions as well—an extremely unsatisfactory solution and one for which most nonanthropologists, including myself, are ill-equipped. Until this deplorable situation is rectified, no Vietnamese research in the behavioral sciences can be accepted with certainty.

No attempt has been made in this research to differentiate between the reputed personality differences to be found in those Vietnamese coming from the North, Central, and South. Although each area was represented, the number of informants from each area did not permit such differentiation. Furthermore, only a limited number of elite were seen. Interviews were conducted in various urban and rural areas from the delta ranging north to Hué and, with the exception of the elite, covered most socioeconomic strata.

I shall attempt to summarize my findings within the following areas: ego structure and identity patterning; the effect of traditionalism on motivation and behavior; stylization of personality and role adoption; institutionalization of affect, perception, attitude, and cognition; and intrafamilial relations and child-rearing practices.

Vietnamese Ego Structure and Identity Patterns

This research, in its broadest statement, confirms the hypotheses that by now, I trust, is firmly established—the ego structure and identity patterns adopted by the individual are a product of, and are consonant with, the parameters established by the society. Thus, the more traditional the society, the more restrictive the parameters, which results in a greater tendency toward sameness within the ego patterning of individual members; the more open the society, the greater are the individuation in ego structure. Concomitantly, it is far more difficult for a member of a restrictive society to break out of the confines of the accepted behavioral and conceptual set than for a member of a society where the boundaries are more flexible so that the individual is permitted greater latitude in the search for personal satisfaction and an individualized identity.

Vietnam is a traditional society that is rapidly being placed into a transitional development sequence by forces beyond its control. As historical patterns become increasingly disorganized by the current conflict, a new set of values is being introduced not only by the United States but also by the impact of modern societies in general. Although many of these values are exogenous to Vietnamese culture, they carry great force because of their proven practical effectiveness and the powerful authoritative position of those who are introducing them.

Not only are these values alien, but many are also dramatically antithetical to the Vietnamese concept of orderly existence. Although an impressive effort is being made by the Vietnamese to retain old values and integrate them with the new, the inevitable and predictable result during this transitional period has been increasing intrapsychic conflict. Although Vietnam is far from a unique case, the complications in ego identity that arise out of this extraordinarily difficult set of circumstances can be anticipated. They are normal for so thoroughly abnormal a situation.

The concept of an individualized, self-determining ego structure—the profound sense of "I am"—is much less clearly established in Vietnam than in most western cultures. Historically, the sense of a unique self that is in essential mastery over one's own destiny has been a concept of severely limited conceivability for the Vietnamese. In a very profound and basic sense, the Vietnamese regards himself as a component within a far greater totality. As such, he is acted upon by external forces, and he expects to be. To be sure, he can and does exert certain controls and direction over his fate, but in the final analysis, he conceives of his capability to establish a personal determination over these external powers as partial. This appears to be a central dynamic within all who were interviewed, a basic aspect of their world view and, as one usually finds in matters of this nature, rarely in conscious awareness. This does not mean that the Vietnamese passively relegate themselves to an unremitting fate; their history provides dramatic evidence to the contrary. Nor do they consciously speak in this vein. In fact, the extensive infrafraternal strife and the maneuvering for position that one constantly encounters seemingly belies this observation. Yet beneath the power struggles, beneath the frequently almost bombastic assertion of self-determination, lies this primary sense of the partial and powerless "I."

The historical sequence has, of course, added measurably to this basic view: Vietnam has repeatedly been invaded; the internal authority structure, both national and regional, has contributed its own extreme dimensions; for long periods of time, the nation and its people have been subjected to the will of more powerful nations. Yet more important than these undeniably potent forces has been the pervasive effect of the conglomerate Confucianism-Taoism-Buddhism that one finds in Vietnam, and the child-rearing patterns within the home and village. The military and political invasions and occupations constitute confirmatory experience rather than primary motivation for a dynamism that is basically set in the home and is a central teaching within each Vietnamese family. In the unconscious self-image of the Vietnamese, he is a component within a broader collective ego structure. As one behavioral scientist with whom the researcher discussed this observation said: "For the traditional-minded Vietnamese, the ego, the 'me' is an illusion—not a reality. One fits into the totality of a family or societal unity; the individual unity is an illusional one; it is not real; it is composed of parts which can react differently and change. There is self-determination, but it is very restricted. It is secondary and limited; it is not a primary force." [1]

The family is seen as the basic unit, and to cut oneself off from the family is to be deeply fractured and incomplete, an intolerable psychological position if one is to function effectively. In the absence of the physical presence of the family—a desirable but not crucial factor—this dynamism is maintained by a particular form of eidetic imagery. I refer to the psychological mechanism by which one reexperiences the incorporated familial and parental attitudes, values, beliefs, prohibitions, areas of permission and validation, etc., into one's own psychic and mental structure. The result is that the individual knows precisely what position his parents and community would take on any issue and on any step that might diverge from the stylized routine pattern of living. A subconscious dialogue ensues, following which a decision is made. This is, again, a universal dimension within all mankind (e.g., one of the primary goals of psychoanalysis is that of minimizing the power of the parental-child dialogue over contemporary behavior). The difference is that the voices of the past are more thunderous and compelling to the Vietnamese, because their primary sense of identity is so indissolubly a part of a unit representing more than one family of which they are merely one segment. It is massively strengthened because all familial units speak essentially the same traditional words with the same traditional views. One hears few echoes in this dialogue of a past that incorporates positions other than the conventional.

This does not mean that the Vietnamese ego structure is necessarily less strong than that found within the Western personality. It does mean that it is different and that it carries more freight. It also means that change is more difficult and that the acceptance of innovation is more restrictive.

Role Adoption

In the absence of a uniquely defined ego identity, one of the more common compensatory mechanisms is that of role playing. Although, again, this is a universal in human behavior and many of the following observations pertain to all, it is necessary that one fully understand the particular breadth and power of this dynamic and Vietnamese personality structure. It is a central security mechanism, and I believe that much of the difficulty that the Westerner encounters in understanding the Vietnamese stems from an inadequate realization of its broad dimensions.

The distinguishing features of role playing among the Vietnamese include the following: (1) it is subtly substantiated and validated by the full community; (2) when it is discovered, it appears subject to relatively minimal criticism; (3) there seems to be extremely little, if any, guilt connected with it; (4) it may be a conscious, as well as subconscious, operation; and (5) the role is frequently and relatively total and often is played out in all dimensions.

In Vietnam, the adoption of a role is not simply a product of insecurity as it frequently is in the West. It appears to be a stylized form that is used by most, although not all, members. One is expected to perform in a particular way and to adopt a particular identity consonant with certain cultural stereotypes. Because of the insistence upon tightly defined traditional patterns of behavior, the Vietnamese are, in effect, forced into adopting a public personality. A Vietnamese who insisted upon defining his own unique position and who acted upon it (assuming it was not in accord with accepted behavior) might find himself in serious difficulty with his fellow Vietnamese. Role adoption is a psychological mechanism that is reinforced, but not consciously acknowledged, by the society; were it to be overtly defined, it would be strenuously denied. In actuality, it conflicts with one of the standards that the Vietnamese consciously hold particularly precious—that one must always be true to oneself. The fact is, however, that although too crass or too unsophisticated an expression may be frowned upon, criticism is, on the whole, minimal. The accuracy of this observation is verified by the lack of guilt that the individual experiences; one has to do something that is disapproved by one's fellows if one is to feel guilty over it.

This pertains not only to the subconscious adoption of a role— something that we all do. On frequent occasions, it also holds true for the deliberate, conscious assigning of an identity and a life history to oneself —something that we do not all do. In addition, although we all assume certain aspects of a role, it is not universal that the role blankets our behavior to the extent that it does the Vietnamese. I do not suggest that there is no room for diversity or individuality within the Vietnamese personality; there is, and it may be fairly considerable as it is increasing as the society becomes less traditionally oriented, but the adoption of a role does cast a much weightier and oppressive shadow, and it is much more difficult to escape than in Western cultures. As an example, in 1966, a student leader with whom I worked stated that, although his family had once been economically well established (the implication was that this was long before his birth), he had grown up severely impoverished and had known hunger much of his life; his father had worked as a coolie for the French and later had made wooden articles which his mother sold in the market while he peddled them from door to door; his father no longer worked, and the informant supported him. In 1967, his history had undergone a remarkable transition, and he said that his father had inherited fairly extensive landholdings which he had sold after World War II; the family had subsisted during some of the more difficult periods on the gold that they had accumulated or inherited; his father had a successful manufacturing business that had suffered because of the war. The informant still maintained that he supported his father, who was retired, and he ended with "to the people in our city [one of the largest in central Vietnam], we were considered wealthy at that time. We were not very rich, but we lived then in easy conditions." This is a far cry from the following original statement. "While living in central Vietnam, being poor, we made wooden articles out in the country; then we would take them to the market in the city. Many times we had to go hungry because we made no sales . . . . My father had to work then as a coolie for the French, but he did not earn enough money. One afternoon, on his payday, my father went to the market to have dinner in a small eating house by the roadside. After not having made even one sale during the entire day, by coincidence I went there at the same time, but I went there to beg the lady owner of the place to give me some food. I did not see my father. My father shared his food with me as with a beggar without realizing that the beggar was his own son." However, the story is not yet complete. The informant had claimed to be from central Vietnam. He was imprisoned for about ten days during the fall of 1966, and after his release, his father insisted that he marry, believing that this would increase his personal responsibilities and decrease his commitment to the political struggle. Another older and very reliable informant attended the wedding, and as he talked to the student leader's father, realized, because of the father's accent, that the family was from North Vietnam. He confronted the student leader with this knowledge and was told, "I adapt easily." The older informant accepted this uncritically and told me that the student leader probably claimed to have come from central Vietnam because he was more like a Southerner (the older informant was a Southerner). "He is more responsible and serious, you can depend upon his words as you can with the Southerner's, and this is why he adopted this identity." The older informant also casually mentioned that the student leader's father had been a minor public functionary in the North, that he had continued this same work after coming South and that he was still employed.

The demonstration leader had constructed an identity and a personal history which fitted the exigencies of the moment and the advantages to be gained. As his goals had changed, so had his construct of his life history. A peasant origin was more advantageous to a popular leader heroically saving the people from oppression; a middle-class background was more advantageous to the Minister of Education, to which position he aspired when I saw him in 1967; and a North Vietnamese background was less desirable than either.

The Vietnamese decide upon a role and create a personal mythos that is based upon an esteemed historical myth. The central fact is that, for the moment, the myth constitutes a superior truth. The actual factual life events that do not fit into it are selectively disregarded, and a life history is constructed that meets with greater approval. The dedication is to the image, not what we in the Western world would call the reality. In appraising this dynamism as found among the Vietnamese, it is necessary that we free ourselves from the constricted vision of our conception of reality. For us, reality is that which can be factually determined—something that can be touched, seen, heard, and experienced in a very direct sense. But there are, in fact, many realities. There is the reality of the dream, the reality of the hidden vision, the reality of a personal truth, the reality of a private morality, the reality of the psychotic experience, the reality of an integration with the past and our ancestors who live above and within us, and, indeed, the reality of a reconstructed life history that more effectively serves the needs of the moment including our dreams and unreached goals. These realities are culturally determined and for the individual may be quite as valid as the reality of a chair, a computer, a factual experience, or a scientifically provable hypothesis. Thus, when we discuss role as it is incorporated by the Vietnamese, we must realize that we are dealing with a conceptual stance that may differ vastly from our own. Although there may be a suppression and reorganization of actual life events, the underlying psychological mechanism is not analogous to that of a Westerner engaging in the same phenomenon.

One additional motivational component, which may underlie the variability of roles within the individual, relates to the changes that are occurring within Vietnamese society. Under the traditional Confucian pattern, a poet was a poet; he knew his position and was held in stabilized regard by the people. In the present society, where there are so many pressures and abrupt changes and where the value of a particular position may change from day to day, the individual is far less certain as to what position may carry the greatest merit with it. The relation between individual role constellation and social values appears to be direct and explicit. Each actively interacts with the other, and as one changes, the other responds. Although one finds that role is more apt to be derived from social stance, the inverse is also constantly occurring. One sees this most dramatically in the impact of a charismatic leader upon his society. Essentially, however, there is point and counterpoint in a thematic interaction between society and the individual, between change and stasis, and between social and personal values.

Institutionalization of Affect, Perception, Attitude, Cognition

To a major extent, attitudes, emotional reactions, perceptions, preferences, and, at times, even cognitive patterns appear to be quite universally institutionalized. There are established stereotyped responses to a given situation, and as one interviews larger numbers of Vietnamese, one is impressed with the similarities with which they perceive both the world and themselves. There is variation within these patterns based upon the psychosocial impact of individual experiences, and there is variation in interpretation among the transmittal agents of the culture (parents, older siblings, extended family members, neighbors, etc.), but one is deeply impressed by the major similarities that are repeatedly found. As would be expected, there is a direct relation between degree of stereotyping and closeness of ties to the nuclear family: the extent of traditionalism within the family; the authority position of the parents; the consistency and continuity of family cohesiveness; and exposure to experiences outside the traditional matrix, to other nationals, and to other cultures through travel. The fact is, however, that this dynamic appears to cross all class lines, and exceptions and major variations appear to be limited.

For example, one young lady, whose father was a former ambassador and a very successful businessman, had just returned to Vietnam after having graduated from a university abroad. Both she and her family had traveled extensively; at the moment, two of her sisters were attending American universities, and another was preparing to leave. All her primary and secondary education had been in French schools, and she spoke excellent English. The university she had attended was one which encouraged independence, yet although she was quietly critical of the limited freedom of the children of the elite in Vietnam, she accepted without question her parents' right to choose her husband or to exercise a veto over her choice. She clearly planned to marry in the near future—not because she had anyone in mind, but because she was of marriageable age, and it was proper for her to do so. She perceived her mother in the accepted manner. "She's such a perfect mother, she's so devoted to her family that you have no occasion to be angry with her—never." Although she had a skilled profession, she agreed that, as a member of the elite, she would have to leave it when she married; it was, however, appropriate to work after graduation prior to marriage but not during summer vacations as a student. "The family would be embarrassed, people would say 'what's wrong with them?'" Regardless of her years abroad, she expressed all the correct attitudes and perceptions.

A further example is the student leader who stated his reaction to imprisonment. "Naturally for a Buddhist, like myself, starvation is very familiar. I, myself, can go on being hungry for three days and even a week— I could only suffer and grin and bear it. The one point was that I missed my family, my parents and also, especially, my fiancee. Especially when thinking of my fiancee it tortured me, it was for her that I worried the most." Immediately after having stated his disagreement with his superior over administrative practices, he said, "But ... I can never forget the Venerable (his present superior), my deep feelings and sympathy toward him are well —eternal." While in prison contemplating his impending marriage that had just been demanded by his parents, he said: "After a time in prison, I felt more strongly about having a family. I have given you many reasons for my parents [directing me to marry]—during my lifetime I am fortunate that on every occasion my parents left me free to decide for myself. I think parents should try their best to guide their children, but leave them free to decide for themselves." His reaction to the birth of his child was to say: "The pain suffered by one's beloved is also our own. If one really loves his beloved, then when he witnesses her suffering he himself suffers more than she does." He described his mother's reaction to the birth of her grandchild in these words: "When I telegraphed her announcing my first child, she hurried down to Saigon. This proved her immense love toward us. I think that we Asian people should be proud of the way we show our love. Saying this we do not mean that European people do not have such love. They do, but, perhaps their way of life is so highly mechanized that true family love, from parents to children, between husband and wife, is not as widespread and deep as ours in Asia."

Further examples were frequent. There was the Viet Cong leader of the major sabotage squad operating in Saigon during 1965–66 who at one point stated that the only truly happy moments he had ever known were when he was killing "American Imperialists." This same man defined his attitude toward Americans differently when he said: "Since I joined the revolution, never for a moment have I thought ill of the Americans. They are good men in their country, but they come here to worsen the situation, and I am sorry for that. But in their country they are good citizens." To the question, "Have any of the Americans mistreated or insulted you?" he replied, "I have so far had no contact with Americans at all."

Conversely, the Buddist Venerable, after he returned from abroad, realized the restraints and narrowed vision in Vietnam. "New ideas came to my mind [when abroad], new attitudes had been received. I have quite a new attitude toward life now, different from the restricted, prejudiced limited view in Vietnam. It is more open and liberal in other countries—I felt myself as a house—when you awaken early in the morning and you open the window the light enters your room and you replace the old light that you had. You feel fresh air coming into your lungs—that was my feeling. At the present time, I need fresh air—that is what I am lacking right now."

With the exception of the Buddhist Venerable, who through his years abroad had realized the restraints imposed upon him in Vietnam and is presented here as an example of someone who had let in the light, all the other responses are sterotyped and determined by traditionalism: perceptions, attitudes, emotional reactions, and thinking. Each can be traced back to a particular revered myth; each represents an identification with a hero or a heroic position; each is held in high esteem by the society and is guaranteed to result in approval; and each has little, if anything, to do with the informant's actual reaction. The wealthy young lady resented her parents' intrusion upon her freedom and in fact, revealed that upon her return to Vietnam, her mother had conducted an intensive reorientation course in Vietnamese morality and proper behavior. The student leader resented his parents' directive to marry; he was frightened by prison; his projective testing and previous interviews revealed his dread of women; and he was extremely unconvinced of his mother's affection. On the Rorschach, he saw his mother as "a ferocious looking hog—looking intensively at someone, and grinding to show his lower teeth"; his father as an animal that had been skinned, "there is only the hide remaining, all the flesh and bones [and visceral] have been removed"; his parents' relation as "two dogs with long white hair—wearing diadems as noble women in the Western world do— and they are facing each other angrily, they are growling at each other in anger, neither is yielding to the other"; and himself, among other self-imagery, as "a small calf—with ass's ears and his eyes are very gentle. He is looking straight at me and I think he wants to be cuddled." He then sees himself as "a three-month old puppy as gentle as the other [the calf but a little more cunning," then as "a scorpion," and finally as "a pony" looking at his reflection on a sheet of ice (the feeling of coldness within himself and lack of parental affection). All of these are a rather far cry from the idealized conscious perception he holds of his mother, father, and himself.

Thus, although a role may be consciously as well as subconsciously assumed, we find that the institutionalization of feelings goes much deeper. The true emotional content is dissociated, and reaction patterns are forced into a universally acceptable mold. This starts very early, and the children are trained from an extremely tender age to perceive and express themselves in highly stylized forms.[2]

Although space does not permit discussion here, it should be noted that the construction of response extends to the perception of nature and that there is an established process for dealing with those experiences that are not covered by traditional interpretation or are not within the scope of Vietnamese experience. In these instances, the exterior aspect is considered a facade, and the assumption is made that it is masking a familiar pattern.

There is a direct relation between role playing and institutionalization of affect. Both are intimately intertwined aspects of the same dynamic. Although certain dimensions of role selection may be on a conscious level, other aspects are far more deeply imbedded. Both role adaption and institutionalization of response are merely the methods used for a much more profound psychological process—the denial of affect. They constitute the machinery through which the culture represses unacceptable emotion with the result being a massive dissociation from true inner psychic experience. The void that is thus created is filled in with dramaticized, consensually validated, stereotyped substitutes. Since one cannot simply do away with one's inner emotional life, the intrapsychic conflicts that are set up between how one really reacts and how one should and must react take a serious toll. When the society remains stable and when the foundations that have been directed to support the superstructure (e.g., family structure, elder status, religious precepts, and community patterning) are solid, the edifice succeeds, though not without sacrifice. When the basic constituent elements are shaken, as in the extended current conflict, and when new societal concepts, behavioral patterns, and values are introduced, a transitional period of profound inner turmoil may be expected to result. In a sense, the Vietnamese do not really have themselves to fall back upon. The "I" is a part of a larger "I," and when that is destroyed, a quantity of one's inner resources is destroyed. In the absence of direct contact, the connection with the family is maintained by eidetic imagery. This is a powerful force, but it does have its limitations when personal identity is so inextricably bound up with, and intensely dependent upon, a larger identity. The identification with village and hamlet has already been destroyed for many, but this was always a secondary source of security, and despite the dramaticized mythos to the contrary, nationalism has never been a strong integrating element as it is in many countries.

Child-rearing Practices

The question with which we are ultimately faced is how do these personality patterns arise? This research can suggest only a partial answer. Further investigation in this area is essential.

When I asked experienced American and European observers how they would describe the child-rearing practices of the Vietnamese, all, without exception, said that they had never known a culture that was so permissive and allowed children so much freedom. When the same question was asked of the Vietnamese about their own childhood, they universally indicated, in one way or another, that they perceived their parents as extremely restrictive. In fact, both sets of observations were correct; in the imposition of parental authority, two levels exist that represent two extremes, and together they constitute a central dimension within parent-child relations and ultimate character formation. The first is that of extreme indulgence and permissiveness. This is observed within the desultory toilet-training pattern, the variable eating and sleeping schedule, the freedom to leave the house, and the absence of censorship for infractions that in many other cultures would be severely punished. On a far deeper level, however, the child is subjected to rigorous absolutes in interpersonal behavior, essential modes of conduct, and a basic value system. Preparatory training for the code of behavior and the traditional forms starts at a very early age; it is intensive, and apparently no deviation is permitted. We have here two levels of behavior. The first, more superficial, is one in which the child is permitted an extreme amount of freedom and self-determination. The second, much deeper in terms of content and psychological impact, is one in which absolute obedience is enforced, and the child is allowed no deviation from a set pattern and no self-determination whatsoever.

Some psychological theory is necessary here in order to understand the importance of these two forces in adult personality configuration. The child's sense of self, as Bettleheim has repeatedly pointed out in his work with autistic children, and as my own and others' experience substantiates, is directly dependent upon his capacity to exert a rational mastery over his own environment. The basis for self-respect and ego strength, the sense of "I am," is directly dependent upon the parents' focus upon satisfying the child's physical, social, and emotional needs. The child's ability to direct his parents to respond to these needs, his capacity to exert a legitimate control over the parents' behavior—in other words, his ability to induce his parents to respond to him, in effect, to serve as vehicles for him—is a crucial determining factor in his subsequent sense of a legitimate and rational self.

In this context, the Vietnamese child is subjected to two widely disparate patterns of authority. On one level, within extremely broad parameters, he is permitted almost unlimited determination over his own needs and desires. On the second level, he can exert almost no influence over his personal destiny. The result is that the first pattern appears to lead to an unrealistic sense of power, while the second appears to lead to a sense of profound powerlessness—both of which operate simultaneously.

The taboos are broad, intensive, and cover an extremely wide range crucial to human behavior. The following are examples: no hostility toward parents or elders and stringently limited hostility toward siblings and peers; acceptance of a formalized code of personal and social conduct; stereotyping of perception, attitude, emotion, and cognition; adoption of a role and acceptance of it as a statement of the true self; and the denial and repression of any emotion that may conflict with culturally approved standards—in other words, the insistence upon dissociation and alienation.

One of the associated personality concomitants is that of extreme dependency upon the father and the mother; there is good reason to believe that this continues throughout adult life. In executing the "you are all powerful—you are powerless" maneuver, the master planner is the mother and, secondarily, the father. It is they who assign the child's position, and, as with any kingmaker, they can also take it away. The Vietnamese clearly establish that children cannot effectively function without the support of parents, and when the child transgresses against an important restriction, the punishment may be dire indeed.

Thus far, this research has established the following interpersonal interactions that the parents employ in controlling the child: (1) direct punishment, (2) the use of guilt, (3) the threat of isolation by withdrawal of support in a dependency-oriented relationship, and (4) the inconceivability of alternate behavior.

In the process of relating to childhood experiences, all informants dissociated hostility as a dimension in their relation with their parents. This not only held true for their memories about their feelings for their parents but also was particularly marked by their absence of recall for hostility on the part of the parents toward them. When pressed, a few blunted and extremely vague incidents were elicited, but none with any sharpness or specificity. The one exception was that of a very sophisticated intellectual who remembered one unjustified attack by his father at age seven.

This mechanism not only applied to incidents relating to the expression of hostility but also extended beyond and included the repression of conscious awareness of hostile impulses and ideation on the part of the parents. Those memories that were elicited under pressure were always hedged with qualifications, justification, and constant self-reassurance as to the intrinsic goodness of the parents and their love for their children. This censorship applied with particular force to the informants' perception of their mothers. All were seen as shadowy figures, amorphous and indistinguishable. Fathers were seen with slightly greater clarity. This stringently restricted awareness of the mothers would suggest either that their negative impact was greater than that of the fathers or that they were more withdrawn and detached or both.

In addition to the interpersonal factors, among the cultural forces that seemed to play a role in the dulled vision of mothers as real people, one stands out as predominant—that of the pervasive effect of Confucianism with its emphasis upon correct conduct, stylized roles, and parent and ancestor worship. These values permeate Vietnamese society and constitute an important base for the dissociative process that was observed. For example, older siblings in Vietnam are expected to assume responsibility for the care and conduct of the younger children. In the traditional Vietnamese family, when the younger misbehaves, it is the older who is punished even if he were not physically present at the time. Understandably, this is deeply resented by the older siblings, because it constitutes a power position on the part of the younger siblings that can easily be exploited and, incidentally, calls forth covert retaliation by the older siblings which probably keeps it from getting out of hand. Yet the blame for this patently unfair situation was consistently directed toward the younger siblings, never toward the parents who had set up and maintained it. The parent was seen as merely acting in the proper culturally accepted pattern of good parenthood.

Whereas the informants themselves have no memories of hostile expression on the part of mothers, and very little recollection of father's anger, the parents themselves freely admit punishing their children, although these admissions are always hedged with qualifications. Thus, a village father gave the following information.

> (When you get angry at the children, how do you discipline
> them?) I hit them. (With what?) A switch. (How do they
> react?) First they cry, then they get up and fold their arms
> across their chest and apologize for having done wrong. They
> then say that they won't do it anymore. (Is this how they
> always react?) Yes, always. (Do you punish them very often?)
> Fairly often, every two or three days one of them gets it.

A leader of the Hoa Hoa sect, in discussing child-rearing practices within his home, first emphasized the rational approach (as did most informants) and the four-fold path.

> You must love the child and you must teach him the four gratitudes: (1) to parents and ancestors; (2) to nation and fatherland; (3) to the three jewels: the Buddha, the Dharma, and the Sangha; (4) to mankind. You must also teach the children not to transgress on anyone else, as we do not want others to do to us. You must teach him that virtue in the right way is more important than anything else—than money, than worldly goods. (Virtue?) By that is meant that we help people who fall upon misfortune, just as should we, ourselves, come upon misfortune, we would want them to help us.

However, when asked what else is done to the child if he misbehaves, he answered as follows.

> We hit him, just like in the United States [laughter]. I don't know how it is in the United States, the fathers here don't hit very often and don't yell very often, but the children are very afraid of the father. The mothers hit and yell very often, but the children are not afraid of them.

Of great interest is the fact that although the parents themselves freely admitted to spanking and occasionally beating their children, none could remember ever being punished by their own mothers—an impressive example of repression and the power of a cultural prohibition. A core motivation underlined the deflection of hostility onto alternate authority figures who do not enjoy the same immunity.

Strengths of Vietnamese Character

There are definitive strengths that constitute a major dimension in Vietnamese character structure, personality assets of impressive consequence upon which individuals have built and will continue to build. Within the tight parameters of traditionalism and the unified group ego, a great deal of individual security is to be found. A narrowly held society severely restricts the freedom of its members, but, if the individual remains within the structure, he shares the strengths of the significant others. The hypothesis may well be held that, under these conditions, the individual member may be stronger than the members of a society in which the individual is a unit unto himself. Although personally I think that this is a rather debatable proposition, I do think that the individual Vietnamese may be less alienated from his fellowmen of the same sex than we. The average Vietnamese and the average American seem both to be equally estranged from their inner emotional life, but in Western societies, there is a more extensive group which does not fall within the compact majority and which can serve as models for others who wish to search for styles of personal relatedness different from their own. The Vietnamese have fewer models and are far less aware of the problem. The stablity that comes from membership in a traditional society is predicated on the stability of the society. It is remarkable that the social turmoil of the past decades has not been more disruptive to the psychological structure of most Vietnamese than it has been. They have proved themselves an amazingly resilient people in the face of a tragic transformation of normal life patterning. Although one finds a profound sense of hopelessness in the older villagers, one is equally impressed by the feeling among most younger Vietnamese, including many of the middle-aged (particularly the women), that if the war were to end immediately, they would very soon reestablish their patterns of family life—economically, socially, and interpersonally.

One is deeply impressed by the integrative strengths and potential that most Vietnamese seem to have as an intrinsic part of their character structure. They have been buffeted and mauled by social and economic conditions completely beyond their control; economically, socially, and geographically their lives have been turned on end. Their mode of accommodation to the reality of dislocation has most often been that of passivity and acceptance. They clearly regard the social cyclone as transitory, although they are fully aware that it may continue throughout the remainder of their own individual lives. This is one of the great compensations to be found within the Vietnamese philosophical system. The individual is one within a total entity, and time carries a greater sense of eternity than does our more frantic sense of the immediacy of the moment and our own individual life span. This is not to be equated with complacency; it is not that for the Vietnamese. It is a sense of generational sequence and of rebirth in the future.

In discussing the strengths to be found within Vietnamese character structure, one primary condition is of overwhelming importance: the parents seem to hold the children in great affection and esteem. I hesitate to employ the term "love"—it is perhaps the most misunderstood and ill-used word in our vocabulary. Whatever the word for it, this feeling is clearly the most crucial aspect of the parent-child relation, and certainly some impressive components seem present in the Vietnamese. The children are essentially happy, gay, and friendly; one sees none of the terror that is found in Haitian children, none of the deadness and withdrawal that one finds in Andean Indian children, and none of the detachment that one sees in certain American subcultures among the children. It seems to me that I rarely heard a Vietnamese child crying. I saw only one instance of a child's whimpering which did not immediately call forth a response from a parent or an older sibling.[3]

One of the reasons that the children are such a delightfully happy lot is undoubtedly because of the security that the traditional family gives to its young. Rebellion is forcefully discouraged from infancy. Alternate be-havioral patterns do not exist. The child is realistically dependent upon the care of the parents who provide compensations for obedience. On the whole, this follows through life. The adolescent rebellion against the parent and home community found in more open societies does not seem to exist at the present time in Vietnam. One of the many questions left unanswered by this research is what happens to the child when, as he grows up, the drive for greater independence and self-initiative begins to appear. The culture must incorporate a means for accommodating these needs. Further research in this area should prove significant. One compensatory cultural form has been determined. As the children grow into adulthood, the father's right of absolute discipline is infrequently exercised. Since traditional patterns are beginning to loosen, this authority is used less in this generation than in the past. Certain forms of parental discipline, such as punishing the child through humiliation and loss of face before peers, are increasingly frowned upon, although they occasionally do occur. As the child grows into adult-hood, the parent, furthermore, tends increasingly to look the other way to avoid noticing infractions. Since many young adults now leave the home community, this is easily accomplished. Hostility, channeled away from the home is always institutionalized. It may be permitted toward foreigners, animals, siblings who have transgressed and been cast out of the family, culturally defined groups such as governing authorities, and certain ab-stractions (e.g., imperialism). Hostility towards one's peers is forcibly dis-couraged, and fights are rare.

Interactions between Men and Women

Both intense heterosexual relations and intimate friendships be-tween those of the same sex appear to be severely constricted among the Vietnamese. Since both are crucial in the generic sequence of psychosocial development and are perhaps the most important forms of compensation for early deficit, the restrictions placed upon their fulfillment are of serious consequence. With one exception (a Vietnamese girl of the elite), all the informants rather wistfully said that they had never had what they would consider a best friend. With one exception, all had many friendly acquaint-ances and positive early group experiences. It is to be noticed that on this level they related with extreme ease.

The dynamic of the all-powerful, all-powerless seems to be actively played out between husband and wife. The women are extremely powerful on one level, virtually powerless on another. For the men, the inverse ob-tains. The women, far more than the men, are aware of their position, and they can be quite verbal about stating certain aspects of it. However, as in most cultures where this dichotomy between status and responsibility is found, the awareness of the pattern is not consciously integrated into a coherent whole in which its full impact is experienced. The culture assigns an almost unlimited determination over familial matters to the male—a pattern consistent, though varying in degree, with other traditional Oriental societies. In the ultimate statement, it is the male who determines the family destiny. This power is assigned, consensually supported, unquestioned. On a deeper and more nuclear level, however, it is far more true than not, that it is the woman who is the primary determinant; exceptions appear to be relatively rare.

The women, although aware, on the subconscious if not the conscious level, of their central position, have almost no rights in the direct assertion of needs and self-determination. The women not only regard themselves as second-class citizens, but as dependent upon the whims and fancies of the males. They complain of their husbands' extramarital affairs; they resent the lack of discussion of matters that directly affect them both; they envy the freedom accorded the male but feel helpless in reorganizing the situation. The result is that the women have compensated for their lack of rational power in controlling those conditions of life, in which they have a legitimate and vested interest, by becoming extremely manipulative—a quality which has evolved into an exceedingly fine art.

One of the unfortunate consequences of this pattern of manipulation, rather than direct assertion, is that it maintains the image of powerlessness in both men and women. The men perceive themselves as pawns, dependent, yet forced to maintain an intact facade without the inner substance that constitutes the core of legitimate power and a sense of self. The women see themselves as bearing basic responsibilities without adequate recognition, having to maneuver deviously in order to achieve what is properly theirs. Neither leads to an increase in self-respect. To a considerable extent, a modus vivendi has been established by the culture, primarily through the assignment of areas of functioning. This is apparently not as satisfactory as it might appear on the surface because certain of the areas that supposedly are traditionally assigned to men are, in fact, actively invaded by the women. Thus, we find Madame Nu and Madame Ky playing an active and often determining role in their husbands' political activities.

It can be authoritatively said that intimacy and closeness between men and women in peer relations are severely circumscribed and subject to serious restrictions. For the men, the mother remains the most important female figure throughout life. There is reason to believe that although the parents, as an aggregate, probably constitute the central significant relation throughout life for the women, the tie to the father is not as focal as is that of the son to the mother. If further research should verify this observation, the reasons may well be found in several cultural patterns. The girl essentially joins her husband's family upon marriage and is expected to live with them for a prescribed period of time, usually one year at present if the situation permits. There is, also, the fact that female children are considered less desirable than male, and, as a result, their ties to parents are less intense. The father is a less significant figure in the household than the mother, and the daughters, having the mother as a stronger figure with whom to identify, are less dependent than the sons.

The Vietnamese male seems to consider the female a dangerous web with whom one must not become deeply entangled. The Rorschach data (Card III) on the student leader rather dramatically bears upon this hypothesis (similar response patterns were obtained from other informants) and may serve to conclude this paper. In his first percept, the informant saw two poodles playing with each other. He remarked upon the clarity with which he saw the figures, and he then mentioned the red areas and stated that he did not wish to consider them at that point. In his second and third responses, the area seen in the first response, now divided, was seen in the following way.

If we look at it this way, I think of a romantic story from India. The story is very long, but I can say it is a love story. Here is the resting place of a princess, the grave of a princess [pointing to an area within the plot]. Now I see steps made of white marble leading to the tower where the remains of the princess are buried; here are two gates of the door. On both sides are dense vegetation. There are pink clouds on a very bright morning; no, afternoon is better, because of the color of the clouds. But if we said morning, it must be at dawn, just before sunrise when we would have clouds of that color. (Can you tell me the story?) Of course, we will imagine it. As you know, in India there are many princely states. In one of the states there is a prince who is very intelligent, very brave, and very strong. He hears that in another state there is a very beautiful princess and he asks permission from his father, the king, to go to the other state. After many hardships, he made it. And in a contest organized in order to choose a husband for the princess, the prince was the easy winner. But as the moment of happiness was nearing, a fiend takes the princess away—a demon—and the prince set[s] out on a long voyage in order to find out where the princess is, and to fight the demon. And, of course, the demon was killed by the prince. But the demon still has enough power to destroy the palace he is living in. In this palace, the princess is kept captive. After the demon is killed, the prince goes into the ruins and finds his lover killed by a crumbling stone. The prince brings the princess back to her princely state, and the prince uses all the resources belonging to himself as well as the princess' father in order to build a palace for the dead princess. And afterwards, the prince leaves for the deep jungle and no one finds him.

In the first reponse, we see the idealization of the parent and the denial of the parents' hostility that is demanded by the culture—two poodles playing with each other, quite harmless. Furthermore, the informant specifically remarks upon the clarity of the image, symbolically attesting to the permissibility of this parental impression, and then adds, "I do not want to pay attention to the red marks now," because, as we later discover, the red symbolizes the blood, and he does not want the initial statement marred. In Card I, his first image is of his parents as two cheerful winged angels, essentially the same pattern as in Card III. Incidentally, the angels are looking away from him (detachment) rather than towards the subsequent percepts that represent himself. The force of the unconscious perception of his parents then breaks through, and he sees his mother as a pig with a severed head (identification based upon subsequent projective material and his repeated characterization of his mother as ignorant and a martyr who insisted upon allowing his father to beat her when he was drunk, despite the entreaties of the children to leave the house with them). He then identifies the parents as two battling lions, their blood pouring over the ground, the first (probably the father) victorious in the gore of the hostile interchange. Thus is the cultural stereotype of the parents as two playful poodles transformed into the reality of the parental interaction and the deep murderous hostility they bear each other. He then tells us the effect that this has had upon him. Using a Vietnamese folktale as a vehicle, he describes the hopelessness that he feels in ever finding love with a mate. The statement is high drama, as myths frequently are, but its essence is a message of despair. He does not perceive himself as totally helpless (the prince slays the fiend), but he cannot defend himself against the power his parents have to destroy his happiness with a woman (the princess), and in the end, he walks alone into the jungle "and no one finds him."

NOTES

1.   Erich Wulff, Psychiatrist, Faculty of Medicine, University of Hué. 1967. Personal communication.

2.   In 1942, a French teacher in Hanoi conducted a simple and revealing experiment in a class composed of twelve-year-old Vietnamese and French boys (Bois, 1942). He presented the following two questions and asked the students to write their reactions.

Question 1: Your friend, a very good student, has become ill; he is absent. What are your impressions?

Results: The answers of the French are various and unpredictable: certain are maliciously happy with his absence, since it will permit them to rank higher in the class; others are sorry for having mistreated the

student . . . . The Vietnamese gave one answer,
essentially: "My friend is sick; I am sad; I think
of him; I hope that soon he will return to us."

Question 2: Which season do you prefer?

Results: Although not specified, preference selection for the
French students apparently ranged over the four
seasons.

Again, although not specified, the Vietnamese
students, with one exception, apparently all chose
spring. (In classical Vietnamese literature, spring is
considered the most beautiful of the seasons.) One
Vietnamese student stated that he preferred summer.
"After the test his father scolded him for what he
considered to have been a bad mistake: he should
have said springtime. He predicted that he will certainly fail for having had an idea so little in accord
with the traditional themes of Oriental literature."

This is an excellent example of how thoroughly indoctrinated the
Vietnamese is at a very early age. Actually, this attitude is found in
those much younger than the students that Bois studied; I have seen
certain of its manifestations in eighteen-month-old children. In the Bois
experiment, the Vietnamese gave traditional, stylized responses with the
exception of the one unfortunate young man who either had been inadequately trained or who attempted to break out of the mold. The
French boys, who had been allowed greater freedom in relating to their
emotions, gave divergent responses based upon their particular preferences and reactions.

3. In comparison with other cultures, a remarkable amount of attention is
paid to young children. One morning I was having breakfast in a small
restaurant in a Delta village. Opposite me, stretched out on a narrow
wooden bench, was a boy of about eight with a baby perhaps one year
of age lying on the older boy's chest. The elder's attention became
focused on us. When the infant started to whimper, a young girl of nine
or ten took the baby in her arms, very obviously impatient at her
brother's distracted mothering. By the time we had finished breakfast,
five older siblings and the mother and father had each held the child,
and each had voluntarily taken the child from the other. Several of
them had kissed him. This type of occurrence is not uncommon, although one must add that the village was in a secure area, and the war
had not seriously disrupted the normal pattern of family and communal
life.

REFERENCE

Bois, G. 1942. Psychologie de la sincerite chez les Extreme-Orientaux. Institut
Indochinois pour l'etude de l'homme, Bulletin et Travaux 5, fasc. 1:7.

MENTAL HEALTH IN THE PHILIPPINES:
THREE STUDIES

9. Mental Disorders in a Philippine Community: An Epidemiological Survey

MANUEL M. ESCUDERO, M.D.
Division of Mental Health
World Health Organization Regional Office
Manila, Philippines

THERE ARE no accurate figures presently available to show the magnitude and extent of mental health problems among Filipinos. Estimates from local and visiting experts tend to point to the relatively low prevalence rates of psychotics and oligophrenics, the easily recognizable institutional patient population. Information on persons with other types of mental disorders of lesser psychopathology who manage to maintain their daily community activities to some degree is unknown. These are the individuals suffering from psychoneuroses, psychosomatic ailments, and other forms of emotional and behavior disorders.

For community mental health programs sensitive to felt needs and built-in resources, assessment of the problems becomes a necessity for administrative and clinical purposes. The etablishment of treatment facilities is only one aspect of a much broader baseline of educational, preventive, early treatment and management, and sustained after-care services close to the community itself. The multiple and complex causal factors in mental illness may be determined by individual or collective studies of families interacting with forces in the community. Persons or families at risk in the community as well as existing variables that may possibly cause mental illness may be brought to the surface.

A review of related studies by Eduardo Krapf (1950), Emma Arce

(1950), Nubla (1955), the Philippine Mental Health Association (1959), Donald Duff and Ransom Arthur (1967), Solon (1964), and Lee Sechrest (1964), all support the hypothesis of a rather low rate of mental disorder in the rural Philippines.

Background of the Study

As early as 1963, the Division of Mental Hygiene made trips to three surrounding provinces (Rizal, Laguna, and Pampanga) to study the feasibility of developing field programs in mental health. Mental hygiene clinics were established in the outpatient departments of the respective provincial hospitals, and a two-way process of contact was maintained between the staff of related agencies and the community. After one year of experience, a decision was made to select the province of Pampanga for an epidemiological survey for the following reasons: expected higher risk of mental disorders in a province historically noted for agrarian and social unrest, Pampanga's accessibility to Manila, and the easy rapport with the Mental Hygiene staff who spoke and understood the dialect. There was support and acceptance for the study by mental health and community leaders in this area.

The objectives of the study were to determine the size and nature of mental health problems in the selected area and possible causes of mental illness as well as to plan appropriate programs for the prevention and control of mental disorders in keeping with local resources. Specifically, the study attempted to answer such queries as: (1) What is the nature and extent of the mental health problems as to age, sex and civil status, education, occupation, clinical features manifested, precipitating factors or stresses, and duration, degree, and severity of the illness? (2) Did these patients seek treatment, and what kind of treatment was given?

The following hypotheses were advanced as a basis for the study. (1) Neurosis, more than any other mental disorder, has the highest prevalence in the community. (2) The factors contributing to poor mental health are physical illness and sociocultural, economic, emotional, and hereditary factors. Interplay of two or more of these factors in a single case is likely to occur.

The scope of the study was limited to a big barrio of Santa Cruz, Lubao, Pampanga, where the greatest number of informants participated with the highest number of reported cases. The community was subdivided with the initial precedence of eight census blocks of urbanized zonification; in a rural area, this is closer to the *purok* system composed of a group of households. For the sample of the study, four *purok* areas were randomly selected along the main road and interior portions of the area. The sample population was 2,360 persons, or 40 percent of the total population of the community. The survey period covered three phases from July 1964 to December 1967.

Follow-ups were maintained to reduce traditional resistances from experiences gained during the preplanning period of the Division of Mental Hygiene staff, the local officials, and survey items. Decision-makers on all levels were integrated during planning sessions to assure collaboration and continuity, because government-sponsored programs create special administrative-political problems where diverse service agencies are involved. Throughout, the office of the Division of Mental Hygiene served, with very limited financial resources, as the coordinating center for the main researchers and planners.

The field study involved three phases, and three methods of investigation were used: questionnaires, interviews, and participant observation. The first phase, in July 1964, had as its purpose the collecting of information, through a preliminary questionnaire, concerning the names, sex, addresses, and overt problems of known mental cases from local informants such as health personnel, teachers, and community leaders. (The questionnaire had been pretested and modified.) The second phase, from March to June 1965, was a house-to-house investigation in the sample area. A sub-team was assigned to each block. The investigators interviewed in depth a responsible member of each household to get data on the physical and mental state of each member. They used a questionnaire consisting of 31 items designed so that the queries gradually led from environmental sanitation, socioeconomic details, maternal and child health practices, family problems, and physical ailments to emotional and mental illnesses. This was intended to identify known and suspected cases. A clinical format was filled out for both active and inactive cases. The home was chosen as the best locale for the interviews in order to encourage a feeling of security in the respondents, but there tended to be less privacy than expected because of visiting neighbors and friends.

The third phase, carried out during the entire year of 1966, was a screening of all the active cases reported in the second stage for the purpose of confirming or excluding the cases. Each case was seen by the team, either at home or in the health center. The interview, using a clinical case record form, obtained detailed information and history to enable the team to assign a diagnosis, identify stress factors, and give indicated management.

Fifty percent of the investigators in the study were permanent residents of the community and may be considered participant observers. They were able to participate in the daily life of the population under study, either openly in the role of investigator or covertly in some disguised role. They observed events, listened to what was said, and questioned people over some length of time.

The Community

Santa Cruz is a large barrio of about six thousand persons in the town of Lubao, Pampanga, situated along the national highway about 86 km north of Manila. It has the appearance of a progressive rural community. A vast cemented flood control structure along the river banks bisects the highway. An old dancehall, reputedly a busy night club at one time, can be seen from the bridge. Houses, made of nipa or concrete, mushroom along the highway where the center of activity rests. One in particular is owned by the town mayor, whose residential site represents extensions of improvements and physical progress for the community. Some dirt streets and feeder roads branch out to the interior, a low lying plain. On the periphery, the houses are scattered with few fences, and animals such as pigs, dogs, and fowl roam freely. The vast fertile lowlands are planted with rice, corn, sweet potatoes, and peanuts, intercropping throughout the year. The lack of electricity, at the beginning of the survey, gave Santa Cruz the atmosphere of a sleepy town of people home at dusk with early bed habits. With the extension of electricity, recreational and leisure time habits changed. Beer joints, dance halls, migrations of seasonal hostesses, and stopovers for hauling trucks penetrated the once quiet town.

The puericulture or health center, situated along the main thoroughfare, is the only government health facility. It is staffed by a physician, three midwives, two sanitary inspectors, and a helper to care for the community's rural health needs. A 25-bed emergency hospital situated three km away, two private medical clinics, and two drugstores complete the picture.

There is a public elementary school with about one thousand pupils enrolled from grades one to six and a private high school of 400 students from the first to the fourth years. The town has one Roman Catholic church, which is being remodeled and renovated under the leadership of a permanently assigned priest, and a smaller church for a minor religious group, the Iglesia Ni Kristo, with no permanent pastor. The busy, old, dilapidated public market continues to cater to surrounding areas amidst large and small stores, a number of dress shops, tailor shops, and beauty parlors. There are a few rice mills and large bodegas of palay where farmers bring their harvest for safekeeping or sale. The two gas stations and one saw mill reflect the business movements.

In general, the people have been quite static, and most families have lived in the same area for several generations. The extended family system prevails. Most residents are well acquainted with all members of their family and with the history of their neighbors. This feature was of great assistance in the field study. The culture of the community is best reflected by a mixture of the extended family system, hero worship, dominant Catholic influence, beliefs in witchcraft, quackery or indigenous healers, and in the supernatural causation and treatment of illness. Cockfighting is the favorite sport among men; home, household chores, and caring of children are the basic concerns of the women. Prayers and visits to church, work as vendors on market days, card games or *panguingue* for the risk-takers, and help in the planting and harvesting season are supplementary activities for the wives. Families are close-knit. Distant relatives from neighboring barrios come to pay visits during seasonal festivities and celebrations. Organization within the family itself is a rank system with father taking precedence over mother, mother over children, and older siblings over the younger ones. Two or more families generally live together. Any member who is employed contributes financially or else meets the collective disapproval of the family clan.

Findings

Number.   A total of 86 active mental cases were identified from the sample population of 2,360. The estimated number of active cases for the entire community was 207, and the prevalence rate per thousand population was 36.44 or a ratio of 1:27.

Age and sex.   The study population was a generally young group, 61 percent among males and 56 percent among females within the age group 0–19 years; the rest were 20 years and over. There was a small difference in age groups by sex. Of the total 86 active mental cases found, there were 24 males and 62 females with a ratio of 1:2.5. In the younger age group, 0–19 years, there were proportionately more males affected than females; while in the older age group, 20 years and over, there were proportionately more females affected than males. Taking all cases together, there were more cases found in the age group 25–49.

Age and sex rates.   The number of cases was noted to increase proportionately with age. The rate per thousand population started to rise from the age group 25–29, reaching a peak at 45–49 years, with secondary peaks at ages 30–34 years and 60–64 years. The trend was the same for both sexes except that the rate for females was higher than males from age 25 and above.

Civil status.   Of the population, 45.97 percent were children (0–14 years), 20.47 percent were single, 29.40 percent were married, and only 3.68 percent were widowed or separated. Among the cases, 16.28 percent were children, 18.60 percent were single, 59.72 percent were married, and 18.06 percent were widowed or separated.

The rates of 86 active mental cases, per thousand population by civil status, showed a high rate of 61.96 per thousand among the married against 33.12 per thousand among the unmarried for both sexes. A significantly higher rate, 105.71, was also observed for married females in comparison with 17.73 for married males. The rate for married females was significantly higher than for unmarried females whose rate was 28.92.

Socioeconomic status.   Income per month per household was established for both the study population and the cases. The income per household of the population was ₱121.16 while that of the cases was ₱148.22. The difference between the two incomes, ₱27.06, was found to be statistically significant.

Occupation.   Occupation refers to the work or activity in which the cases were engaged prior to becoming ill. Among female cases, 41.94 percent were housekeepers; 25.80 percent had no activity at all; 19.36 percent were merchants and vendors; and the remaining 12.90 percent were engaged in other activities. Among the male cases, 41.67 percent were jobless; 33.33 percent were students; 16.66 percent were farmers; and the remaining 8.34 percent were engaged in professional and military work. Combining both sexes, there was a high percentage distribution of cases in the categories of the unemployed and housekeepers.

Education.   More than three-fourths of all cases had no schooling or had reached only the elementary school level and less than one-fourth had reached the high school and college level.

Disturbance or symptom pattern.   Each case presented more than one disturbance or symptom pattern. The most frequently cited complaints of both sexes were disturbance of physical functions and emotional disturbances. Males and females presented contrasting features in terms of other categories. While the males showed marked disturbance in behavior, verbalization, physical and mental growth, and school performance, the females showed marked impairment in thought and social relations.

Diagnosis.   The mental hygiene team, during the second and third stages of the survey, obtained the medical and social history by means of psychiatric interviews, physical examination, and observation of behavior. They then diagnosed each case according to a broad diagnostic classification. Definition of each diagnostic category has been taken as criteria for labeling each case. The most frequent diagnosis found for both sexes was psychoneurosis. There were six times more females than males suffering from this disturbance. The other diagnostic categories, found more among males, were mental deficiency, epilepsy, and personality disorder. Other organic, affective psychoses and menopausal syndromes were found more among females than males.

Psychoneurosis is a disturbance encountered in all stages of life but is most marked during adult and middle age. Mental deficiency is more frequent in infancy, childhood, and adolescent life, and epilepsy is found among adolescents and adults. Other organic syndromes are found among adults in middle and advanced age groups. Menopausal syndromes occur among women in the middle age group. The schizophrenias and affective psychoses are found among adults.

Onset of mental illness.   Onset of illness in this study means the age in years or the period of life that the first symptoms occurred among the cases. The survey apparently shows that among the 86 active mental cases found, the onsets occurred more frequently among females in the adult and middle ages and among males in the preschool and adolescent period.

Duration of illness.   Duration means the number of years that a mental case had been suffering from the disease from the time of onset up to the time of the survey. There seems to be a difference between the sexes in regard to the duration of illness. Among males, 33.33 percent had the symptoms for less than a year, another 33.33 percent from over a year to three years, and the remaining 33 percent had the disease for four or more years. Among females, 9.68 percent had the symptoms for less than a year, 43.54 percent for a year to three years, and 45.17 percent for four or more years. Findings suggest that the female cases among the 86 active cases had the disease for longer periods than the males.

Severity of illness.   Severity is based on the individual's ability to carry on his usual occupational, social, and physical activities in spite of the disturbance. Of the 86 active cases, 16 percent were severe and 84 percent were mild. It appears that while the majority of disturbances for both sexes was generally mild, the proportion between the sexes differed. Females developed relatively milder forms, and males tended to develop severe disturbances as shown by the fact that 39 percent of the male cases suffered from severe disturbance in contrast to 8 percent of the female cases.

Positive family history.   Fifty-six percent of the cases in both sexes had positive family histories of mental illness, some three generations removed. This finding will be studied in depth as a follow-up.

Nature of stress factor.   Physical illness was found to be the leading factor in influencing mental disturbance in 55 percent of the males and 63 percent of the females. Emotional stress ranked second for both sexes. Other influential stresses were: (1) Intellectual or educational stress which affected more males than females and (2) sociocultural and economic stress which affected more females than males. These stress factors were found in a combination of two or more in 58.5 percent of all cases. In 35 percent of all cases, only one stress factor was found to influence the illness. In 5 percent of all cases, stress factors could not be identified.

Kind of treatment.   Only 10 percent of the cases received psychiatric help. Others consulted general practitioners (44.4 percent), native healers (5 percent), or both (15 percent), and the remaining 25.6 percent did not receive any treatment.

SUMMARY OF FINDINGS

1) The study community is typically rural with estimated population of about six thousand in 1965. The population was generally young and equally distributed by sex.

2) A prevalence rate of 36.44 active mental cases per one thousand population was found. There were more married female cases found, 45–49 years of age and over, suffering from psychoneuroses.

3) The income of families having cases was higher by ₱27 a month than those families without cases.

4) The active cases were mostly not gainfully occupied.

5) Majority of the active cases found have not had sufficient schooling, having invariably reached the elementary level only.

6) Appraisal of the problems in terms of symptoms or disturbances involves physical functions and emotions for both sexes. Disturbances of

behavior, verbalizations, and impairment of physical and mental growth also were found prominent among men but not among women, while disturbances of thought and social behavior were found prominent among women but not among men.

7) Female cases were suffering mostly from psychoneuroses, while males were found to have mental deficiency, personality disorder, epilepsy, and schizophrenia.

8) Among the married, the most common diagnosis was psychoneuroses; among the unmarried, mental deficiency and affective psychosis, among the youngsters psychoneurotic reactions.

9) The six groups of mental disorders found with the highest frequency of occurrence are:

Psychoneurosis	15.2 per one thousand
Psychosomatic disorders	6.8 " " "
Mental retardation	5.9 " " "
Psychosis	3.9 " " "
Personality disorders	2.5 " " "
Epilepsy	1.8 " " "

10) A big proportion of the cases had the symptoms for more than three years; however, the symptoms were mild, the individuals were able to continue working, and interaction in the community activities remained uninterrupted.

11) There were proportionately more cases with positive history of mental illness in the family.

12) The most important stress factors identified were physical, emotional and social in nature, in the order of their frequency, often occurring in combinations in a single case.

13) Only ten percent of all cases had availed themselves of psychiatric services.

14) More male cases began having symptoms at preschool age and adolescence, while more female cases showed symptoms during their adult and middle age.

Analysis

There are varied and complex biological, social, and psychological factors involved in mental illness. In this study, some of these factors were identified, usually in combination in each case. It is clear that certain factors are predisposing or precipitating in some cases, and, in other cases, merely attributes which are useful as clues for a more detailed study.

Demographic attributes such as age and sex are fundamental variables in the comprehension of the development of disease. Age is an index of the accumulation of life experiences and of the likelihood of greater exposure to disease agents and disease processes. The generally accepted statement that mental disturbance increases with age is proven in this study. The rate of cases increased from age group 25–29 and reached a peak at 45–49 years. With advancing age, however, there was a slight decline, but still the rate is much higher than the younger age groups of 0.24. The period of middle age marks the recession of physical agility and intellectual ability for many persons. The stresses and strains of living become more manifest with anxiety. Menopause in females commonly presents symptoms, the severity of which depends upon the degree of decrease in activity of the endocrinal and reproductive glands. Increasing concern over body functions and perception of body image predisposes the person to hypochondriacal worries.

The impact of mental illness on each sex is an important factor in epidemiological investigation, as the relation of sex as a variable in mental illness is of much interest. Studies of hospital patients have shown higher rates for males. In community surveys, no consistent findings have been established. Some, such as the Baltimore study (Miller and Barhouse, 1967), reported higher mental disorder rates among females. In that study, more women than men were found to be suffering from mental disorders, with a ratio of 1 male to 2.5 females. A woman is more likely to be the expressive leader in the family; therefore, it would seem likely that wives would define their crises in affective or interpersonal terms. Of the 86 active mental cases which we studied, 50 percent were married; 37 of these were females, and only 6 were males. In the marital state, individual partners are compelled to adjust to an environment and interpersonal relation quite different from those in which they were brought up. Mental illness is, in some cases, precipitated by factors concerned with sexual function, such as anxiety in pregnancy, childbirth, abortion, motherhood, and love-making.

In contrast to the findings of the Baltimore study, we found three times (18 to 6) as many unmarried males as married males, correlated with a high frequency and percentage of mental illness. One explanation is that marriage is a relation which demands a most highly sustained adaptation so that a premorbid person or a male who is basically unstable or "difficult to live with" is prone to be unmarried.

Surprisingly, the income of families having mental illness was higher by ₱27 a month than that of the general population under study. The community is typically rural, the way of life simple, and cost of living low, so that income is more a characteristic of patients rather than a factor influencing the occurrence of the disease. Over 60 percent of the cases were jobless or nonworking housewives. Job satisfaction is one of the indices for good mental health. On the other hand, unemployment is a sign that all is not well with the person. Emma Arce's study (1950) of the mentally ill at the then National Psychopathic Hospital stated that housewives who were confined mostly in the household tended to be bored and dissatisfied, i.e., they were higher mental health risks. It is apparent that housewives like to get out of household chores and prefer to be more gainfully employed. They need outside interests and respite from routine and monotonous chores. In this community, recreational outlets are neglected. The less educated are prone to develop mental illness. This finding is similar to Tsung-yi Lin's study (1953) on the incidence of mental disorders in Chinese and other cultures.

The emotional and mental disorders were manifested in a variety of symptom patterns. Why are there variations in symptom patterns? Are they indicators of differences in psychiatric disorders or of personality patterns? These are some questions for exploration in future studies of the known cases. Quite prominent is the expression of psychological distress in physiological terms for both sexes. Physical disease is easily accepted by all. Patients can openly discuss physical complaint with others without stigma.

Psychoneurotic disorders were the most prevalent in the population under study and had a positive relation with the income of the cases. It appears that the higher the income, the higher the rates for most types of neuroses. As in comprehensive community surveys done elsewhere, we can safely assume that neuroses are among the common ailments. The other categories of mental disturbances were of low frequency compared to psychoneuroses. This finding alone is important for countries with limited financial and manpower resources like the Philippines. The administrative planning of preventive-educational-early management programs has to shift from the traditional priority of building mental institutions to the upgrading of diagnostic and treatment of skills of existing health personnel in rural health units. The persons suffering from psychoneuroses seldom expressed need for hospitalization. They continued to function in their community activities with a minimum of disability.

The onset of mental illness occurred at any age but more often in adulthood and middle age for the female cases and in preschool children and adolescents among the males. This distribution underscores the need to support and strengthen the maternal and child health programs. Since most of the cases had been suffering from their illness for at least three years, one may attribute this state to ignorance or absence of health facilities or tolerance for aberrations in the community. The nature of the illnesses was generally mild so that hospital care was not needed in most instances, and the afflicted could perform their tasks with minimal discomfort. This implies the negative aspect of long, untimely separation from the security of the family in the community when placements in distant hospital centers for the mentally ill are designed by health planners.

Upon closer scrutiny of the community studied, the prevalence rate of 36.4 per one thousand population contradicts past studies or estimates that a low rate of mental disorders exists in the rural Philippines.

Conclusion

The survey findings provide baseline data showing, more or less, an extensive description of the mental health problems in the community studied. There are many more aspects of the problem to be explored, and longitudinal follow-up study of the 86 cases living with 65 families may clarify related research questions.

The available data as it stands now can provide administrators with information for planning community mental health programs wherein education, prevention, and early treatment of disease can be programed within available personnel resources and facilities of the rural health services. Some indicated guidelines as suggested by the findings are:

1) Integration of mental health into public health practice.

2) Training of public health workers on aspects of mental health.

3) Strengthening mental health aspects of maternal and child health services to facilitate mental health education on a broad base.

4) Undertaking similar surveys in selected rural and urban centers to make some valid comparison on the epidemiology of different geographical settings to acquire a dynamic perspective of the country's pressing mental health problems.

REFERENCES

Arce, E. 1950. A survey of the mentally ill in the National Psychopathic Hospital. Manila, M.A. Thesis, National Teachers College.

Duff, D. and R. J. Arthur. 1967. Between two worlds: Filipinos in the U.S. Navy. American Journal of Psychiatry 123:836–48.

Krapf, E. E. 1950. A survey of mental health conditions in the Philippines. World Health Organization, Western Pacific Regional Office Consultant Report.

Lin, T. 1953. A study of the incidence of mental disorders in Chinese and other cultures. Psychiatry 16:313–36.

Miller, D. and R. C. Barhouse. 1967. Married mental patients in crisis: a research report. American Journal of Phychiatry 124:364–70.

Nubla, H. C. 1955. Sociological aspects of insanity in the Philippines. M.A. Thesis, University of Santo Tomas.

Sechrest, L. 1964. Mental disorder in the Philippines. University of the Philippines. Research Digest 3:5–9.

Solon, F. S. 1964. The presenting symptoms of first 150 cases from the Cubao Mental Hygiene Clinic. Manila, Unpublished Term paper, University of the Philippines, Institute of Hygiene.

10. Stresses, Resources, and Symptom Patterns in Urban Filipino Men

ANTHONY J. MARSELLA, Ph.D.

Social Science Research Institute
University of Hawaii
Honolulu, Hawaii

MANUEL ESCUDERO, M.D.

Division of Mental Health
World Health Organization Regional Office
Manila, Philippines

with the assistance of
PAUL GORDON, M.A.

University of Hawaii
Honolulu, Hawaii

IN THIS STUDY we have sought to explore the relation between culture and mental disorder through a multivariate analysis of various culturally related stresses and resources upon the development and expression of various symptom patterns. Four broad premises governed our research: (1) Man and his sociocultural environment are interdependent systems which reflect the attributes of each other. (2) Consideration must be given to the interdependencies of the situation and to the individual (as a total organism) if behavior is to be understood; this is probably best accomplished through multivariate data-processing procedures. No organism exists apart from an environment, and no behavior is independent of the environment in which the organism finds itself. (3) All behavior is influenced by the sociocultural experience of the individual since behavior is modulated by such learned factors as an individual's conception of time and space (Hall, 1959), causality (Greenfield, 1966) and even sense reliance (Segall, 1966). (4) Maladaptive behavior is continuous with adaptive behavior and assumes forms and patterns consistent with the individual's culturally conditioned life style; thus, disordered behavior in any culture can be considered to be culture-specific. This position can be contrasted with disease models which discern universal regularities due to man's physical similarities.

Our research utilized three basic variables: stress, resource, and symptoms. Stress was defined as a state of tension arousal fostered by operationally assessable concepts such as conflict, frustration, discrepancy, or anger. Its occurrence was explored in the following content areas: marriage, child-rearing, employment, housing, interpersonal relations, values, physical health, safety, and nutrition. For example, it was felt that employment stress might be indexed by such measures as the degree of discrepancy between ideal and real attributes of the subjects' employment situation (we later learned of the Parker-Kleiner [1967] study of the urban Negro in which this same concept was effectively implemented); or, stress might be indexed by the reported frequency of being angry, worried, or sad regarding the interpersonal processes.

Resource was defined as any aspect of the organism's functioning which could be viewed as a mediator of stress. Resources were indexed by a number of methods, including the subject's philosophies for coping with stress, his responses to a 24-item philosophy-of-life questionnaire, and his reports of behaviors in crisis situations.

Lastly, efforts were made to identify symptom patterns or clusters as an index of mental adjustment which is influenced by the interaction of stresses and resources. The term symptom is used guardedly because of its association with disease interpretations of mental disorder. Our colleagues have strongly advocated substitution of the term "complaint" for symptom, since the population was a normal one in which self-report rather than medical examination was used. Since, however, the study was conceived and carried out with the term symptom, its use has been continued throughout the paper, but the reader should bear in mind that "complaint" can be used in place of symptom.

Method

Subjects. The subjects were 96 males, married Filipinos residing in the Sampaloc municipal district of Manila. Each subject was recruited by interviewers from among individuals encountered in the street. In addition, subjects were also sought out in their business offices, e.g., barbers, physicians, etc. The subjects were assigned to one of six groups based upon age—young, 30–42; middle, 43–55; and old, 56–68—and social class position, high or low, thus permitting a 2 x 3 research design with an N = 16 per cell. Social class was determined by the subject's reported monthly income, occupation, educational achievement, father's occupation, and a judgment by the interviewer. For inclusion in the high-class group, a subject was required to have a monthly income of ₱900 (U.S. $225), an administrative, business, or professional occupation, a minimum of a B.A. degree, and to be born to a high-class family. For inclusion in the lower-class group, a subject was required to have a monthly income below ₱400 (U.S. $100), a labor or clerical position, a maximum of a high school diploma, and to be born to a lower-class family.

Procedures and materials.   Each subject was administered an extensive interview schedule by a team of two supervisory-level social workers from the Manila Department of Social Services over a period of four sessions for 8 to 12 hours in order to decrease fatigue and increase subject-interviewer rapport. All interviewers underwent a period of training in the use of the interview schedule and interviewing techniques prior to the investigation. A total of four interview teams participated with each team interviewing four subjects in each of the six conditions. Interviewers alternated in the roles of observer and interviewer. In addition to administering the interview schedule, the main source of data, the interviewers were also required to submit a qualitative report of their interview experiences. The interview schedule consisted of ten general sections designed to identify and assess stresses, resources, and symptoms through the use of open-ended questions, incomplete sentences, adjective checklists, forced-choice statements, and a number of other quantitative and qualitative response-scaling tasks.

Specific task variation.   For purposes of the present paper, only the tasks utilized in the present data analysis will be summarized—these tasks include the interpersonal stress measures, the discrepancy stress measures, the 24-item philosophy-of-life questionnaire, and the 60-item symptom checklist.[1]

1) Interpersonal stress tasks. For these tasks, subjects were asked to report the frequency (often, sometimes, seldom, never) of their being upset (angry, sad, worried) in 12 different interpersonal situations across 5 different interpersonal relations (immediate family, relatives, friends, superiors, and strangers). Thus, 60 situational-relation units were produced for analysis. Of the 12 interpersonal situations, 5 were self-oriented and 7 were other-oriented in that the locus of the fault was either internally focused or externally focused. Therefore, it was possible to assess interpersonal stress from both of these loci.

2) Discrepancy stress task. For these tasks, the subjects were asked to rate the degree of felt importance (very important, somewhat important, a little important, not important) of various qualities in spouses, employment, and housing. Following this, they were asked to report how closely (very much like, somewhat like, a little like, not like) the qualities were met in their real-life situation. Discrepancy stress was assessed by the difference between the reported felt importance and the reported real-life situation. For example, if a subject indicated that high wages was very important (scaled 4) to him in his assessment of an occupation but that high wages was not like (scaled 1) his real-life job, he received a discrepancy score of 3. If the subject reported that high wages was a little like (scaled 2) his actual job, he would have received a discrepancy score of 2. If he said somewhat like (scaled 3), his score would have been 1. Discrepancy scores were assessed for each quality on the three measures, and a total discrepancy score was then assigned to each subject for the various areas of marriage, employment, and housing.

3) Psychological resources task. For this task, subjects were asked

to indicate the extent of their agreement or disagreement with 24 philosophy-of-life statements. The statements were derived from a pilot study and a review of previous publications on Filipino values and beliefs.

4) Symptom report task. For this task, subjects were asked to report the frequency (often, sometimes, seldom, never) of particular symptoms which they might have experienced during the previous six months. The 60 symptoms included examples from four areas of functioning (cognitive, affective, behavioral, physiological) and were derived from pilot research and other symptom questionnaires.

Data Analysis. In seeking to understand the relations among the various behaviors which we termed stresses, resources, and symptoms, we employed factor analysis. First, the symptom checklist was subjected to a factor analysis in order to identify various patterns or clusters. Owing to skewness in the response distributions, the symptoms were treated as dichotomous data with an endorsement of often, sometimes, or seldom, scored 1 and never scored 0. Phi correlational co-efficients were computed between all possible pairs of variables, and the resulting matrix was analyzed by the principal axes method followed by a varimax rotation (Harman, 1967). An eight factor solution was employed with at least the ten symptoms registering the highest loadings used to interpret each factor. Only three symptoms did not meet the complete requirements for factor analysis because of their infrequent endorsement (somnabulism, kleptomania, and suicidal thoughts); however, because these were so few in number, they were all included in the final factor analysis. Following the derivation of the factors, the subject's demographic characteristics and his scores on the stress and resource measures were rotated through the patterns to determine their loadings (Mosier, 1938).

Finally, mention should be made of the use of self-report methods, since this was the primary alternative for obtaining the present data. It is well known that self-report measures are influenced by many factors, and the present ones are no exception. The issue of validity is a real one, and we do not wish to ignore it; however, it is hoped that procedural variations which we have used, such as effective rapport, intensive interviewer-interviewee contact, and cross-checking of responses have offset many of the limitations of the self-report method so that the validity of our findings is increased.

Results

Results of the factor analysis are presented in Table 1. The table is designed so that each factor can be reviewed in terms of its related demographic, stress, and resource variables and its symptom (complaint) patterns.

In varimax rotation procedures, the signs (positive or negative) are unimportant. However, it should be understood that positive and negative

Table 1:   Factor Analysis of Symptom Checklist and Associated Demographic, Stress, and Resource Measures

Factor I

Demographic variables:
1. None

Stress variables:
1. Other-oriented interpersonal stress   -.2044

Resource variables:
1. Some people were born to suffer, others to succeed.   +.2393
2. People really have little control over the things which happen to them in life.   -.2074
3. A person's life after death is all that really counts.   -.1907

Symptom pattern:
1. Feels very tense and irritable for no apparent reason.   -.6012
2. Feels like running away from home to get away from troubles.   -.5925
3. Sleep very poorly and frequently wakes up in the night.   -.5599
4. Dislikes being around other people.   -.5595
5. Feels very sad and depressed.   -.5259
6. Memory seems very poor.   -.5250
7. Has severe headaches.   -.5250
8. Feels very afraid for no reason.   -.4914
9. Has too much energy and cannot slow down.   -.4602
10. Faints.   -.4571
11. Cries alone by himself.   -.4446
12. Has pains in his stomach.   -4430
13. Spends a great deal of time thinking of how things used to be.   -.4145
14. Stays in bed a lot even though well rested.   -.4113

Table 1: (Continued)

	Factor II
Demographic variables:	
1. Low social class	+.4922
2. Number of people in the dwelling	+.2242
Stress variables:	
1. Self-oriented interpersonal stress	+.2527
Resource variables:	
1. Some people were born to suffer, others to succeed.	+.2109
2. Things always happen according to the will of God.	+.2225
Symptom pattern:	
1. Loses feeling in hands, arms, or legs.	+.7063
2. Feels dizzy for no apparent reason.	+.6812
3. Suffers from excess gas or belches.	+.5129
4. Talks out loud to himself.	+.4688
5. Suddenly feels like laughing for no apparent reason.	+.4624
6. Has hot flashes.	+.4553
7. Feels like committing suicide.	+.4358
8. Hands and feet feel cold and moist.	+.4114
9. Has very bad dreams.	+.4082
10. Heart beats very hard even though has not exerted himself.	+.4029
11. Feels very lonely even when other people are around.	+.3749
12. Has pains in stomach.	+.3548
13. Cries alone by himself.	+.3615
14. Feels very afraid for no reason.	+.3560
15. Bites fingernails.	+.3061

Table 1:   (Continued)

Factor III
(Bipolar)

III A

Demographic variables:
1. Young age   +.7027

Stress variables:
1. None

Resource variables:
1. None

Symptom pattern:
1. Sees visions of such things as animals, spirits, or people.   +.4410
2. Loses temper over little things.   +.3412
3. Stays in bed a lot even though well rested.   +.2887
4. Talks out loud to himself.   +.2883
5. Feels other people are trying to harm him.   +.2576

III B

Demographic variables:
1. Middle age   −.4360
2. Old age   −.2566

Stress variables:
1. None

Resource variables:
1. God always looks after those who trust and love him.   −.2592
2. It is better to worry only about today and let tomorrow take care of itself. −.2226
3. Some people were born to suffer, others to succeed.   −.2102

Symptom pattern:
1. Has trouble with diarrhea.   −.4943
2. Feels weak all over for no apparent reason.   −.4570
3. Has trouble with constipation.   −.4016
4. Suddenly feels like laughing for no apparent reason.   −.3014
5. Has too much energy and cannot slow down.   −.2604
6. Has convulsions.   −.2574

Table 1:   (Continued)

Factor IV
(Bipolar)

IV A

Demographic variables:
  1. None

Stress variables:
  1. None

Resource variables:
  1. None

Symptom pattern:
1. Feels like God has abandoned him.	−.5649
2. Stutters when he tries to speak.	−.5630
3. Hands tremble.	−.5263
4. Feels like people are trying to plot against him.	−.5098
5. Feels like hurting other people.	−.4780
6. Feels other people are trying to harm him.	−.4321
7. Feels unattracted to the opposite sex.	−.4204
8. Suffers from shortness of breath even though has not exerted himself.	−.4163
9. Suffers from excess gas or belching.	−.3492
10. Has convulsions.	−.3478
11. Has difficulty concentrating or keeping attention.	−.3054
12. Hands and feet feel cold and moist.	−.3047
13. Feels tense and irritable for no apparent reason.	−.2864
14. Heart beats very hard even though has not exerted himself.	−.2853
15. Has trouble with constipation.	−.2846

IV B

Demographic variables:
1. Middle age	+.2314

Stress variables:
  1. None

Resource variables:
1. All that is needed in life are the simple things like a comfortable house, food, and health.	+.2073

Symptom pattern:
1. Has convulsions (interpreted as excessive vomiting).	+.3478
2. Talks out loud to himself.	+.2819
3. Likes to drink alcoholic beverages.	+.2279

Table 1:   (Continued)

	Factor V
Demographic variables:	
1. Number of people in the dwelling	+.2958
2. Lower social class	+.2813
Stress variables:	
1. Housing discrepancy	+.2867
2. Employment discrepancy	+.2311
Resource variables:	
1. All that is needed in life are the simple things, like a comfortable house, food, and health.	+.2668
2. A person must constantly try to improve himself, no matter how many troubles he faces.	−.2521
Symptom pattern:	
1. Feels like breaking things in anger.	+.6881
2. Bites fingernails.	+.6487
3. Feels like everything in life is just a dream—not really true or real.	+.4811
4. Feels like has too much energy and cannot slow down.	+.4365
5. Has difficulty concentrating or keeping attention.	+.3444
6. Stays in bed a lot even though well rested.	+.3350
7. Heart beats very hard even though has not exerted himself.	+.2935
8. Suffers from shortness of breath even though has not exerted himself.	+.2786
9. Has pains in stomach.	+.2720
10. Likes to drink alcoholic beverages.	+.2368

Table 1: (Continued)

Factor VI
(Bipolar)

VI A

Demographic variables:
1. Middle age +.5210

Stress variables:
1. None

Resource variables:
1. None

Symptom pattern:
1. Has difficulty concentrating or keeping attention. +.4085
2. Skin breaks out with rashes or pimples. +.3870
3. Spends a great deal of time thinking of how things used to be. +.3103
4. Hands and feet feel cold and moist. +.2798
5. Feels other people are trying to harm him. +.2698
6. Cannot get certain thoughts out of his mind even though he tries. +.2141
7. Cries alone by himself. +.2015

VI B

Demographic variables:
1. Old age −.6685

Stress variables:
1. None

Resource variables:
1. Knock and it shall be opened, seek and you shall find, ask and it shall be
   given you. −.2852

Symptom (complaint) pattern:
1. Takes medicines and pills such as aspirin and laxatives. −.2710
2. Hears voices or sounds even though there is nothing around to cause them. −.2492
3. Has a very poor appetite for no apparent reason. −.2421
4. Feels like everything in life is just a dream—not really true or real. −.2307
5. Cannot control certain muscles and they seem to jump or twitch. −.2301
6. Feels very afraid for no reason. −.2240
7. Feels weak all over for no apparent reason. −.1898

Table 1: (Continued)

Factor VII
(Bipolar)

VII A

Demographic variables:
    1. Number of people in the dwelling   +.4774

Stress variables:
    1. None

Resource variables:
    1. None

Symptom pattern:
    1. Feels like running away from home to get away from all his troubles.   +.3450
    2. Feels very afraid for no reason.   +.3221
    3. Skin breaks out with rashes or pimples.   +.2219
    4. Loses temper over little things.   +.2205

VII B

Demographic variables:
    1. None

Stress variables:
    1. Other-oriented interpersonal stress   −.2881
    2. Self-oriented interpersonal stress   −.2216

Resource variables:
    1. Most peoples' troubles are usually the result of other people.   −.2875
    2. People really have little control over the things which happen to them in life.   −.2268
    3. People must demonstrate their faith and must suffer before gaining happiness.   −.2235
    4. Many troubles in life are caused because people don't have equal chances.   −.2201

Symptom pattern:
    1. Stares blankly at things.   −.4460
    2. Feels people are trying to plot against him.   −.4385
    3. Cannot control certain muscles and they seem to jump or twitch.   −.4102
    4. Feels an uncontrollable urge to take something which does not belong to him.   −.4079
    5. Feels other people are trying to harm him.   −.3796
    6. Has a very poor appetite for no apparent reason.   −.3380
    7. Suddenly feels like laughing for no apparent reason.   −.2422
    8. Feels like everything in life is just a dream—not really true or real.   −.2314
    9. Loses feeling in hands, arms, or legs.   −.2270
  10. Heart beats very hard even though has not exerted himself.   −.2198
  11. Spends a great deal of time thinking of how things used to be.   −.2056
  12. Faints.   −.2054

Table 1:   (Continued)

	Factor VIII
Demographic variables:	
1. None	
Stress variables:	
1. Marital discrepency	−.2651
2. Housing discrepancy	−.2159
Resource variables:	
1. God always looks after those who trust and love him.	+.2787
2. All that is needed in life are the simple things like a comfortable house, food, and health.	+.2234
Symptom pattern:	
1. Smells things which other people cannot smell.	−.6243
2. Feels like eating even though not really hungry.	−.5997
3. Feels inadequate and not able to do things as well as others.	−.5627
4. Has great difficulty trying to make up his mind or make a decision.	−.5557
5. Hears voices or sounds even though there is nothing around to cause them.	−.5138
6. Loses temper over little things.	−.5037
7. Stutters when he tries to speak.	−.5015
8. Feels very lonely even when around other people.	−.4990
9. Perspires a great deal even though it is not hot.	−.4724
10. Cannot get certain thoughts out of mind even though he tries.	−.4537
11. Suddenly feels like laughing for no apparent reason.	−.4176
12. Feels very sad and depressed.	−.3809
13. Body has hot flashes.	−.3661
14. Likes to drink alcoholic beverages.	−.3452
15. Thoughts are all confused and jumbled.	−.3423

loaded items within the same factor indicate bipolarity. The present analysis yielded four bipolar factors (III, IV, VI, VII). In these cases, items with opposite signs indicate inverse relations. For example, in Factor VII, the symptom, "feels afraid for no apparent reason," has a positive loading, while the symptom, "feels people are trying to plot against him," has a negative loading. In interpreting this factor, these two symptoms should be seen as "opposites." That is to say, if one is found in a pattern, we would not expect to find the other. In the case of the example, this is quite logical, since one item indicates no awareness of the fear source and the other indicates that people are the fear source.

Interpretations

In the following paragraphs, we will focus on each symptom pattern in terms of its associated demographic, stress, and resource variables. It should be recalled that the present analysis does not contain all of the stress and resource variables explored in the study; owing to data-processing delays, only the tasks cited previously are employed.

Factor I. Symptom themes: agitated depression (1, 3, 5, 6, 7, 8, 9, 11, 12) and withdrawal (2, 4, 10, 13, 14); Demographic variables: none; Stress variables: other-oriented interpersonal stress; Resource variables: "people really have little control over the things which happen to them in life"; "a person's life after death is all that really matters"; "some people were born to suffer, others to succeed" (inverse).

The presence of other-oriented interpersonal stress suggests that this pattern would probably be found among individuals who see "others" as the locus of their interpersonal difficulties. The resources which loaded on the pattern are somewhat consistent with the "other" theme of the stresses and the symptoms, since they appear to reflect a fatalistic or deterministic sort of orientation in which individual control over events is absent and a person must simply try to bear up and try to live for his "life after death." The inverse loading of the philosophy of life, "some people were born to suffer, others to succeed," implies this belief to be uncharacteristic of individuals evidencing the other variables. This poses an interesting problem since the belief seems to reflect the same deterministic theme of the other resources. However, a distinguishing characteristic of the "suffer-succeed" belief is its emphasis on being born to do this, and it is possible that the individuals characterized by this constellation of variables feel things are out of their control not because of some birth determinancy but rather because of the influences of "others" on their lives. This interpretation is somewhat supported by the loading of other-oriented interpersonal stress on this pattern since these statements imply that the locus of difficulties resides in others.

The agitated depression and withdrawal themes of the symptom seems to make much clinical sense in relation to the chief stress and resources. For example, interpersonal stress in the Philippines is something which is mediated against by idealized, normative values which emphasize "smooth interpersonal relations" (Lynch, 1964). In reality, of course, interpersonal stress does occur, although all normative rules operate against it. The individual is caught in a bind in which he must try to repress interpersonal hostilities, and the symptoms seem to imply efforts to do this by withdrawal tactics and depressive behaviors—the latter possibly have secondary advantages. The interesting feature of this cluster is that the individuals seem to be consciously aware of others as the source of their difficulties, but they are limited in their capacity to resolve things ("little control over what happens") and must turn to such fictions as "life after death" to reduce their stress.

One question which it seems logical to ask at this point is why we have construed this pattern in an all-or-none (acting out or depression and withdrawal) manner with no attention to other possibilities such as cognitive mediation of hostile impulses and resolution within this framework. Specifically, it is our contention that Filipinos in general are not introspective and prefer not to solve problems cognitively. The comments of others support this belief. For example, Constantino (1967, 20) observed that the Filipino is unreflective, and when he does engage in reflection it is largely "autistic" and determined by "needs, wishes, and conflicts as distinct from external stimuli."

Our personal experiences support Constantino's observations. The Filipino child is taught not to think or reason why but merely to unquestionably obey his elders. There are numerous Filipino expressions used by the parents to reinforce this. Children are told, "If you think too much, you'll go crazy" or "You think too much, what does it get you; it doesn't solve your problem." On the other hand, a trust in one's own emotional cues is encouraged, especially in interpersonal situations. If a Filipino tried to be cold, objective, and intellectual in an interpersonal situation, he would soon find himself ostracized and castigated by others.

Other cultural forms also condition anti-reflective or anti-introspective patterns of behavior. The Catholic religion emphasizes absolute obedience and an unquestioning attitude from its members while simultaneously encouraging a subjective or intuitive validation of experience in which emotions and not intellect play the important role. The Filipino language structure also leads to highly concrete and subjective thinking rather than to objective and abstract thinking, and this may reduce the effectiveness of problem solving via cognitive methods.

In summary then, this pattern of symptoms seems to be related to high frequencies of other-oriented interpersonal stress and philosophies of life which center upon lack of internal control over events and concern for a life hereafter rather than the present. In our opinion, all of these factors are also a function of Filipino limitations in handling experiences cognitively which reduce the alternatives for resolving tension to all-or-none patterns of depression/withdrawal or explosive acting out.

Factor II. Symptom themes: psychosomatic (1, 2, 3, 6, 8, 10, 12) and alienation anxiety (4, 5, 7, 11, 13, 14, 15); Demographic variables: lower social class; Stress variables: self-oriented interpersonal stress; Resource variables: "some people were born to suffer, others to succeed"; "things always happen according to the will of God."

In this pattern, the picture which emerges is one of a lower social class individual who mediates his stresses by commitment to highly deterministic beliefs which emphasize externalized control of events in a manner somewhat similar to Factor I. These beliefs might be conceptualized as somewhat fatalistic but, nevertheless, of positive value in preventing individuals from completely breaking down in the face of the extreme environmental deprivation which characterizes life for the lower class in Manila. Guthrie (1967) coined the term "optimistic fatalism" to cover beliefs such as this. It is also to be noted that the stress variable associated with this pattern should be self-oriented interpersonal stress, since items on this task were geared to assess an individual's tendency to blame himself for difficulties rather than others. Lower-class subjects apparently must shoulder the burden of stresses incurred not only from environmental deprivation but also from acknowledged interpersonal limitations stemming from the self. Perhaps they tend to see themselves as the source of interpersonal difficulty because living in overcrowded conditions makes it difficult for them to focus their anger upon others, since hostility in Filipinos, as indicated in Factor I, often leads directly to violence. Being upset over one's limitations may well be a protective mechanism which evolves under crowded living conditions to prevent interpersonal aggression.

The fact that the demographic variable, number of people in the dwelling, is loaded on this pattern in combination with lower social class suggests the possible influence of space limitations (population pressure) for the symptoms. Specifically, much as animal research (Snyder, 1968) has demonstrated that overcrowding leads to severe somatic difficulties, the present pattern of symptoms seems to suggest that the same problem may occur for humans. The present factor provides a demonstration of the ill effects of overcrowding for both physical and mental adjustment. In the case of the latter, it appears that even though there are numerous people sharing a dwelling, alienation is still a danger.

The particular pattern of symptoms associated with this pattern seems to be characterized by somatic and alienation anxiety subgroupings. Of special interest in the pattern is the presence of suicidal thoughts and defective interpersonal supports ("lonely around others," "cries alone," "talks to self"), for the Filipino culture has long been considered to be group-oriented and to value smooth interpersonal relations (e.g., Lynch, 1964). Bulatao (1964) has contended that the Filipino ego-structure is "unindividuated" or group-based, and Lynch (1964) stated that a Filipino seeks his security through "interdependence rather than independence." To be alienated from the group would be tantamount to nonexistence and complete insecurity for a Filipino, and this may be what occurs within this pattern.

Laquian (1967) has claimed that life among the lower-class Filipino is "warmer and more supportive," but our results seem to suggest that the lower class is confronted by considerable interpersonal as well as environmental burdens, and their reliance on deterministic beliefs does not signal an easy escape. Perhaps the crux of the issue in this particular case is the breakdown in traditional life which urbanization fosters and the failure to establish new patterns as adequate substitutes. The result for the poor is a cultural vacuum in values, with consequences for the development of alienation and possibly even more serious forms of mental and emotional disorder. We can almost imagine the following sequence: "Everything is God's will— we must accept our burden—yet what can I do to solve my family's problems —to whom can I turn—things seem so hopeless." The dilemma is apparent, and its resolution is obviously difficult.

Factor III (Bipolar). (A) Symptom themes: seclusiveness (all items); Demographic variables: younger age; Stress variables: none; Resource variables: none.

Like some of the other patterns, this pattern yielded no associated variables other than age. The theme of the symptoms suggests seclusiveness which leads us to speculate about this pattern as an alienation syndrome in young men in which there is withdrawal from the world and subsequent mistrust of people. We wonder if the confusion wrought by social change in Manila finds the younger man in an especially vulnerable position—caught between the old and the new—and perhaps forced to withdraw in the face of the pressures. This is but conjecture, and more research is required to test the accuracy of the idea.

(B) Symptom themes: physical deterioration (1, 2, 3, 6) and affective lability (4, 5); Demographic variables: middle age and old age; Stress variables: none; Resource variables: "some people were born to suffer and others to succeed"; "it is better to worry only about today and let tomorrow take care of itself"; "God always looks after those who trust and love him."

The theme of the resources in this pattern may be interpreted as deterministic or fatalistic, for the philosophies imply little opportunity for change as a function of individual effort and a reliance upon God for any assistance. We wonder what other alternatives are available to middle-aged and older men whose futures are fairly well determined by this point in their lives. A commitment to the views, "some were born to suffer and others to succeed" and "God will take care of those loyal to him," probably does much to reduce any tensions which might spring from negative evaluations of one's social-economic position. Similarly, the emphasis upon "worry only about today" possibly slows the clock a bit and postpones, at least psychologically, the aging process. It may also reduce the stress of uncertainty about one's future.

The symptom pattern itself reveals no particular cultural influences, although the two polarities (diarrhea-constipation and fatigue overenergetic) tend to reflect the theme of restraint versus arousal which characterizes many of the patterns. The resources suggest a fatalistic orientation and resignation to life which one associates with growing old and often mislabels as wisdom instead of despair.

Factor IV (*Bipolar*). (A) Symptom themes: paranoid fear (all items); Demographic variables: none; Stress variables: none; Resource variables: none.

Of all the symptom patterns derived in the present study, this pattern appears to have the clearest theme—paranoid fear. Not only were the typical paranoid complaints present, "others plotting against me" and "others trying to harm me," but even the endorsed somatic items appear to reflect frightened bodily states, e.g., 2, 3, 8, 9, 10, 12. However, in spite of this clarity of themes, the absence of demographic, stress, and resource variables makes it difficult to relate this pattern to sociocultural factors. Some speculation on a possible cultural basis for this pattern may be made. We would contend that fear levels and interpersonal suspicions are abnormally high in the Philippines. Reasons for this are many, including Filipino folk views (Constantino, 1966) of the world as a harmful place filled with dangerous forces capable of great harm to people unless all sorts of obsessive, ritualistic practices are employed. A case can also be made that the Catholic Church perpetuates and encourages these fears through its emphasis on spirits, death, mysticism, and ritualistic observances.

Another source of fear conditioning is the very real problem of personal safety in the Philippines. It is well known that crime rates in the Philippines are unrivaled across the world, and personal safety is of great concern to most Filipinos. What especially adds to this concern for personal safety is the explosive nature of crime in the Philippines where seemingly peaceful and harmonious situations often suddenly erupt into serious violence ending in death. These are not infrequent occurrences, and the daily headlines on violence foster views of the world as a hostile, unfriendly place in which one must always be on guard.

The "unindividuated" ego structure of the Filipino personality (Bulatao, 1964) offers another vantage point for understanding this paranoid fear pattern. Specifically, the lack of an autonomous and independent ego results in feelings of insecurity, isolation, and fear with even minor social rejection. In the case of the present pattern, it is also to be noted that the key symptom is the feeling that "God has abandoned him." To be rejected and abandoned by one's social group is terrible enough, so one can imagine the fear produced by abandonment by God.

Lastly, it is also possible that the fear complex is generated out of one's concern for his own hostile potential. In this case, it is possible to envision a man who is truly frustrated and angered by the world about him, but who must repress rather than express his anger. Here, we once again get into the notion of Filipino limitations in handling experiences through conscious cognitive activity. Sechrest (1969, 321) has contended that "hostile feelings may be inadequately labeled and poorly understood or responded to in the Philippines—thus, even when only a minor disagreement occurs, hostility might 'escalate' into violence because of no 'intermediate levels' of expression." Sechrest (1969) also saw paranoia as being related to projection of repressed hostility derived from various interpersonal relations, and he suggested that the Filipino (in the generic sense) may be unable to handle hostilities effectively with resulting paranoid behavior. The paper by Dr. Lapuz in this volume also provides an excellent example of the Filipino's frequent fear of losing control over hostile feelings.

Although our data failed to yield any relation between specific stresses and the paranoid fear pattern, we may speculate upon the role of traditional beliefs, religion, personal safety fears, Filipino ego-structure, and management of hostility as factors in (B) Symptom themes: alcoholism (1, 2, 3); Demographic variables: middle age; Stress variables: none; Resource variables: "all that is needed in life are the simple things like a comfortable house, food, and health."

The inverse relation of the pole to the paranoid fear pattern indicates that this cluster of variables is diametrically opposite. Individuals manifesting these behaviors would not be expected to evidence any of the paranoid fear behaviors. This constellation is related to being middle-aged and implies a problem with alcoholism. The philosophy of life which is part of this grouping conveys a passive individual who attenuates his discontents by setting limited goals. One conclusion which might be reached is that this pattern is reflective of a middle-aged man who is possibly undergoing a change-of-life and who must reevaluate his situation. After years of working, he may feel he has accomplished little, and thus he adjusts by limiting his goals and turning to drink.

Factor VI, pole A, also represents a middle-age pattern and, the items which loaded suggest that this period is also a stressful one. In other data, not included in the present paper, middle-aged men reported significantly more concern for family welfare than did the other two age groups. This extra concern may pose an added stress at a time which is already critical because of numerous other pressures of life.

Factor V. Symptoms themes: physical and psychological arousal (1, 4, 5, 7, 8), withdrawal (3, 6), and orality (2, 9, 10); Demographic variables: lower social class and number of people in the dwelling; Stress variables: employment and housing discrepancy; Resource variables: "all that is needed in life are the simple things like a comfortable house, food, and health"; "a person must constantly try to improve himself no matter how many troubles he faces" (inverse).

This factor was one of three factors related to the number of people in the dwelling, suggesting the possibility of population pressure as a variable related to the symptom. This in itself is only part of the picture, since, in this factor, lower social class status and several stress and resource variables also loaded highly.

Judging from the configuration of variables, it appears that individuals manifesting this pattern are poor, live in overcrowded quarters, and have large discrepancies between their hopes and aspirations regarding housing and employment and their real-life situations. In coping with these stresses, they employ a philosophy of life which is consoling because of the limits it sets on getting ahead in a world which makes it impossible to do so. The negative loading of the other philosophy-of-life variable (i.e., "a person must constantly try to improve himself," etc.) indicates that this latter belief is uncharacteristic of individuals evidencing the other variables. Being content with the simple things in life is opposed to a belief which emphasizes constant effort to improve one's status. As a pattern, the demographic, stress, and resource variables offer a picture of a person overwhelmed by the pressures of poverty and the limited chances of ever getting ahead. To handle these pressures he sets his goals low and asks only for the simple things. Perhaps he is reconciled to his fate as a poor man in an affluent world.

The symptoms associated with these variables reflect themes of arousal, withdrawal, and passivity. The arousal-type symptoms in part convey feelings of anger, hostility, or at a minimum, agitation. However, the others seem to suggest that efforts are made to control the anger or agitation by withdrawal and internalized containment rather than explosive outbursts. This can be partially seen in terms of the bed retreat, the fingernail biting, and the drinking, to mention only a few of the reported symptoms. It is obvious that the individual's health will eventually suffer over periods of time (e.g., heart palpitations, shortness of breath, stomach pains).

The withdrawal and orality themes are consistent with the overcrowded living conditions. In animal research on overcrowding, Snyder (1968, 126) reported that as rat populations in confined spaces increased, social organization changed and some rats became withdrawers and recluses. Our Filipino subjects cannot physically withdraw to a "perch high atop a cage," but they can turn to fantasy and dreams. But this may not solve the problem and may only add to the frustration as even small castles in the air crumble in the face of continued poverty and unrealistic aspirations.

Factor VI (Bipolar). (A) Symptom themes: cognitive arousal (1, 3, 5, 6, 7) and somatic arousal (2, 4); Demographic variables: middle age; Stress variables: none; Resource variables: none.

The absence of any stress or resource variables in this factor suggests that understanding must be sought in variables other than those assessed, but the loading of middle age implies that variables associated with age-class membership may be related. Being middle-aged, with all the biological, psychological, and sociological changes this entails, can possibly be viewed as a time of great stress for the urban Filipino male. It may be speculated whether this period is as stressful among Filipino men as it is among males in the Western world where it often signals the change-of-life theme. A man characterized by this pattern might say, "I want out" (symptom 2) but "my hands and feet are tied" (symptom 4)—"how am I going to resolve anything; I'm so confused, I can't think straight." This is only speculation, and additional study is warranted.

(B) Symptom themes: physical deterioration (1, 3, 5, 7) and reality contact deficit (2, 4, 6); Demographic variables: old age; stress variables: none; Resource variables: "knock and it shall be opened, seek and you shall find, ask and it shall be given you."

In our opinion, this cluster of symptoms represents the older-aged male urban Filipino—his body failing and his mind no longer able to cope with the press of realities. Even his resource ("knock and it shall be opened," etc.) is a highly religious, quasi-mystical dictum that is probably limited in functional utility since the words probably lack any realistic counterpart. The saying itself reflects a passivity of old age which seems to be consistent with the symptoms. Krapf (1953) commented that the aged in the Philippines do not suffer the same frequency and extent of old-age disorders because of the important social role the aged are given in the family. However, family ties and obligations in the urban setting are not the same as those in the more traditional rural settings of which Krapf was speaking, and with the breakdown in these ties and obligations, the stress of growing old may be much greater.

Factor VII (Bipolar). (A) Symptom themes: anxiety (6, 8) and eruptive violence (12, 13); Demographic variables: number of people in the dwelling; Stress variables: none; Resource variables: none.

Unlike Factors II and V, which were also characterized by the presence of the number-of-people-in-the-dwelling variable, this pattern is not related to any other stress or resource variables. Any attempts at linking this pole of the factor to sociocultural factors must be speculative. The fact that lower social class status did not load on the pattern suggests that the symptoms are not strictly related to space availability since both classes are characterized by large extended family units although the higher income groups have much larger dwellings providing more space per occupant. This suggests that the symptom grouping might be more directly related to particular interpersonal processes developed within the context of large numbers of people residing in the same dwelling. The number of people in the dwelling, independent of space, may have implications for a particular style of life as well as a particular set of values and attitudes. Perhaps there are more obligations to be met, more individual desires to be suppressed, more roles to be assumed, and fewer rewards to be obtained.

It might logically be asked why the pattern is not characterized by high loadings on the interpersonal stress variables. As the results indicate, this factor is bipolar, and the interpersonal stress variables loaded on the opposite poles which implies that interpersonal stress is uncharacteristic of the pattern. Let us review the other pole and then offer a possible solution to the dilemma.

(B) Symptom themes: withdrawal (1, 10, 11, 15, 16), paranoia (2, 5) and impulse control (3, 4, 7, 9); Demographic variables: none; Stress variables: self-oriented and other-oriented interpersonal stress; Resource variables: "most peoples' troubles are usually the result of other people"; "people must demonstrate their faith and must suffer before gaining happiness"; "people really have little control over the things which happen to them in life"; "many troubles in life are caused because people don't have equal chances."

This pole of Factor VII is associated with individuals who consciously report interpersonal difficulties—individuals who consciously indicate their relations with people to be a source of difficulty in their lives. The related philosophy-of-life items endorsed reflect basic themes of "others" being the locus of stress rather than one's own limitations (i.e., "most peoples' troubles are usually the result of others"; "people have little control," etc.; "many troubles in life are caused . . . equal chances.") and the need to "suffer before finding happiness." It appears as if individuals manifesting these variables see others as the source of their troubles but simply try to bear up under the stresses and accept things as they are. The symptom themes mimic these thoughts in that they reflect withdrawal, paranoia, and impulse control. Perhaps the stress of the paranoid-type feelings and the social pressures against any overt antagonism lead to the withdrawal and impulse-control symptoms.

Turning to the other pole of the factor, it might be speculated that it is the conscious awareness of interpersonal discord which determines the symptom patterns. If you live in a dwelling with many other people, e.g., extended family, the pressures upon you may be extensive, but you cannot respond in a hostile way toward others. You must suppress antagonisms and perhaps even deny the possibility of any difficulty being due to interpersonal relations. Once you consciously come to see others as a source of difficulty, a completely different set of symptoms and resources enters the picture, i.e., Pole B.

In summary, Factor VII is a bipolar pattern characterized by the independent constellations of variables. One is related to the number of people in the dwelling and is associated with anxiety and eruptive disorders evidencing no consciously identifiable reference to interpersonal discord although this would seem to be important. The second is related to consciously reported interpersonal stresses and associated behaviors which include projective-type philosophies of life and paranoid, withdrawal, and impulse-control symptoms.

Factor VIII. Symptom themes: cognitive confusion (1, 4, 5, 10, 11, 15), somatic disruption (2, 9, 13), and depression (3, 6, 7, 8, 12, 14);

Demographic variables: none; Stress variables: housing and marital discrepancy; Resource variables: "all that is needed in life are the simple things like a comfortable house, food, and health" (inverse) and "God always looks after those who trust and love him" (inverse).

The inverse relation of the two resources and the high loadings of the housing and marital discrepancy stresses suggest that this pattern would probably characterize an individual who is discontented with his life and strongly motivated to change; however, whether the alternatives for change are available is quite questionable and this may account for the particular symptoms which were found.

The large number of hallucinatory and cognitive confusion complaints of this pattern may suggest psychoticism; however, it should be understood that the Filipino culture often encourages its members to see, hear, or smell things which are not there, both through the rewarding of prestigeful roles to such individuals and through direct reinforcement (Jocano, 1969, 104). For example, we are personally aware of families in which children were encouraged to hear deceased relatives and of individuals who were asked to intercede with spirits because of their extra-sensory powers. In addition, the Catholic religion, especially as practiced in the Philippines, fosters a mystical attitude toward life which sometimes makes the limits of reality somewhat indistinct. Constantino (1966) described the Filipino mental makeup as a highly subjective one which was limited in handling experiences in an objective manner. Rather than mediating experiences in a detached scientific manner, the emphasis is upon emotional subjectively validated actions in which more objective cues are ignored.

Certain of the symptoms also suggest an inadequate, alienated individual who has turned to drink to cope with his loneliness and depression. Perhaps in the face of insurmountable problems regarding marriage and other socioeconomic issues, alcohol enters the picture as one of the few sources of gratification.

Conclusions

As noted previously, one of the primary purposes of this study was to explore the relations of various demographic, stress, and resource variables to the development and expression of symptom patterns. In the absence of any theory which might systematically relate these variables, or even one which provides a rationale for believing a relation exists, we turned to our intuition and to speculation. To be sure, there is a commitment to certain basic premises, such as those stated in the introduction; however, numerous gaps remain and further study is warranted. We believe that our approach holds promise for the future in that a limited rationale and a number of methodological techniques have been evolved for relating cultural variables to adjustment patterns. Although this is only a beginning effort, it

appears from the present findings that some understanding of the interdependencies among the variables investigated is now available.

ACKNOWLEDGMENTS

This study was facilitated by assistance from the Philippine Mental
Health Association, The Foundations' Fund for Research in Psychiatry,
the Fulbright-Hays Program of the Philippines, and the Social Science
Research Institute (NIMH Grant no. 09243), University of Hawaii,
which we gratefully acknowledge. We also wish to express our appreciation for the invaluable assistance of Mrs. Carmen Santiago, Maryknoll
College, Quezon City, Philippines, in serving as field research director
of the project and adviser to the authors. The authors thank the staff
of the Manila Department of Social Welfare, Mrs. Lilly Pablo, Assistant Director, for serving as interviewers. Within this group, special
recognition is due to Aimee Albino, Pilar DeGuia, Madeleine Flores,
Carole Maglaya, Rosaria Marasigan, Lulu Pablo, Evelina Pangalanan,
and Lydia Valdez. Final appreciation is extended to Dr. Howard Blane,
Dr. George Guthrie, and Miss Karen Essene for their helpful comments
and assistance in data processing.

NOTE

1.   Complete copies of these questionnaires may be obtained from the
senior author.

REFERENCES

Bulatao, J. 1964. Hiya. Philippine Studies 12:424–38.
Constantino, J. 1966. The Filipino mental makeup and science. Philippine Socio-
logical Review 14:18–28.
Greenfield, P. 1966. On culture and conservation. *In* Studies in cognitive growth.
J. Bruner, ed. New York, John Wiley and Sons.
Guthrie, G. 1967. Philippine temperament. *In* Six perspectives on the Philippines.
G. Guthrie, ed. Manila, Bookmark.
Hall, E. 1959. The silent language. Garden City, New York, Doubleday.
Harman, H. 1967. Modern factor analysis. Chicago, University of Chicago Press.
Jocano, L. 1969. Growing up in a Philippine barrio, New York, Holt, Rinehart
and Winston.
Krapf, E. E. 1953. On aging. Proceedings. Royal Society of Medicine 46:957–64.
Laquian, A. 1967. Slums are for people. Manila, Bustamante Press.
Lynch, F. 1964. Social acceptance. *In* Four readings on Philippine values.
F. Lynch, ed. Institute of Philippine Culture Papers No. 2. Quezon
City, Philippines, Ateneo de Manila University Press.
Mosier, C. 1938. A note on Dwyer: the determination of the factor loadings of a
given test. Psychometrika 3:297–99.

Parker, S., and R. J. Kleiner. 1967. Mental illness in the urban Negro community. New York, Free Press.

Sechrest, L. 1969. Philippine culture, stress, and psychopathology. *In* Mental health research in Asia and the Pacific. W. Caudill and T. Y. Lin, eds. Honolulu, East-West Center Press.

Segall, M., D. Campbell, and M. Herskovits. 1966. The influence of culture on visual perception. New York, Bobbs-Merrill.

Snyder, R. L. 1968. Reproduction and population pressure. *In* Progress in physiological psychology. E. Stellar and J. Sprague, eds. New York, Academic Press.

11. A Study of Psychopathology in a Group of Filipino Patients

LOURDES LAPUZ, M.D.

Department of Psychiatry
University of the Philippines
Manila, Philippines

THE SUBJECTS OF the study reported here were patients seen by me in my private office. Excluded were all cases of psychoses, functional or organic. No patient was included who was younger than 13 years or older than 60. Only Filipinos, born and raised in the Philippines, whose parents were also Filipino, were considered. Many Filipinos count Chinese and Spanish forbears in their immediate or remote ancestry. Where the parents were preponderantly foreign in extraction and mode of living, the patient was excluded. Individuals who came for a psychiatric evaluation for license or compensation purposes were not included. Patients with serious physical illnesses in advanced states, such as cancer or decompensated heart disease, were likewise omitted.

The resulting group, numbering 130 males and 289 females, or a total of 419, are Filipinos between the ages of 13 and 60 years whose psychiatric illnesses fall into categories of neurotic reactions, personality disorders, psychophysiologic reactions, or situational adjustment difficulties.

Tables 1 and 2 indicate the breakdown of the sample along various lines.

The patients in this study belonged to the middle and upper-middle classes with a few in the upper economic class. These patients were very much involved in the economic tensions of the times. The acquisition of

Table 1: Sample Breakdown according to Age

Age by Years	Males	Females
14-20	31	46
21-30	43	97
31-40	35	89
41-50	15	39
51-60	6	18
Total	130	289

Table 2: Sample Breakdown according to Occupation

Males	N	Females	N
Students	51	Housewives	128
Executives	14	Students	56
Businessmen	13	Office workers	27
Skilled workers	13	Teachers (all levels)	22
Government employees	9	Business	15
Salesmen	5	Unemployed (single)	8
Politicians	4	Executives	7
Bookkeepers	3	Bank employees	5
Teachers (college & h.s.)	3	Dentists	4
Unemployed	3	Nurses	3
Doctors	2	Doctors	3
Lawyers	2	Lawyers	3
Engineers	2	Social workers	2
Clergymen	2	Nuns	2
Farmers	2	Movies and TV work	2
Musicians	2	Salesgirls	1
		Chemists	1
Total	130	Total	289

material comforts and the prestige that goes with money and position were leading preoccupations.

The writer feels that focusing on neurotic and personality disorders will provide greater information as to the relevance of social and cultural factors in emotional illness. The following symptom categories, listed in the order of frequency, were the most outstanding: (1) somatizations; (2) depressive phenomena; (3) difficulty in mastery of aggressive impulses; and (4) phobic states. Each patient in the entire sample had symptoms falling under one or more of the above categories. Nearly all the patients presented one or more bodily complaints for which no organic cause was demonstrable and which proved to be an expression of the psychological problem. The somatic symptoms afforded generous secondary gains for the patients in terms of attention from loved ones and doctors as well as release from responsibility. Once in a while, a patient would be accused by the family of putting on an act or imagining things, but this tended to be the exception. Somatic symptoms were readily given credence and were therefore greatly effective in eliciting concern from others.

Symptoms which tended to be confined to one sex rather than the other were the following: In men, poor balance when standing or walking, eye pains, low back and groin pains, urinary disturbances such as difficulty in starting the flow and pain during micturition; in women, numb feelings over various parts of the body, tremors, tingling sensations, hot and cold sensations not related to menopause, feeling feverish or chilly, unusual sensations over the tongue, choking sensations, foreign body sensation in the throat, body weakness, fatigue, urinary frequency. The lips, tongue, and throat seemed to be particularly vulnerable organs in women, while the eyes, legs, and lower trunk seemed to be the counterpart of these in men.

Some patients described the body disturbance in bizarre-sounding phrases. The following are examples of bizarre-sounding descriptions of somatic disturbances:

> My flesh is falling off.
> The back of my head has solidified.
> My head is being pulled up and the rest of my body, too.
> The organs inside my body are falling.
> Something inside my abdomen is breaking.
> My throat is closing up.
> I feel warm sensations from the back to the front of my tongue.
> My eyes seem to be falling out.
> Lines go back and forth in front of my eyes.
> The skin on the sides of my nose is decaying.
> I wear dark glasses when I go out; otherwise I feel like falling or stumbling.
> There is a foul smell from my scalp on the left side.
> A vein on my left temple feels so tight it's going to break.

My head feels compressed and flattened on one side.
My veins are like rope—hard and tight.
A cold feeling stabbed me right in the middle of my back and
slowly went up the back of my neck. Now my neck feels tight.

It has been suggested by many workers that as a population grows
more sophisticated and knowledgeable about body morphology and physi-
ology, there will be less somatic conversions and more psychophysiological
conversions. The latter approximates scientific notions about how the body
works more closely. A trend in that direction is apparent in this study.
On the other hand, it may take more than knowledgeability and sophistica-
tion to bring about a decline in conversion reactions or in the marked
readiness to utilize somatization to express emotional conflict. Many of the
patients in this study who had finished college education had a facility for
using body language in most unscientific ways.

In addition to 17 males and 38 females diagnosed as cases of reactive depression, I found significant depressive features in a large percentage of the rest of the patients. The patients in this study employed an
array of defenses to conceal their depression from themselves. The people
around them also helped to reinforce this denial. Thus, they were mislabeled
as merely sad-looking, lonely, disappointed, or feeling low because of
physical illness. Clinically, the equivocation with which a Filipino patient
was diagnosed as depressed stemmed from two factors: his various ways of
disguising the depression, as mentioned above, and the consequent absence
of a prolonged siege of guilt feelings and self-castigation that one encounters
in other depressions, particularly those found in Western culture. In the
cases of reactive depression in this study, the patient spoke not so much of
feeling guilty as of having committed a sin. Depression in these Filipino
patients was combined with ways and means to help him avoid totally self-
annihilative attitudes. Nonetheless, the patient felt just as wretched and just
as rent with ambivalence as his Western counterpart and, with his regressive
devices, sometimes ended up by paying a dearer price for recovery.

In at least 50 percent of the male patients, the fear of losing control of oneself was expressed clearly, directly, and early in the psychiatric
encounter. The patient's statement or first association to losing control was
that of "doing something terrible," "hurting somebody," "running amok," or
"going crazy, shooting people." A blank wall then appeared with the patient
having no idea whatsoever, in his conscious mind, of who would be his
prospective target and why. Many times the patient expressed regret at
having even admitted the problem. He would then start to backtrack with a
laugh and, in a joking tone, would state a quick denial of any serious intent,
saying, "Of course, I would never do anything like that."

There were two frequent ways of displacing aggressive impulses—
via somatizations and phobia formations. After a particularly difficult interpersonal encounter which generated hostile feelings, the patient quickly

developed chest pains, headaches, gastric distress, or some somatic disturbance. A visit from parents towards whom hostile feelings could not be expressed or a recurrent problem with the wife with whom confrontation was either impossible or dangerous are examples of incidents which brought on a flurry or exacerbation of somatic complaints. The patient also suppressed anger by rationalizing that it would be bad for his health—his heart, his blood pressure, etc.—to let go of his feelings.

Women did not seem to find as much difficulty as the men in verbalizing irritation, resentment, and even anger. The hysterical outburst seemed to be the ace up a woman's sleeve when tensions became unbearable and she had to let go. At least 80 women in the group mentioned having had one or more hysterical outbursts. Western (American) female patients are not completely exempt from this type of behavior, but from my knowledge, they show it less frequently. Their tendency is to be better controlled and to give verbal expression to their anger.

Phobias and phobic states were numerous in both groups. The phobic state pertained more to a generalized fear of venturing into certain situations, while the phobias singled out certain specific objects or situations as evocative of great fear. Phobic states rode on waves of anxiety attacks, and they disappeared as the anxiety subsided. It was quite usual, however, to find that even after the acute phase of the illness had passed, with the patient declaring himself well, one or two phobias continued to persist. As it turned out, these remaining phobias had been there long before the illness but had never been an object of concern to the patient. Other phobias were mentioned accidentally or casually during treatment; they caused hardly any discomfort and, at most, a bit of embarrassment or amusement. Those who were forced by circumstances to seek help had the phobias shown in Table 3.

There follows a list of phobias mentioned by patients. The first ten occurred in over 50 percent of these patients; the rest were encountered in sporadic cases. The last two—fear of public speaking and fear of reciting in class—were also quite frequent; they were found in almost all the adolescents and in many adults as well. Phobias included fear of: death; being alone; looking at dead people; ghosts, Dracula, monsters; heart attack; falling asleep; harm coming to children; cancer; illness; collapse; going near funerals, funeral parlors; darkness; hospitals; injections; medicines (all kinds); chemicals, DDT; allergy to certain foods; germs; traveling outside Manila; riding buses alone; walking alone; going downstairs and upstairs alone; falling while walking; heights; crowds; elevators, closed spaces; crossing the street; planes; being robbed, attacked, raped; being trapped in a traffic jam; water shortage; going hungry; swimming; rain, thunder, and lightning; fire (including pilot flame of gas ranges); animals (lizards, snakes, dogs, and cats); public speaking and reciting in a classroom.

Listening to the Filipino patient in this study, one was led to conclude that the patient's interpersonal world was his primary source of

Table 3:   Phobias of Males and Females
          Forced by Circumstances to
          Seek Help

Phobias of Males	N
Fear of planes	2
Fear of riding any vehicle	1
Fear of walking downtown alone	1

Phobias of Females	N
Fear of going out alone	3
Fear of injections	2
Fear of planes	2
Fear of elevators	1

emotional gratification, superseding that of personal satisfaction from individual achievement or mastery. His successful negotiation of interpersonal affairs with family and friends brought him reassurance, recognition, and material reward. Reassurance pertained to his need for security and acceptance. Recognition assured him that he could produce an impact on another person and helped fulfill his own need for power and prestige. These two results were significant rewards in themselves. If his material needs were still unmet, propitious interpersonal relations were more than half the battle toward their fulfillment. Such attitudes were evident not only in his behavior but also in his fantasies. The latter were replete with actual people toward whom he directed his libidinal and aggressive strivings. He was not inclined to do retrospective analysis of upsetting events or to dig into past relations to illuminate the problems of the present. This was due, in large part, to the fact that, in many instances, patients had never completely left behind their pasts, their childhood, and significant childhood figures. The significant people in their pasts were likely to be the same as the people important in the present. In a figurative sense, and often in a literal sense as well, patients had not traveled far in the choice of love and hate objects.

In all females diagnosed as cases of depressive reaction, separation was invariably one of the factors leading to the illness. The causes which combined to bring the woman to the brink of depression were several and varied. The last straw might be quite trivial or too obvious to be ignored— an unwanted pregnancy, a fight with her in-laws, a surgical operation, a sister ailing with a fatal disease, a religious retreat, a prolonged illness of a child, or a neighborhood burglary. As one traced the history, one noted that the patient had been adjusting at an optimal level until something happened.

This something was on the order of a separation from loved ones, either in a literal or symbolic way. An interesting observation was that the depression occurred after the separation had terminated, and reunion with the loved one had taken place. Often, several months or a year elapsed before the symptom became obvious. When the women were asked to recall their emotional states during the separation, it became evident that they had successfully repressed all the anguish and feeling of emptiness during that period by keeping busy with work, housekeeping, or a hobby, while friends and relatives dropped in all the time. With pain and effort, they recovered memories of the terrible strain of the separation and the agonizing attempts they made to minimize or assuage it directly.

The clinical picture in adolescents was most frequently that of an acute failure in ability to function in school in the face of what was perceived to be an overwhelming challenge. The consequence may be a grossly disabling psychophysiological reaction or an acute phobic state. The excessive protection and gratification that the boys had received from a maternal figure must be mentioned as a significant factor. Nearly all of these patients had been emotionally close, until puberty or the prepuberty period, to mother, an unmarried aunt, or grandmother to whom they were quite special. A few, who were father's pets, received similar kinds of nurturing and protecting from father. Problems in adult males had to do largely with ambivalent attitudes towards failure and success. The conscious fear was always that of failure; yet the pursuit of success was so impeded by anxiety that failure was virtually courted. There were 16 patients in whom a clear-cut encounter with success was directly related to the onset of the illness.

Table 4 shows a simple diagram giving, at a quick glance, the interrelation of recurrent dynamics. Each one is a site of psychopathology, representing an area of ego weakness. The pathways shown by the arrows indicate the general directions of pathogenesis. The diagram is oversimplified, as one can readily see. For example, the backward flow of processes, such that the

Table 4:   Interrelation of Recurrent Dynamics

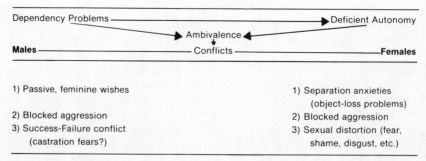

resulting pathology often reinforces the original disturbances, is not indicated. Thus, the conflict areas generated in men and women can reinforce and entrench further the basic dependency problem. In addition, conflicts between men and women, with already compromised segments of their personalities entering into further incompatible interactions, will give rise to other forms and pathways of pathology.

Ambivalence was a key conflict in these patients. It was present in practically every sphere of the patient's emotional life, but most flaringly manifested at the height of the illness. When the acute illness subsided, the ambivalence retreated behind repressive or rationalization defenses. In the character neuroses, wherein no acute illness brought the ambivalence to awareness, patients remained complacently convinced that there were no contradictions in their attitudes and actuations.

Points of difference between the depressed Filipino patient and his Western (American) counterpart may be speculated upon. Rather obvious are the differences in philosophies of child-rearing practices; one encourages dependence while the other encourages autonomy. Less obvious are the differences in unconscious fantasies behind what appears to be very similar ambition-driven behavior in the two cultures. The Western patient fantasizes that, with success, he may regain happiness through symbolic recapturing of the love of people he left behind. He finds out that success brings nothing of this and, in fact, can actually bring about an even lonelier position. The feeling of emptiness recapitulates the original feeling of rejection through early independence, and this leads to vicious self-hate.

American culture places a premium on accomplishment and success. Success is then defined in these terms. Filipino culture does not give unequivocal support to these goals. One must, first and foremost, be a good son devoted to his parents; then, and only then, may one also be successful. The fantasy of the Filipino patient driven by ambition is that he is pursuing self-enhancement at the price of renouncing emotional bonds.

The Filipino patients in this study drove themselves in the interest of self and, in their minds, over their parents' entreaties. Their driving ambition was fueled by a symbolic rejection of their parents which enabled them to get away from home and establish a separate identity. Success was therefore achieved, symbolically as it were, over their mother's dead body. The theory of "pathognomonic introjection," as Fenichel (1945) labels it, is not quite applicable to these Filipino patients. The formulations of ego psychologists, who see depression as an ego experience, may be more apropos of our patients. These familial and cultural experiences lead to somewhat different psychological formulations. In the Filipino patient, internalization of parental figures does not occur as completely and thoroughly as in Western patients, and they continue to be very much a part of his present reality. Moreover, he sees other people close to him—spouse, uncle, employer—as part parent or part superego. A Western patient who regresses in his depression is giving up the internalized loved object, liberating self-destruction instincts, and in a severe clinical situation, he succumbs to a psychotic depression. In the Filipino patient, since internalization of parental figures is incomplete, the regression seeks to reestablish the libidinal ties by coercing the superego representatives, wife and family, to be loving. Thereby, the ego is saved from further invasion of sadistic destructive elements from the superego.

In my opinion, there is a significant correlation between contradictory attitudes as they exist in the culture and the psychological ambivalence that played a key role in the emotional disorders in this study. In these patients, illness grew out of ambivalence in relation to dependency conflicts, guilt over success, tenuous controls over aggression, and in women, an inability to separate from parental objects and to fully accept their sexual role. Although the themes are similar in the culture and in these patients, and the possibility of their mutual derivation is strongly suggested, the lines of correlation are neither clear nor direct.

The patients in this study have led me to consider the importance of the following four cultural situations in contributing to psychological conflicts: (1) belongingness and what economics is doing to it, (2) the problem of aggression in men, (3) dilemma of women, and (4) adolescent crisis. It appears that changes in the social and cultural scene are forcing previous ambivalence to a head, forcing confrontations and a start towards resolution. These areas are trouble spots and will clamor for decisions to be made on the basis of value choice and psychological reality. One can only speculate as to what still remains, what appears to be undergoing transition, and how these might interplay with psychological factors.

Typically, the Filipino still denies that he has taken steps to make the break from old ties. This is largely due to efforts by the older generation —the parents—to deny what is happening. It is their children, now grown up, who are making all the moves to attenuate the old bonds. Curiously, much of this attenuation has been helped by geographical separation. Perhaps, some day, the time will come when a Filipino no longer has to cross miles of ocean and continent to emancipate himself from his parents. But for now, the lure of economic success in foreign lands has conspired successfully with wishes, unconscious or not, to be on one's own so that many Filipinos have been able to move away from home.

The coming of an industrialized technological society focuses on the Filipino as an individual. The support of his family and of the group are still important, but where he has to make a choice between them and his individual ambitions, likely as not, he will favor the latter. "To be" is replacing in primacy the old ethic of "to belong."

Cultural studies with more detail and depth, dealing with hostility and aggression in the Filipino male and sexuality in the Filipino female, would be greatly relevant to the kinds of psychological conflicts encountered in this study. By singling out these areas, I am neither excluding nor minimizing others but merely regarding these two as predominating.

In my experience with an admittedly limited number of American patients in psychotherapy in the United States and in the Philippines, I have heard quite often the lament of the patient, "I feel like a phony" or "I feel like such a fake!" This seems to stem from his constant struggle to fit into a certain mold, to better himself, as well as from his dismay when his real self announces itself in other ways. Autonomous and free, he is nevertheless driven and compelled by some force to achieve, to succeed, to be strong, and to be self-sufficient. Somewhere along the way to mastery of himself and of his environment, he suspects he may have lost the joy and essence of living.

In this study, I did not encounter one patient who felt lonely, isolated, or alienated, except in transient situations. However, it was a threat which hung over many of them, particularly adolescents. Instead of this kind of complaint, the Filipino patient's lament is apt to be, "I am not loved!" or "They have rejected me; I am not in!"

As the Filipino moves towards a modern technological and industrialized society, will he be merely trading a headache for an upset stomach?

REFERENCE
Fenichel, O. 1945. The psychoanalytic theory of neurosis. New York, Norton.

COMPARATIVE APPROACHES

12. Maturity in Korea and America

DONGSE HAHN, M.D.

Department of Psychiatry and Neurology
Seoul National University Hospital
Seoul, Republic of Korea

IN THE REALM of Western psychiatric theories, a person's maturity has been equated largely with his mental health. Neurotic problems are considered to be a measure of resorting to an immature level adjustment in the face of difficulties with reality; psychotic reaction is regarded as a further regression to an earlier immature level; and personality disorders, of course, signify immaturity of personality (Noyes and Kolb, 1968; Ewalt and Farnsworth, 1963). This theory does not seem to incorporate cultural factors. What happens to an otherwise mature Western man's mental health when he is placed in a non-Western culture? Does his culturally syntonic behavior become fragile and even break down when he is faced with culturally alienated environmental difficulties? What about a Korean man's mental health when he experiences the rapid changes in the process of his nation's modernization, and what happens to his dependency need when his family system breaks down? A still further question would be: since modernization in Korea largely means Westernization, are the problems which a Korean man faces, when he begins to adjust to a nuclear family system, similar to those of an American? The author would like to examine some of these problems in this paper and attempt to reach some understanding.

Dependence and Korean Adults

Independence is highly valued in American society as a criterion for measuring an individual's maturity (Noyes and Kolb, 1968; Ewalt and Farnsworth, 1963). If one tries to use this concept of maturity in evaluating the mental health of a Korean, it will be totally inadequate, since the Korean family system incorporates mutual dependency among its extended family members in a healthy attempt to enable each member to deal with his environment. The point of difference is clearer when one considers the difference in the social unit of the two societies. In Korea, the basic social unit is the family which, as the group with its collective identity, functions as a social norm. In contrast, an individual is a social unit in American society with emphasis on independent individual identity (Hahn, 1968).

Because of the high value placed on independence in America, children are taught to say "I love you" to parents, but the behavioral expression of love is not allowed. Because children's dependency on parents, including affectionate behavioral expression, is discouraged, an affectionally immature and inwardly conflictual personality makeup may result in the adult. The working of this pattern is exemplified in the following account.

A 51-year-old American male who has been residing for several years in Korea with his wife and two daughters received psychotherapy because of chronic marital discord. He described his relation with his wife as that of "a dog on a leash," the dog being himself. About two months after the psychotherapy began, the patient separated from his wife and was admitted to the hospital as a night patient. At that time, he had been impotent with his wife for several years but was having relations with a young Korean girl. When he was bedridden for four days with influenza, the girlfriend visited him daily, but his wife, whom he had been seeing much more frequently than his girlfriend, did not come to see him. When questioned as to whether his wife had come to see him in his sickbed, the patient answered that he neither asked her to come nor had she asked to visit him. It took some time for the patient to realize that this episode meant that a natural loving male-female relation did not exist between him and his wife but did exist between him and his girlfriend. When the patient had come to an understanding of this, he mentioned that American psychiatrists would have had a more difficult time comprehending his feelings than would a Korean psychiatrist, whose culture is a male dominant one. The patient complained that his wife was a domineering woman, despite her insistence that she was very feminine and therefore submissive.

The English language seems to be poverty-stricken in words of love, while the Korean language is affluent in expressions of love but is limited in terms that express the conceptualization of hostility. Whenever a child expresses fear, Korean parents comfort and protect him in such a way that he need not be fearful as long as he is dependent on the parents (Vogel,

1961). Korean parents will alternately tease children about ghosts and animals and then comfort them. A crying baby will stop when parents threaten him by mentioning a tiger, mouse, cat, or ghost. Expressions of anger or disagreement, however, especially toward superiors, are not culturally sanctioned. A Korean father can say that he will "kill the child" if his son hits him.

In American society there is a culturally sanctioned outlet for aggression—a free competition—which is somewhat deficient in a hierarchically ordered society such as Korea. This difference in handling aggression and competition in the two cultures is well illustrated in the daily greeting, one of the most frequently used verbal communications of human beings. In America, people say, "How are you?", and nine out of ten answer to this by saying, "Fine," possibly implying, among other things, "I win." One out of ten may say, "Wonderful!" or, rarely, "Feel like a million dollars," possibly implying, among other factors, "I am stronger, bigger, richer than you." Such are the distinctively competitive American greetings. Korean greetings differ greatly. To "How are you?", nine out of ten Koreans say, "So-so," and one out of ten say, "Simply staying alive," implying, "You win, I won't compete with you." The general implication is one of withdrawal and resignation which leaves the competition unmet. In contemporary society, this old-fashioned greeting of the absentee landowner is changing to one of the pretense of "busy, busy" greetings, at least in some quarters among the new organization men.

The lack of a culturally sanctioned outlet for aggression is made obvious in the next section which discusses the consequences of this lack. A 38-year-old married Korean male came from a town near Seoul University Hospital with complaints of headache, dizziness, insomnia, and indigestion of two and one-half months' duration. A medical checkup revealed no organic basis for his symptoms, and he was referred to psychiatrists for examination. The internist to whom the patient finally resorted after repeated futile visits to a local clinic was a professor at Seoul University Hospital and was also a war refugee from the patient's native village in North Korea. All the symptoms suddenly began two and one-half months before, following coitus with his wife. He stated that he was drunk on that day, and the following morning felt dizzy and headachy. He frequented the local clinic thereafter and finally went to Seoul. His decision to go to Seoul University Hospital was apparently motivated by a dream on the previous night. His mother appeared in his dream and told him not to have intercourse, since it would be hazardous for his health. In the dream, he followed his mother's advice and began to clothe himself, and there appeared a strange man. Seeing this, the mother uttered, "Obscene!" The patient awoke from this dream feeling depressed. He wept bitterly when speaking of his mother.

A digression here to relate briefly the patient's history may present clues to his behavior. He was born and raised in North Korea and graduated from a local high school. When he was 21 years old, the South Korean

Army occupied his village, and he subsequently went to work for the South Korean police. Some months later, he left his village with the retreating army. He left behind his widowed 60-year-old mother and his married brother and sister. He believed that his family might have been tortured by the North Korean police, because he had worked for the South. After evacuating to the South, he joined the army. With the Korean armistice in 1954, he was discharged from military service and married a local girl whose family also migrated from the province of Chungchongnamdo. Thus, neither his family nor his wife's family were nearby. His major social contact was limited to close friends at the prison, where he had been working as a warden for the past ten years. He tearfully related that his work imprisoned him, and this was the punishment he deserved because of his desertion of his family.

In psychiatric examinations, the patient did not think that he had overt marital discord, and his potency was average until the onset of symptoms. His mother had appeared in his dreams once before, when his wife had given birth to their first baby. She gave him her suggestion for the baby's name, and the boy was named according to her wishes. His latest dream, however, was incomprehensible to the patient at this point.

Obviously this patient was a tragic product of the Korean war. He was torn between childhood ties to his family, particularly to his mother, and social upheaval to which he had to adjust. He had come to identify his wife with his mother and had attempted to solicit some consolation from the identification. Because he felt sorry for his mother, he dreamed of her, and this dream also served as an excuse for his impotence. In turn, he was sorry for his wife because of his impotence. Therefore, he began to suspect his wife's fidelity. The deep-seated dependency need of this patient conflicted with his need to adapt to his changing environment so that neurotic symptoms resulted. His last resort of consulting the internist from the same native village was a clannish choice, a remnant of the longing for his family.

Man's behavioral characteristics seem to become more prominent when he goes to an unfamiliar environment, and his immaturity may manifest itself when he goes to a foreign land. There have been many descriptions of conspicuous behavioral patterns of Korean and American soldiers stationed in Vietnam. One of these is the notion that Korean troops are good fighters, while Americans show other than aggressive combat characteristics. Many Korean soldiers in Vietnam are so aggressive that they put the notorious Japanese Kamikaze pilots to shame. An American, on the other hand, can be said to be fairly mature in controlling his aggression and to adjust well in a competitive organization but to be fairly immature in romantic endeavors. An American soldier might treat a prostitute as a date thereby evidencing some emotional investment, and, at the same time, he may have difficulty in detaching himself from his date. An American officer in a deserted outpost in Vietnam does not hesitate to join a long line of enlisted men in front of a brothel and wait his turn, but such behavior would be unthinkable for his Korean counterpart. As Caudill and Doi (1963) said of the Japanese, the Korean also seems to have difficulty in controlling his aggression and is immature in aggression, while the American is immature in terms of affection.

Sexual deviation is a serious and frequently occurring problem in American society but not in Korean society. Korea has relatively few homosexuals, and homosexual panic is unheard of among Koreans. Although potency is a major concern of Koreans, sex offenders and adultery problems are negligible. Instead, Korea has problems which might be called aggressive deviation. Reckless driving and fearless pedestrians on Korean streets are two of the most striking phenomena impressing foreign visitors. Untreated Korean psychotic patients seem to display more aggression—exhibiting destructiveness, wildness, and homocidal and suicidal tendencies—than similar American patients.

In the case of suicide, there is a peculiar Korean phenomenon which reflects the Korean's family centered-ness and aggressive drive; this is the so-called family suicide. The father of the family confers with his wife about the family dying under a given circumstance; the wife, of course, agrees with her husband. Then, the father first commits homocide by killing the children and then the wife, who are part of his collective identity, and finally commits suicide. The family suicide can be termed as suicide deviation.

Love stands out as the most important theme of native American novels (Hsu, 1968). Themes of American art are inner conflicts of love, and the characteristic behavioral pattern is contractual fair play. Korean art shows no preoccupation with sex, but the Korean exhibits behavioral characteristics of intrafamilial dependency and interfamilial aggression. A major problem in Korean psychopathology is that which has to do with meeting family obligations, whereas the key issue in American psychopathology seems to be that of inner conflict of which the greater part centers around sex.

REFERENCES

Caudill, W., and L. T. Doi. 1963. Interrelations of psychiatry, culture and emotions in Japan. *In* Man's image in medicine and anthropology. I. Galston, ed. New York, International University Press.

Ewalt, J. R., and D. L. Farnsworth. 1963. Textbook of psychiatry. New York, McGraw-Hill.

Hahn, D. 1968. The oriental concept of freedom. Unpublished paper. Mimeo.

Hsu, F. L. K. 1968. Americans and Chinese. *In* Asian Psychology. G. Murphy and L. E. Murphy, eds. New York, Basic Books, Inc.

Noyes, A. P., and L. C. Kolb. 1968. Modern clinical psychiatry, 7th ed. Philadelphia, Saunders.

Vogel, E. F., and S. H. Vogel. 1961. Family security, personal immaturity, and emotional health in a Japanese sample. Journal of Marriage and Family Living 23:161–66.

13. A Comparative Study of Patienthood in Japanese and American Mental Hospitals [1]

KAZUO YAMAMOTO, M.A.

Division of Eugenics
National Institute of Mental Health
Ichikawa, Japan

THIS STUDY ANALYZES some of the problems of the roles confronting mentally ill patients in a Japanese mental hospital. It is based on the psychosocial conception of "problematic role issues and role conception of patienthood" as put forth by Pine and Levinson (1961). We also examine cultural differences in interpersonal relations and in patterns of need expression between Japanese and American mental patients, using, in part, data presented by Levinson and Gallagher (1964) concerning the Massachusetts Mental Health Center.

Caudill and Doi pointed out in several papers characteristic aspects of Japanese interpersonal relations based on insightful observations and clinical experiences in small psychiatric hospitals and psychotherapeutic interviews (Caudill, 1959, 1961; Caudill and Doi, 1963; Doi, 1962). In the present study, we tried to analyze by systematic questionnaire method the role conception of patients who were admitted to spend some parts of their lives under the control of the mental hospital social system. This role conception of patients exhibited many characteristic aspects of Japanese psychiatric values, interpersonal relations between patients and hospital staff, and Japanese personality.

Hospital Organization and the Situation of the Patients

Our research was carried out at Konodai National Hospital in Ichikawa, a suburb of Tokyo. The hospital has about 350 psychiatric beds, distributed in seven psychiatric wards, two of which are open, and the other five closed. Konodai is a general hospital but was an army mental hospital before World War II. The department of psychiatry is composed of a chief psychiatrist, seven ward psychiatrists (each of whom runs a ward), two psychiatric social workers, and a clinical psychologist. The six or seven nurses appointed to each of the seven wards are trained as general medical nurses rather than as psychiatric nurses, although some of them have long term experience with psychiatric patients.

The psychiatric wards in this hospital are decentralized, both administratively and in terms of orientation to patient care. There is little interchange among the wards. For example, a patient who requires hospitalization and who has had contact with one of the psychiatrists in the outpatient service will be admitted to that psychiatrist's ward. When he is discharged, he will be discharged to the same psychiatrist's care. This closeness between doctor and patient occurs frequently in Japan and assures a continuity of care that is often missing in the United States.

Medical policy in all of the wards is oriented to somatic treatments, especially drug therapy and, to a lessening extent, electroshock therapy. This is not to say that the doctors have no interest in or do not feel the necessity of psychodynamic and psychosocial orientation. Our National Institute of Mental Health psychological research staff has been accepted by some of the doctors to engage in psychotherapy with some patients in their wards (Saji, Dendo, and Yamamoto, 1965). Nevertheless, psychodynamic and psychosocial orientations have not become a part of the central policy, due to shortages of hospital staff and to strong Kraepelinian orientations of most of the psychiatrists in this hospital. Systematic programs of rehabilitation do not exist except for a small program created by the social workers.

Most of the patients come from the middle and lower class families in Tokyo or Chiba Prefecture, and most of their hospital charges are met by Japan's well-established medical insurance system. Seventy-six percent of the inpatients are diagnosed as schizophrenic; the remainder suffer from neurotic or psychopathic disorders. The length of stay is long—three or four years on the average—although recently the term has become shorter. Patients sleep in rooms of two to eight western-style beds and do not stay alone except when their illnesses are severe. There are no cells for solitary confinement in the hospital.

In addition to eating, sleeping, taking care of personal hygiene, and receiving medicines, the patient's everyday life in the hospital consists of engaging in group activities organized by the nurses. These include the assembling of boxes, decorating souvenirs, dancing, group discussion, taking walks, and so on. However, these ward activity programs are not completely consistent, and sometimes there are periods when patients are inactive and left to their own devices. Most doctors and nurses are groping in the dark to find the most suitable administrative and psychosocial activities for the wards.

Sample

We obtained a sample of 100 patients (50 men and 50 women), including 30 open-ward patients (15 men and 15 women) and 70 closed-ward patients (35 men and 35 women) from two closed wards. Initially, we intended to obtain our sample from all seven wards, but when we realized that it was difficult to establish an understanding about our research aims from all seven ward psychiatrists, we decided to limit our sample to three wards whose psychiatrists had close contact with our research staff and understood the purposes of our research. However, the ratio between the numbers of open-ward and closed-ward patients in this sample is approximate to the distribution ratio of all the patients in this hospital.

The sample patients in these three wards were selected by the ward psychiatrist and the chief nurse on their potential to participate in a research interview. Patients who possibly would disturb their ward and who might be resentful of the interview as well as new patients and patients suffering from severe symptoms were omitted. Thus, the sample of 100 patients contained 88 patients with schizophrenia, 7 with neurosis, and 5 with other diagnoses. The sample had a greater number of schizophrenics than the ratio of the total hospitalized, .76 percent. The average total duration of hospitalization of the sample was three years and seven months. The range of the duration was from one week to 19 years.

The mean age was 31.6 (SD = 5.60); 16 patients were under 20 and over 8 years of age. Most subjects were in the age range of 20–40. Our group was approximately the same age as Levinson's sample at the Massachusetts Mental Health Center. Each patient's social class position was assessed by means of the Hollingshead Two-Factor Index (Hollingshead and Redlich, 1958) combining occupation and education. More of our patients were in the lower class than was the case in the Massachusetts sample, although there is not a significant difference (Table 1).

Procedures

We adopted the Role Conception Inventory developed by Levinson and Gallagher (1964) which includes the following seven topical areas of patienthood: (1) orientation to psychiatrists (2) orientation to nurses and aides (3) orientation to patients (4) nature and causes of illness in self (5) conception of treatment (6) conception of cure (7) orientation to the hospital as an institution. We made fairly literal translation of the entire

Table 1:   Class Composition

Social Class Level	Massachusetts Mental Health Center	Konodai National Hospital
	Number of Patients	
I, II	20	21
III	38	26
IV	28	32
V	14	21
Total	100	100

x²=2.816, df=3, not significant

scale except for Item 32 on race which was inapplicable, because our interest lay, at that time, in making a direct comparison between Japanese and American concepts of patienthood.[2]

Interviews were individually conducted with the tester orally reading a statement from single cards. He then handed the card to the patient who placed it in one of six trays. Three trays indicated three degrees of agreement with a statement (given a score of 5, 6, or 7), and the other three trays indicated three degrees of disagreement (given a score of 3, 2, or 1). In rare cases when a subject could not take a stand on an item, he was allowed to put the card aside; it was given a score of 4, the middle of a seven-point scale. The interview required about 60 minutes, and data collection covered a period of about four months, June to September, 1967.

The responses of 100 subjects to the 116 inventory items were factor analyzed by the Thurston centroid method, and the six significant rotated factors[3] were extracted by the Varimax rotation method. In Levinson and Gallagher's analytical procedure, three primary orthogonal factors and four fusion factors were extracted. From a statistical point of view, fusion factors differ from the Varimax rotated factors. However, our discussion requires the psychosocially meaningful factors for comparative examination, so we may neglect the difference in the statistical procedures.

When we tried to derive the meaning of each factor in the Japanese data, we used the items that had over ± .30 factor loadings. In this study, with a sample of 100, loadings of ± .35 or above were relatively high (significant at well beyond the 0.1 percent) and loadings of less than ± .20 were negligible (not significant at the 5 percent level). The previous study, an attempt to make factor scales, used the items having factor loadings of ± .35 or above (Yamamoto et al., 1968), but in this discussion, we adopted more items to determine cultural differences.

Results and the Meaning of Factors

The results of factor analysis (rotated factors) are shown in the appendix in which the item number and contents are identical with those of Levinson and Gallagher (1964). Table 2 presents the summary of interpretations of the six factors. We will describe the contents and presumed meaning of each factor as it relates to the structure of patienthood in Japan, following Levinson and Gallagher's conception of problematic role issues and role conceptions in mental hospitalizations. The items that showed over ± .30 rotated factor loadings in each item factor are seen in Tables 3–8. Our interpretation of each factor was based on the significant factor-loaded items.

Factor I.   While the content of this set of items showed great variety as seen in Table 3, it does present an answer to the problematic role issue: "What constitutes an ideal mental hospital and an ideal patient on the way to recovery?" This question, which confronts all patients, is one of the significant role-tasks of patienthood. Thrust into a new and alien world, the patient finds it imperative to develop a meaningful concept of his own hospitalization that will aid him in interpreting this world and what he may expect from it. The question, of course, is very much related to the values

Table 2:   Problematic Role Issues and Role Conceptions of Patients in a Japanese Mental Hospital

Factor	Issues* and Conceptions†
I	1) What constitutes an ideal mental hospital and an ideal patient on the way to recovery?
	2) Preference for being submissive to paternalistic autocracy and being dependent on warm and sympathetic nurture.
II	1) What do I need in my everyday life?
	2) Emphasis on the importance of strict but dependable support from my hospital staff, especially my doctor.
III	1) How do I feel about this hospital?
	2) Feelings of this hospital staff as punishing me and not helping me.
IV	1) In what ways is this hospital good or bad?
	2) View of this hospital staff as having deep interest in me (+) versus having no interest in me (-).
V	1) Am I mentally ill?
	2) Denial (+) versus acknowledgment of mental illness (-).
VI	1) How do I wish to be in my everyday hospital life?
	2) Need for withdrawal (+) versus being encouraged and active (-).

* 1)=Problematic role issues

† 2)=Role conceptions

and policy held by the hospital staff which, also, merits inquiry. However, my data deals primarily with patient concepts.

The items in the first factor, which I have called "Preference for being submissive to paternalistic autocracy and dependent on warm and sympathetic nurturance," delineate one dimension of response concerning the good hospital and the good patient on his way to recovery. Several items illustrate a conception of the characteristics of the helpful staff member. A good nurse, for example, "treats all patients alike and is always gay and cheerful with the patients." "A sympathetic nurse, especially, can do more to help a patient get well than a doctor can." On the other hand, the main job of nurses is "to see that the patients stay in line" and, in cooperation with doctors, "to teach each patient the grown-up, right ways of living." These items suggest that patients prefer warm, sympathetic care from the hospital staff.

The implications of control, reeducation, and resocialization are further emphasized in the items referring to the hospital as a school for learning about private feelings, how to live with oneself in a framework of strict rules and discipline. Recovery through learning rather than through medical treatment per se has a dimension of passive relinquishment of self to the authority of the doctor-teacher in that the patient puts himself in the hands of the doctor, does what the doctor tells him, and does what he is supposed to do. Within an interpersonal context, the doctor was viewed as being kind, gentle, encouraging, and helpful. Patients appeared to be very concerned with developing and maintaining strong, benevolently paternalistic ties with both the doctor and the nurses. They also showed their concern for how much they are loved by these staff members by alternately denying and affirming their need for kindness and warmth. If the doctor and nurses assumed, in a patient's mind, aspects of good parents, then the other patients appeared as helpful brothers. Patients felt a sense of community, and the hospital was like a resort for resting and enjoying themselves.

In summary, the patient conceived of himself as a child in a family. He wanted a hospital environment that would induce the development of warm and sympathetic human relations. He preferred to be submissive and passively dependent in the hopes of obtaining a good standing with his doctor and nurses; with other patients, he desired a helpful sibling relation. All of these relations are permeated by paternalistic ideas and feelings.

Factor II. Whereas Factor I is generalized in terms of ideal expectations, Factor II emphasizes the patient himself as he pursues his life in the ward: what he finds detrimental or beneficial, the impact of doctors and nurses upon him, and what he wants concretely from members of the hospital staff. This group of items is addressed to the problematic role issue: "What do I need in my everyday hospital life?" The role conception portrayed in Factor II emphasized the importance of strict but reliable forms of support from the hospital staff, especially the doctor (Table 4).

Table 3:   Factor I: Preference for Being Submissive to Paternalistic Autocracy and Being Dependent on Warm and Sympathetic Nurture

	Factor Loading	
Item	Factor I	Other Factors
20. The job of the nurses and doctors is to teach each patient the grown-up, right ways of living	580	—
18. If a patient does what he's supposed to do around here getting well will take care of itself.	568	—
31. The best way a patient can tell how he's coming along is by what his doctor tells him.	483	—
70. The best thing a patient can do here is to put himself into the hands of his doctor and hope for the best.	425	—
25. Most doctors here are quick to give encouragement and help to the patients.	412	367(IV)
112. My doctor is a very kind and gentle person.		
33. I feel I should always put my best foot forward when I see my doctor.	410	466(IV)
50. Whenever I see my doctor, he always seems to know exactly what he's doing and what would be best for me.	334	518(IV)
21. A good nurse is one who is always gay and cheerful with the patients.	710	—
81. In many cases, a sympathetic nurse can do more to help a patient get well than a doctor can.	520	—
1. A good nurse treats all the patients alike.	498	315(IV)
51. The main job of the attendants and nurses is to see that the patients stay in line.	444	—
96. I would enjoy helping the nurses care for the other patients.	376	−443(VI)
34. The nurses here are very generous about sharing cigarettes with patients.	315	—
36. It is very important for the hospital to keep strict rules for the patients.	595	—
85. This hospital is like a school for learning about your feelings.	536	—

Table 3: (Continued)

Item	Factor Loading	
	Factor I	Other Factors
65. Living in the hospital gives me a better chance to learn to live with myself than I ever had before.	459	—
83. The best help for me is in talking and thinking about my personal problems.	412	—
5. What I need most is for people to show love and sympathy toward me.	382	−392(II)
69. It would be easy for a patient to get so used to this place that he'd want to stay here a long time.	380	—
68. What I need most is for people to be strict with me and keep me out of trouble.	346	—
26. The best thing the hospital can do for me is to get me back to the normal state I was in before the breakdown.	307	—
54. This hospital is like a resort hotel for resting and enjoying yourself, if you are able to.	300	—
111. A mentally well person is one who is liked and appreciated by everybody.	552	—
37. A mentally well person is one who never needs help from anybody.	478	—
3. Patients can often help each other get well.	463	—
115. Patients should stick together because we are all in the same boat.	405	−414
114. A mentally well person is one who keeps his feelings and emotions to himself.	348	—
6. A mentally well person doesn't care whether other people like him or not.	342	334(IV)
79. If a patient is cheerful and doesn't complain about things, he's as good as well again.	322	—

Table 4:   Factor II: Emphasis on the Importance of Strict but Reliable Forms of Support from the Hospital Staff, Especially the Doctors

	Factor Loading	
Item	Factor II	Other Factors
39. My doctor expects too much of me.	-447	368(III)
2. My doctor can tell what's going on in my mind just by looking at me.	-439	—
33. I feel I should always put my best foot forward when I see my doctor.	-404	396(I)
16. Most doctors here are too young to know just what they are doing.	-356	307(III) 376(IV)
97. A good doctor will try hard to find out things the patient wants to keep to himself.	-325	—
46. If a nurse allows herself to joke and kid with the patients, she will lose their respect.	-559	—
62. If the nurses want you to do something, they will keep after you until you do it.	-352	425(III)
7. The main reason for mental hospitals is to give sick people a place to blow off steam.	-502	—
60. The hospital should stop being so soft with the patients and make them do more work.	-333	372(III)
5. What I need most is for people to show love and sympathy toward me.	-392	382(I)
108. This hospital is like a prison for keeping people locked up.	-316	317(V)
9. Most patients want to be left alone.	-515	—
113. I wish people would leave me alone.	-304	510(VI)
84. The patients who talk a lot in ward meetings and Patient Government are the sort of people who like to boss and run things.	-483	—
47. I try to stay away from patients who use dirty language and act vulgar.	-419	—
72. You have to be careful with the other patients because they might hurt you or take advantage of you.	-381	—
43. If a patient was feeling bad and then gets to feeling better, he would be foolish to wonder about why he felt so bad.	-517	—
13. Medicine and shock are the only real treatment that patients get around here.	-448	—
23. A lot of the patients here could snap out of it fast if they really wanted to.	-388	—
53. Any patient who goes around talking about his personal problems must be pretty sick.	-335	308(III)
63. I expect to be working on my personal problems even after I leave the hospital.	340	—

Table 5: Factor III: Attitudes that This Hospital is Punishing Me and Not Helping Me

	Factor Loading	
Item	Factor III	Other Factors
82. If a patient does wrong, it is the duty of the doctor to have him punished.	531	—
39. My doctor expects too much of me.	368	−447(II)
16. Most doctors here are too young to know just what they are doing.	307	−356(II) −376(IV)
88. It bothers me to see nurses sitting around and talking when they could be tidying up the ward.	527	—
62. If the nurses want you to do something, they will keep after you until you do it.	425	−352(II)
104. It gripes me, the way the nurses watch you and keep an eye on what you're doing.	362	—
73. This hospital may help some patients, but quite a few are discharged without real improvement.	520	—
61. To get out of the hospital fast, a patient had better keep quiet about any strange experiences he may have here.	372	−333(II)
29. Patients come and go so fast here that it is useless to try to make friends with them.	515	−329(II) 346(VI)
105. With the sort of things that go on here, a patient's moral and religious standards are likely to be weakened.	449	—
4. Almost every patient I've seen around here seems to be sicker than I am.	340	—
32. When a patient is sick, it is extra hard for him to live in a ward with patients of so many religions.	320	—
86. I have trouble keeping myself from doing things I know I shouldn't do.	369	—
35. To be really well, I will have to go through a big change in myself.	368	−447(II)
53. Any patient who goes around talking about his personal problems must be pretty sick.	308	−335(II)

The patients felt unable to control inner anxiety which may have been triggered by any excess of inner or outer stimulation. Thus, they appeared to seek situations where they were able to express anxiety safely as well as situations where they could avoid stimulation, for example: "the main reason for mental hospitals is to give sick people a place to blow off steam," but, on the other hand, "patients who go around talking about their personal problems are considered pretty sick," and the patients avoided other patients "who use dirty language and act vulgar." Stimulation that threatened a patient was seen as coming primarily from the other patients who might have hurt him. That the patient liked to encapsulate himself in order to avoid intimacy with other patients is expressed in the wish to be left alone in his everyday life.

His greater inner anxiety, which he tried to control by himself partly by withdrawal from other patients, needed strict control and dependable support from the doctor, hospital staff, and nurses. The nurses must be strict. "If a nurse allows herself to joke and kid with the patients, she will lose their respect," but she should not push them. "If the nurses want you to do something, they will keep after you until you do it." The patient expressed a particular wish to gain perfect control and warm, dependable support from his own ward doctor in the thought that "the doctor can tell what's going on in one's mind by looking at him." However, his wish for control and support is frustrated in the doctor-patient relation. The patient expressed a desire for more strict and active contact with the doctor, feeling that the hospital policies should not be lenient. Furthermore, patients should work more, and the good doctor should be conscientious in learning about things that the patient appears to want to keep to himself. This view of the doctor as all-seeing is complicated by contradictory feelings of hostility and unreliability; doctors, for example, "are too young" and "expect too much." Total hostility is expressed in the endorsement of the statement, "This hospital is like a prison."

In short, the patients in Factor II expressed a strong wish for their doctor to apply strict, active, and dependable controls and supports which would augment the control of inner anxiety and discomfort. Actually, they were unsatisfied in this regard and expressed a lack of confidence in and hostility toward doctor and hospital.

Factor III. In Factor II the patients showed an unfulfilled need for dependency upon their doctors. This means that patients were disappointed in the expectations that were expressed in the items of Factor I. The third problematic role issue may be viewed as a result of these unsatisfied processes. The answer to the question, "How do I feel about the hospital?" is that the patients "view the hospital as punitive and not helpful."

The items in Factor III (Table 5) portrayed feelings of hopelessness, guilt, and hostility in the patients' view of the hospital. For example, the patients felt that the hospital may help some people but that quite a few are discharged without real improvement. This may express the patients' sense of deprivation of their dependency needs. Associated feelings of guilt were expressed explicitly or implicitly in beliefs that the doctors should punish them and that their moral and religious standards are likely to be weakened, as well as in their difficulties with self-control.

The patients were, nevertheless, stubborn or negativistic as shown by the following comments. It bothered them "to see nurses sitting around and talking," "the way they keep an eye on what one is doing," "the doctors are too young," and "expect too much of one," and "the patients come and go so fast that it is useless to try to make friends with them." In short, the patients felt that the hospital was not helpful and was punishing them. This feeling seems to be related to a paranoiac projection of inner anxiety and hostility.

Factor IV. The item-family of Factor IV offered a concrete evaluation of the extent to which the hospital staff, especially doctors, take a deep personal interest in the patients (Table 6). As we have seen in the previous factors, paternalistic relations between the hospital staff and the patients were typical. In such relations, the concern of the patient was his standing in favor with the doctor and nurses. Generally, we can say that the problematic role issue in the Factor IV is "In what ways is this hospital staff good or bad for me?"

The items with positive factor-loadings described the doctor and nurses as having deep personal interest in the patients. The patient felt that his doctor was the best and that he was the doctor's favorite. Thus, he believed that the doctor took a deep personal interest in him, was kind and gentle, always seemed to know exactly what he was doing and what was best for the patient and was quick to give encouragement and help. The nurses were also kind and gentle to the patient and "go out of their way to do little things that the patients want."

The items having negative factor-loadings took the opposite position, describing the doctor and nurses as having no interest in the patient. The patient thought of himself as being unfavored by the hospital staff, feeling that no one cared about him; the doctor saw him as very ill; the nurses lacked interest in him; and the other patients cared only for themselves. In short, the role conception in Factor IV is regarded as the patients' view of this hospital staff as "having deep personal interest (+) versus having no interest in me (−)."

Factor V. Whereas the preceding factors dealt primarily with ideas about the hospital, staff, and the patient's life, the focus here, as seen in Table 7, is on the patient himself and his internal state. The central issue of Factor V can be stated simply: "Am I mentally ill?" This is a question every patient puts to himself, even if it is left unanswered. By virtue of being hospitalized, he has been defined by society as being different in some sense. The hospital staff devotes its efforts to diagnosis of his difficulties and to helping the patient confront his problem. But each patient has his own opinion about his difficulties which may have little or no bear-

Table 6:   Factor IV: View of This Hospital Staff as Having Deep Interest in Me (+) Versus Having No Interest in Me (–)

Item	Factor Loading	
	Factor IV	Other Factors
8. My doctor takes a deep personal interest in me.	546	—
50. Whenever I see my doctor, he always seems to know exactly what he's doing and what would be best for me.	518	354(I)
112. My doctor is a very kind and gentle person.	466	410(I)
25. Most doctors here are quick to give encouragement and help to the patients.	367	412(I)
116. The nurses here are very gentle and kind to the patients.	679	—
58. Most of the nurses here will go out of their way to do the little things the patients want.	581	—
16. Most doctors here are too young to know just what they are doing.	–376	–356(II) 307(III)
66. My doctor feels very bad about my troubles.	–307	—
28. The nurses here spend too much time with a few pet patients.	–444	—
11. I wish the nurses took a stronger personal interest in me.	–421	—
98. A lot of the patients here will get away with everything they can.	–312	—
107. No one here cares about me.	–304	—

Table 7:   Factor V: Denial (+) versus Acknowledgment of Mental Illness (–)

Item	Factor Loading	
	Factor V	Other Factors
99. I am healthy in body and mind.	651	—
90. I am well enough to be discharged today from the hospital.	602	—
71. I may have a nervous condition, but my mind is OK.	519	—
24. The day I walk out of this hospital I will know I am well.	386	—
108. This hospital is like a prison for keeping people locked up.	317	–316(II)
77. In my opinion, I am mentally ill.	–644	—
17. Sometimes my feelings get out of control.	–644	—
30. There are times when I feel very low and depressed.	–598	—
78. I am restless and nervous most of the time.	–511	—
115. Patients should stick together, because we are all in the same boat.	–414	405(I)

Table 8: Factor VI: Need for Withdrawal (+) versus being Encouraged and Active (–)

Item	Factor Loading	
	Factor VI	Other Factors
94. I like to take care of my own business and stay out of the affairs of other patients.	537	—
113. I wish people would leave me alone.	510	–504(II)
101. Most of the work the patients do around here helps the hospital more than it helps the patients.	377	—
102. I try to stay away from patients who feel low and depressed all the time.	367	—
29. Patients come and go so fast here that it is useless to try to make friends with them.		515(III)
6. A mentally well person doesn't care whether other people like him or not.	346	329(II)
109. I would resent it if the nurses wanted to know about my personal difficulties.	334 330	342(I)
19. I am very close friends with some of the patients here.	–530	—
100. I often talk to other patients about my personal troubles.	–490	—
45. I like to go to lots of hospital activities, such as O.T. and dances and patient government.	–481	—
96. I would enjoy helping the nurse care for the other patients.	–443	376(I)
74. I wish my doctor would give me more advice and guidance.	–336	—
41. The nurses should encourage a patient to act up if he feels it coming on.	–336	—
38. Keeping active and busy is the main thing that helps me.	–316	—
80. I like it best when I know just what the rules are and what I am supposed to be doing every minute.	–316	

ing on a professional diagnosis. Thus, the items in Factor V present the denial (+) versus the acknowledgment of mental illness (−).

The items having positive factor-loading portrayed an attitude of denial of mental illness, as the following items illustrate. "I am well enough to be discharged today from the hospital"; "I am healthy in my body and mind"; and the classic, "I may have a nervous condition, but my mind is OK."

The opposite attitude was described in the items having negative factor loadings. Patients acknowledged their difficulties as mental in origin and expressed their inner turmoil. They made frank statements of mental illness and feelings of loss, restlessness, nervousness, and depression.

Factor VI. The final factor shows another problematic role issue: "How do I wish to be in my everyday life?" The need described in the items of Factor VI seems to be related to daily life activities in the wards (Table 8). Factor II was similar to Factor VI, but related to a more general need for strict but dependable supports from the hospital staff.

The items having negative factor-loadings expressed the patient's desire to receive more active encouragement and guidance from the doctor, to participate in hospital activities, and to have close relations with other patients. He also wanted his activities to be bound by rules that would guide him at all times. The items having positive factor-loadings showed that the patients expressed negative attitudes toward hospital work, the nurses, and other patients. They seemed sulky and negativistic, wanted to be left alone, kept problems to themselves, and avoided other patients who might be like themselves.

The role conception in Factor VI, then, presents a dimension of the need for withdrawal (+) versus being encouraged and active (−). It seems, by clinical impression, that this dimension is related to the extent of gratification and dependable supports the patient receives from his doctor and nurses.

Discussion of Japanese Patienthood

Our discussion of the patient's role issues and conceptions in this hospital is based on the six significant factors mentioned above.

1) The patients in this mental hospital saw as an ideal a hospital where they are shown benevolence by the hospital staff if they are submissive and passively dependent and where they receive sympathetic, warm regard and nurturant reeducation. Therefore, the responses to the inventory focused on effective and dependable vertical ties with the hospital staff—ties expected in a benevolent patriarchal family rather than in a place organized for functional effective recovery.

2) In this sense, the patients clung to the doctor-patient relation as a means of maintaining strict and dependable supports for controlling inner anxiety. Their need of support, however, was not satisfied by the

doctor, and they expressed hostile and nontrusting feelings to the hospital staff.

3) The patients felt the hospital was not helpful and saw hospitalization as punishment, not treatment. These feelings are, in all likelihood, related to the persecutory symptomatology seen in schizophrenic patients. As most of the patients in this sample are schizophrenic, we can assume that the feelings arose from the characteristics of schizophrenia. However, it is noteworthy that the paternalistic, family-like ties strengthened the projection of paranoid feelings in the patients.

4) One of the most important considerations of the patients was whether members of the hospital staff take a deep personal interest in them. In other words, the patients always concerned themselves with whether they were the favorite of their hospital staff. This concern is reflected in the typical Japanese personality characteristic of passive dependence, *amae,* which means "to be dependent and presume upon another's benevolence" (Doi, 1962). The paternalistic staff-patient relation seemed to accept and encourage *amae.*

5) In everyday hospital life, the dimension of "withdrawal versus being encouraged and active" was prominent. The attitude of withdrawal is characteristic of Japanese schizophrenic patients (Schooler and Caudill, 1964) and may be seen as a manifestation of *suneru* which, according to Doi (1962), is a common term "describing the behavior of a child or adult who pouts and sulks because he is not allowed to *amaeru* as much as he wants to." The opposing attitude of being encouraged and active also related to *amae.* Here the patients indicated that they wanted more encouragement and strong, warm interest from their doctor in order to maintain their activities in hospital life.

6) The patients were also concerned with whether they were mentally ill. The label of mental illness was threatening to them. This concern is characteristic of the attitudes of both chronic schizophrenic patients and those held by the hospital staff, attitudes which can affect the staff's behavior toward patients. The hospital staff, particularly doctors, were concerned with *byō-shiki* which literally means illness (*byō*) and acknowledgment (*shiki*)—that is, whether the patient could acknowledge his deviant and abnormal thought or behavior. Although the interplay here is subtle, one can say with some assurance that patients with *byō-shiki* tend to be more favorably regarded by doctors than patients without *byō-shiki.*

Some Impressions of Cultural Differences

Our observations of the cultural differences between the Japanese and American patient's patienthood are based on the Levinson and Gallagher data (1964). Although the social structure and policy of the Konodai National Hospital differ from those of the Massachusetts Mental Health Center, so that we are unable to compare them directly with each other, we have some general impressions of cultural differences, particularly in terms of interpersonal relations and patterns of need-expression, that range beyond the differences between the hospital settings.

1) Americans, like Japanese patients, showed a preference for benign autocracy and conventional facade as the answer to the question of an ideal hospital and an ideal patient. However, the meaning of the autocracy that is reflected in the consciousness of patients from each country differs. American autocracy means the controlling function of a social system toward recovery, so their doctor-patient relations are less emotionally toned than those in the Japanese hospital. The American doctor-patient relation is more like a contractual one, as may be seen in this item: "as long as my doctor knows his business, it does not matter whether he likes me personally or not." The Japanese autocracy means a paternalistic relation that includes more effective interpersonal components; the patient expects, and is expected, to be passively dependent. When patients are submissive and passively dependent, they can expect to get help and benevolence from their superiors—doctors and nurses.

2) In this context, the American patients brought up another problematic role issue concerning the way to recovery. While the Japanese patients expect their recovery only within the paternalistic relation, American patients make a distinction between the doctor's competence and their dependence on him. The Japanese patients, on the other hand, do not judge the talent of their doctor but simply want to put themselves into his hands.

3) The Japanese patients are deeply concerned with whether the hospital staff has a personal interest in them. This concern with gratification remains within the vertical structure of the hospital staff and patients and is not expressed in the horizontal structure of the patient-patient relation due to the strong effective control of the paternalistic doctor-patient relation. American patients seek gratification in smooth relations among patients in the ward.

4) The Japanese patients express their passive dependent needs more directly than American patients. They expressed *amae* in the need for nurture, the need for encouragement, the need for dependable supports, and the attitude of *suneru*. On the contrary, the American patients express their individual needs by criticizing other patients' babyish dependent attitudes. The difference stems from the fact that American culture disapproves of the admission of dependent needs, particularly in men; conversely, the Japanese culture accepts—and sometimes encourages—the expression of dependent needs (Doi, 1962; Caudill and Doi, 1953).

5) Japanese patients in this hospital are less expressive of inner turmoil, sometimes denying mental illness, than American patients at the Massachusetts Mental Health Center. This difference may come from sample differences between both research studies. However, another reason may be in the social control of Japanese hospitals with regard to characteristic symptoms of Japanese schizophrenic patients. Schooler and Caudill (1964) point

out that the symptom of physical assaultiveness has the highest incidence of any symptom among Japanese schizophrenics; it is also significantly greater compared to American schizophrenics. Such assaults are most likely to be made against members of the family and, in the case of male patients, against the mother in particular. The Japanese hospital in this study is like a family group. If a patient were allowed to express his emotions and turmoil freely, he would express aggression and violence against the hospital staff, as if it were his own family. Therefore, Japanese hospital staffs suppress the patients' assaultiveness by administering tranquilizing medicine, so that ward activities will not be disturbed. The expression of aggression is punished by the hospital staff.

Summary

In this paper we have presented six significant factors relating to the problematic role issues and the role concepts of patienthood in a Japanese mental hospital. We have also discussed cultural differences of interpersonal relations and patterns of need-expression between Japanese and American patients. In Japan, staff-patient relations are paternalistic and family like; Japanese patients always turn to the hospital staff to satisfy their passive dependent needs. They put their trust in the staff's benevolence as the way to recovery. In the United States, staff-patient relations are less affective and more functional than in Japan. American patients tend to have a contractual view of their relation to the hospital staff and have less direct expressions of dependency. These cultural differences can be understood, in part, as reflecting differences in the control and acceptance of dependent needs by the general social culture in Japan and America.

ACKNOWLEDGMENTS

The author wishes to express his gratitude to Mr. Takao Murase, National Institute of Mental Health, Japan; Miss Michiko Adachi, Tomobe Hospital of Ibaragi Prefecture; Mr. Yutaka Akiyama, Rissho Women's College; and Miss Kumiko Kiyohara, National Hospital of Shimoshizu for their energetic cooperation in developing the research design and data collection. Grateful acknowledgment is also made to Dr. Howard T. Blane of Harvard Medical School and Massachusetts General Hospital for his helpful suggestions and advice regarding factor analysis.

Appendix: Mean, Standard Deviations, and Factor Loadings of
Each Item in Role Conception Inventory

Item No*	Mean	SD	I	II	III	IV	V	VI
1	6.30	0.59	498	32	-158	315	-117	-65
2	4.03	1.86	220	-439	12	258	92	18
3	5.06	1.65	463	-260	-138	0	37	-57
4	3.20	1.60	92	-192	340	-131	261	-17
5	3.66	1.95	382	-392	-22	-179	70	-3
6	5.13	1.88	342	-116	15	99	50	334
7	2.53	1.69	195	-501	152	87	25	82
8	5.73	1.14	277	-44	139	546	-37	-247
9	3.80	1.80	-34	-515	166	187	131	55
10	5.10	2.00	54	129	32	-79	-25	46
11	3.83	1.93	99	-272	138	-421	206	-188
12	5.06	2.06	142	-202	120	47	-69	-75
13	3.50	2.09	-11	-448	98	-89	33	107
14	5.70	1.48	297	-50	43	87	140	-152
15	4.60	2.12	92	-126	137	175	-167	-20
16	2.53	1.52	-93	-356	307	-376	35	216
17	5.00	2.03	46	183	72	-32	-644	22
18	4.40	1.88	568	-231	106	132	80	-91
19	5.00	1.92	264	-139	-62	22	102	-530
20	5.26	1.61	580	-60	131	117	-176	-52
21	5.36	1.51	710	-92	-57	108	95	89
22	4.20	2.18	106	-54	-30	27	-16	-14
23	3.16	1.66	180	-388	-76	-20	255	-141
24	5.50	1.40	223	-106	-206	288	386	-189
25	5.26	1.68	412	-164	-114	367	99	-63
26	5.80	1.15	307	-112	8	76	-1	-205
27	5.06	1.72	-35	-37	-145	3	65	46
28	2.23	1.16	101	-259	127	-444	-148	45
29	3.03	1.77	43	-329	515	-44	78	346

* This sequence and its respective contents are identical with those of Levinson and Gallagher (1964).

Appendix: (Continued)

Item No.	Mean	SD	I	II	III	IV	V	VI
30	4.46	2.01	35	-80	214	-80	-598	64
31	5.00	1.83	483	-229	96	229	54	-115
32†	3.26	2.06	200	-193	320	-56	-10	104
33	3.93	2.06	396	-404	21	-91	172	-39
34	4.56	1.85	315	-46	206	280	124	-43
35	5.36	1.71	293	177	315	179	-126	-47
36	5.90	1.26	595	194	182	170	-17	-166
37	4.10	2.17	478	-87	189	104	20	217
38	4.90	1.70	188	-248	144	166	78	-316
39	3.03	1.71	51	-447	368	17	25	-72
40	3.23	1.79	177	-185	168	-163	-8	-151
41	5.50	1.40	271	-213	-38	-56	-30	-336
42	2.70	1.62	-10	-209	216	-157	-259	86
43	2.90	1.78	46	-517	59	81	58	185
44	4.86.	1.87	270	-148	169	18	173	-76
45	4.36	1.92	158	-120	82	21	130	-481
46	2.83	1.85	144	-559	207	94	105	-19
47	3.83	2.00	171	-419	-97	-146	11	-55
48	4.33	2.15	122	-127	89	-66	-75	61
49	3.06	1.89	111	-159	264	-195	-283	-8
50	5.00	1.72	334	-229	173	518	71	-81
51	4.96	1.82	444	-279	-12	165	-59	84
52	2.90	1.66	-11	-83	247	-68	84	202
53	4.20	1.84	197	-335	308	91	29	14
54	4.83	1.91	300	-75	35	65	-50	-149
55	5.53	1.45	85	-93	74	79	34	201
56	5.10	1.86	61	-171	11	279	131	-118
57	5.46	1.25	278	21	-59	158	169	5
58	5.36	1.58	94	-62	-74	581	16	67

† This item was revised from, "When a patient is sick, it is extra hard for him to live on a ward with patients of so many races and religions," to, " . . . to live on a ward with patients of so many religions."

Appendix: (Continued)

Item No.	Mean	SD	I	II	III	IV	V	VI
59	5.86	.81	220	52	-99	205	-105	-181
60	3.16	1.76	124	-487	228	-203	67	-222
61	3.06	1.81	255	-333	372	26	218	55
62	3.06	1.77	67	-352	425	-45	14	-68
63	6.26	1.01	157	340	89	52	0	-222
64	5.50	1.50	229	59	8	112	36	-270
65	5.13	1.77	459	191	148	18	-34	-192
66	3.16	1.74	-1	-26	42	-307	-238	221
67	3.66	1.89	-173	-222	291	167	149	171
68	4.76	1.85	346	-287	156	126	-60	-184
69	4.16	1.96	380	-116	265	-60	-219	-97
70	5.10	1.88	425	-101	-49	172	-43	212
71	4.23	1.97	215	-184	207	-22	519	-71
72	2.96	1.86	63	-381	59	-266	259	106
73	4.13	1.97	4	23	520	-63	-14	59
74	4.83	1.85	201	-72	159	-50	-51	-371
75	1.83	1.53	29	-271	219	-193	43	177
76	5.63	1.65	71	-105	81	100	-221	-107
77	5.10	1.93	84	101	-45	-46	-644	-164
78	4.80	2.00	-90	-87	58	-128	-511	-91
79	4.76	1.75	322	-255	-48	78	198	47
80	5.56	1.38	233	-71	65	104	-47	-316
81	4.76	1.88	520	-119	-116	-122	122	-156
82	4.40	2.23	121	-134	531	242	36	50
83	5.10	1.68	412	-49	108	17	21	-153
84	3.60	1.88	186	-483	42	-152	-118	92
85	4.16	2.10	536	-156	183	49	71	-99
86	3.30	1.87	222	-66	369	18	-28	-106
87	5.10	1.80	68	73	57	39	-22	224

Appendix: (Continued)

Item No.	Mean	SD	I	II	III	IV	V	VI
88	3.20	1.73	42	-28	527	-147	-35	-70
89	4.86	1.59	107	-28	71	46	-143	-24
90	3.60	2.07	1	-231	250	-110	602	-91
91	4.56	1.88	-29	-17	-200	127	19	8
92	5.26	1.55	278	-224	-82	-70	258	20
93	4.06	1.68	-144	-68	295	-275	-257	151
94	4.63	1.79	68	-179	185	-54	101	537
95	3.86	2.02	255	-135	235	4	-159	149
96	5.73	1.17	376	-22	-69	38	2	-443
97	5.03	1.67	132	-325	-21	58	-281	-178
98	4.70	1.76	124	-10	114	-312	-121	43
99	3.60	2.09	239	-97	204	72	651	-74
100	5.20	1.64	-119	46	58	110	15	-490
101	2.73	1.77	-56	-295	243	-190	125	377
102	3.06	1.83	86	-66	135	-148	83	367
103	6.20	1.15	249	124	92	90	-109	159
104	3.26	1.99	103	178	362	-266	158	19
105	3.90	1.98	-16	-91	449	-120	-52	-6
106	4.40	2.04	5	-91	267	122	50	106
107	2.30	1.41	-17	-202	258	-304	9	274
108	2.20	1.73	-30	-316	287	-193	317	128
109	2.56	1.50	19	-97	186	-138	171	330
110	3.40	1.79	48	-221	139	-49	-157	67
111	4.93	2.06	552	-94	42	59	36	80
112	5.83	1.28	410	96	13	466	-17	-26
113	3.16	1.94	-84	-304	73	-138	-79	510
114	4.46	1.87	384	-205	-7	-29	91	-19
115	4.53	1.90	405	-82	192	119	-414	-205
116	5.73	1.28	113	-26	-100	679	22	-119

NOTES
1. The first Japanese publication of the patienthood study (Yamamoto, Murase, Adachi, Akiyama, and Kiyohara, 1968) described the psychosocial characteristics of the Japanese mental hospital. In the present paper, the author reanalyzed his data for a comparative study.
2. In a later study, for which we are collecting data in two other private mental hospitals, we made a substantial revision of the scale so that its items would be more relevant to the situations of the mental patients and mental hospitals as they exist in Japan. Also, Yamamoto and Kiyohara (1969) made the scale for the patienthood of gastroenteritis and tuberculosis inpatients based on the experiences of this study and the interview materials in a general hospital.
3. We extracted seven significant factors in the Japanese paper (Yamamoto et al., 1968). However, when we reexamined these factors for this paper, we decided to omit the fourth factor, because its meaning is unclear.

REFERENCES
Caudill, W. 1959. Observation on the cultural context of Japanese psychiatry. *In* Culture and mental health. Marvin K. Opler, ed. New York, Macmillan.
———. 1961. Around the clock patient care in Japanese psychiatric hospitals: the role of the tsukisoi. American Sociological Review 26:204–14.
Caudill, W., and L. T. Doi. 1963. Interrelations of psychiatry, culture and emotion in Japan. *In* Man's image in medicine and anthropology. I. Gladston, ed. New York, International Universities Press.
Doi, L. T. 1962. A key concept for understanding Japanese personality structure. *In* Japanese culture; its development and characteristics. R. T. Smith and R. K. Beardsley, eds. Chicago, Aldine.
Hollingshead, A. B., and F. C. Redlich. 1958. Social class and mental illness. New York, John Wiley and Sons.
Levinson, D. J., and E. B. Gallagher. 1964. Patienthood in the mental hospital. Boston, Houghton Mifflin.
Pine, F., and D. J. Levinson. 1961. A sociopsychological conception of patienthood. International Sociological Review 28:963–72.
Saji, M., H. Dendo, and K. Yamamoto. 1965. A study on the therapeutic relationship with schizophrenic patients. Japanese Journal of Mental Health 14:21–39. [In Japanese]
Schooler, C., and W. Caudill. 1964. Symptomatology in Japanese and American schizophrenics. Ethnology 3:172–78.
Yamamoto, K., et al. 1969. A structural analysis of the patienthood in mental hospital. Japanese Journal of Clinical Psychology 4:243–55. [In Japanese]
Yamamoto, K., and K. Kiyohara. In press. A structural analysis of the patienthood in a general hospital—on the gastroenteritis and the tuberculosis inpatients. Japanese Journal of Clinical Psychology. [In Japanese]

14.   A Cross-Cultural Comparison of Psychiatric Disorder:
       Eskimos of Alaska, Yorubas of Nigeria,
       and Nova Scotians of Canada

JANE M. MURPHY, Ph.D.

Department of Behavioral Sciences
Harvard School of Public Health
Boston, Massachusetts

DURING THE PRESENT CENTURY a good deal of attention has been attracted to culture as a determinant of psychiatric disorder. Culture, thus, holds a position parallel to heredity and organic damage in stimulating thought and generating research.

Some of the main ideas about the relation between culture and psychiatric disorder can be summarized briefly in the following outline.[1] (1) Culture may be thought to determine the pattern of specific psychiatric disorders such as latah, witiko, and koro. (2) Culture may be thought to produce basic personality types, some of which are especially vulnerable to psychiatric disorder. (3) It may be thought to produce disorders through different kinds of child-rearing practices. (4) It may be thought to affect disorders through types of sanctions such as shame and guilt-inducing differences. (5) It may be thought to perpetuate disorders by rewarding them in certain prestigeful roles such as shaman or artist. (6) It may be thought to produce disorders through certain stressful roles such as "barren woman" or "second son." (7) It may be thought to affect disorder through indoctrination of its members with particular kinds of sentiments such as excessive fear or jealousy. (8) Cultural change may be thought to produce disorder through rearrangements and disjunctures in values, beliefs, or practices which occur at a speed to tax the ability of personalities to cope

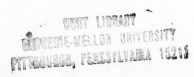

and adapt. (9) Culture per se may be thought to produce disorder; that is, the process of socialization in all cultures may damage the resources of personality for spontaneity and self-expression. (10) Culture may be thought to affect the distribution of disorders through patterns of breeding or hygiene.

Despite the general support given the notion that there is a relation between culture and psychiatric disorder, there is lack of agreement as to what kind of relation it is. There is, however, a fairly large number of people who believe that the relation is one of such tight interdependence that the difficulties posed for adequate research are almost insurmountable. According to this view, psychiatric disorders, unlike many of the physical disorders, are so inextricably linked to the context in which they are found that it is impossible to identify them separately from culture. An extreme cultural relativist might suggest, for example, that inadequate testing of reality can be considered a psychiatric symptom only if the culture defines reality-testing as valuable. Certainly, the definition of reality varies from culture to culture. Certainly, also, the value of an objective and scientific approach to reality is characteristic of some cultures and not of others. This line of thinking, expanded to all symptoms identified in Western psychiatry, would make comparison among cultures impossible.

During the last two decades, while the above ideas have been in the wind, the Harvard Program in Social Psychiatry [2] has had opportunity to conduct psychiatric epidemiological studies in communities of different cultural orientations. An explanation of our approach is given as a Methodological Note at the end of this chapter. Our main concern has been to discover the relevance for epidemiology of social processes within a given cultural group. Despite the relativist viewpoint, we have been interested in the question of cultural difference and have looked at the problem of comparison from many points of view. As will become apparent in the following paragraphs, we ultimately came to the position that cross-cultural comparisons are to some extent feasible and are worthy of investigation.

The members of the Social Psychiatry Program, under the direction of Alexander H. Leighton, began this research in the early 50's. The first site was Stirling County, a rural and maritime area of Nova Scotia.[3] The county has a population of 20,000 which is about equally divided between French-speaking and English-speaking. One reason for selecting Stirling County was the opportunity it provided for investigating social process in a rather small geographic area where two distinct subcultural and language groups are contiguous. At the same time, the French and English differences are not of a magnitude to make very difficult the translation of questions and identification of symptoms. Our findings showed marked similarity between the two groups in prevalence rates and only a few minor differences in types of symptom patterns. It seemed reasonable to attribute this similarity to the fact that the French and English, though having some genuine differences, are both in the mainstream of Western culture. This suggested that an adequate exploration of the relation between culture and psychiatric disorder would require choosing populations of much greater contrast.

The three contrasting cultural groups I will discuss are Eskimo, Yoruba, and Nova Scotian. Among them we have examples of two non-Western cultures and one Western, three racial groups, three very different zones of habitat, and three groups undergoing different rates of change.

The Eskimo study comprises 178 individuals (the total adult Eskimo population) living in Sivokok Village on St. Lawrence Island in the Bering Sea during the year 1954–55.[4] Background work was done to obtain the Eskimo view of psychiatric disorder so that it could be taken into account during the course of evaluating the data. A systematic review of each member of the population was carried out with a key informant, and the records of the town council meetings and of the public health nurse were checked in order to compile dossiers on physical illnesses and behaviors of psychiatric interest. In addition, we administered a structured interview questionnaire to 21 individuals, a 12 percent systematic sample of the adults.

The Yoruba study refers to a group of Egbas (a subtribe of the Yoruba) living in fifteen villages near the city of Abeokuta in Nigeria during 1961.[5] A probability sample was drawn from heads of households (alternating male and female), and 245 adults were observed and interviewed by a team of psychiatrists using the same questionnaire as was employed among the Eskimo sample.

The Novia Scotia study consists of the same kind of probability sample—254 subjects drawn, in this case, from ten communities in 1962.[6]

Results

At this point in the work, we can say with considerable confidence that in none of the groups was psychiatric disorder randomly distributed in the populations. The intracultural processes we have investigated consist of community integration, rapid change, social stratification, and role functioning as mediated through age and sex. In each cultural group some of these turn out to be significantly related to the prevalence of psychiatric disorders.

We were also interested to see whether there are recurrent patterns of association between psychiatric prevalence and these processes in all three of the groups studied. At times we have been struck by the consistency of one or another finding from culture to culture and have been tempted to think that possibly we were on the track of a universal relation. In fact, however, an intriguing exception has always come to light demanding a new look at the specific cultural situation. For example, numbers of epidemiologic studies, our own as well as other's, have shown a relation between aging and increased prevalence.[7] In the Yoruba study, however, this was not true, and we were led to give consideration to the fact that, among the groups we are comparing, the Yorubas stand out in the degree to which they socially reward those who hold positions of seniority with age being a major route to seniority. Perhaps this kind of cultural arrangement offers sufficient protection against the problems of aging to account for the relative health of the Yoruba elders. In sum, we have found no association of disorder prevalence and sociocultural process that holds up across all of these three cultures.

As the work progressed, we became increasingly impressed by the fact that cultural relativity was not as great a stumbling block as we had expected. By and large, the same kinds of psychiatric disorder were found in these different groups and were recognized as such by the culture-carriers themselves and by our psychiatrists. For example, the standard we used to identify sociopathic deviance was the standard of the culture in which the deviance was found. The cases were identified from within rather than without, but when we moved on to the next cultural group, we found that virtually the same standard was put forth and, also, that it was virtually the same as the psychiatrists'. "Why similarity?" became the interesting question rather than "Why difference?" Because we found that we were identifying and counting the same kinds of psychiatric phenomena in the three cultures, it seems appropriate to offer comparative findings among cultures; that is, between culture comparisons in addition to within culture comparisons.

I wish it were possible to say that the three studies followed exactly and absolutely the same methodology. In large measure this is true. However, the Eskimo study, done 15 years ago, was a pilot effort, and what we learned from exploration we applied in subsequent investigations. In order to minimize distortion attributable to variation in methods, I decided to focus exclusively on "definite" cases. We call these Type I and Type II cases as explained in the Methodological Note. The findings in these terms are given in Table 1.

The first point to be made in giving these figures is a statement of recognition that the samples are small and that this work was not carried out in the light of an advance theory or with a view to testing a hypothesis. The figures describe what we found, and the results of testing the differences by chi-square are given as a matter of interest.

Focusing on definite cases means presenting individuals whose symptom patterns are sufficiently clear-cut that a clinician would recognize these people as similar to his patients. These cases show the greatest amount of abnormalcy and are, by nature, the most noticeable. Thus, I believe we are in a position to make an accurate estimation of the number of definite cases among the 677 individuals who comprise the same populations of the three cultures.

In the table of findings, phrases such as "psychotic pattern," "psychoneurotic pattern," and "mental deficiency pattern" are used to indicate behavior commonly found in people who have been given these diagnostic labels.[8] It is important, however, to stress that the words are descriptive of phenomena and are not diagnostic. It has been a fundamental principle of

Table 1:   Percentage of Types I and II Psychiatric Cases in Three
Cultural Groups

| Symptom Patterns* | Cultural Groups | | | |
	Stirling County (N=254)	Yoruba (N=245)	Eskimo (N=178)	Significance of Difference
Psychoneurotic pattern	12	10	14†	Not significant
Psychophysiologic pattern	11	9	10†	Not significant
Psychotic pattern	0.5	4	0.5	Significant 0.01 level
Mental deficiency pattern	4	0.5	2	Significant 0.05 level
Senility pattern‡	4	6	4	Not significant
Personality disorder pattern	4	2	1	Not significant
Sociopathic pattern	2	0.5	4	Not significant
Epilepsy pattern§	0.5	0.5	1	Not significant
Total percentage of Types I and II cases	18	15	19†	Not significant

* "Symptom patterns" as utilized in our method are divided into "major symptom patterns" and "detailed symptom patterns." This division is more fully explained in the Methodological Note. For the studies reported here, eight major symptom patterns serve as a comprehensive categorization: psychoneurotic, psychophysiologic, psychotic, mental deficiency, brain syndromes, personality disorders, sociopathic, and generalized motor disturbances. These are the categories presented in this table with the exception of senility which is a detailed pattern in the major pattern of brain syndrome and epilepsy which is in generalized motor disturbances.

† These figures are the results of the systematic sample studied among the Eskimos. Other Eskimo findings refer to the total adult population.

‡ The percentages for senility have been age-adjusted, using the number of individuals 60 years and over in each group as the denominators. Senility accounts for most of the cases with a brain syndrome pattern, and the differences among the cultural groups regarding brain syndromes other than senility are also nonsignificant.

§ In the major pattern of generalized motor disturbance, the detailed patterns other than epilepsy are also nonsignificant when the three cultural groups are compared.

our research that the psychiatric findings be given in this descriptive sense without a priori commitment to etiological assumptions since discovering causal relations is the ultimate purpose of the research.

In keeping with the descriptive approach, it should be noted that different symptom patterns can be found in the same individual. For example, the presence of a senility pattern does not rule out the presence of a psychoneurotic pattern. Thus, the sum of the percentages of all the kinds of symptom patterns among the Yorubas, for example, exceeds the percentage of Yoruba individuals who are classified as definite cases. In line with the focus on definite cases, all symptom patterns that were judged by the psychiatrists to be minimally impairing or in which they had low confidence have been eliminated from these findings. Even under these stringent conditions, it is extremely rare to find a person with only one symptom pattern.[9]

A final explanatory note regarding the table is that the Eskimo figures are a mixture of the results of studying the total population and those of the 12 percent systematic sample (where the latter are used, they are noted by an asterisk). The reason for combining the two is to give the most accurate picture possible. The self-report of symptoms through the questionnaire interview has proved to be the best way of gaining information about psychoneurotic and psychophysiologic patterns. If in the Eskimo cases we relied only on the key informant and public records data for these categories, they would be considerably underrepresented—5 percent as compared to 14 percent for psychoneurotic and 3 percent as compared to 10 percent for psychophysiologic. Where the other symptom patterns are concerned, we have looked mainly to sources outside the subject for evidence. In all three studies, these sources included key informants and knowledge about events that are usually recorded in public documents, such as hospital, school, and court records.

Interpretation

The most striking aspect of the results given in the table is the lack of difference in the number of cases and the distribution of symptom patterns among the three cultural groups. Thus, not only did we find that we were counting the same kinds of phenomena from group to group, but also we found a remarkable similarity from group to group in the number of individuals who can be classified as psychiatric cases.

With regard to the frequency of symptom patterns, again there is more similarity than difference. In broad outline, psychoneurotic and psychophysiologic patterns are relatively common (with about 10 percent to 15 percent of the definite cases in each group exhibiting such symptoms), while all the other patterns are relatively infrequent in occurrence (roughly 5 percent or fewer of the cases having the psychotic, mental deficiency, senility, personality, sociopathic or epileptic symptom patterns). It is also to be noted that no symptom pattern is unrepresented among the groups.

The main point to be made from this analysis is that the groups are more alike than different from each other in psychiatric features despite the degree of contrast they represent in cultural characteristics. It is, however, worthwhile to look at the differences that did appear. I will discuss three of these: psychotic pattern, mental deficiency, and sociopathic pattern. I have included the first, because it seems a genuine result worthy of further research, the second, because it is, I believe, spurious, and the third, because it is suggestive.

The psychotic differences are not only statistically significant but also of interest in terms of the interpretation of epidemiologic findings. Psychoses have been given considerable attention in cross-cultural investigations, generally through the use of hospital records. Although methodological problems are involved, there is some evidence that psychoses have a low and rather stable rate from population to population. In the studies reviewed by Lin, for example, the psychoses rates (when converted from per thousand to per hundred) vary from less than 1 percent to 1.5 percent (Lin, 1953; Mishler and Scotch, 1965). The results of the Stirling Study are in line with this trend. In the 1952 data for Stirling County as a whole, .9 percent of the respondents were evaluated as having a psychotic symptom pattern; in the 1962 findings from selected communities as reported in this paper, the rate was .5 percent.

In view of the above, we anticipated that the psychotic pattern rate in these three cultural groups living in natural communities would not vary greatly and that it would be only slightly lower than the rate would be had we included hospital residents. Yet, we found that the Yorubas had a significantly higher prevalence of the psychotic pattern (4 percent) as compared to the two North American groups (Eskimos, .5 percent and Stirling County, .5 percent).

In trying to assess whether or not this is a genuine difference, several questions come to mind. Have we simply measured the availability of hospitals to the communities selected or have we found a difference in psychiatric characteristics? Are the individuals with psychotic patterns from Nova Scotia and Alaska in hospitals and, therefore, not in the community population to be counted? In other words, is the Yoruba rate simply due to lack of hospitals and a relatively large number of people with the psychotic pattern being in the community?

As it turns out, the Yorubas we studied live closer to a mental hospital than either of the other groups. As far as we were able to determine, the Yorubas in this area have as good a chance of receiving hospitalization as do people in Nova Scotia and probably a better chance than the Eskimos. The Yoruba rate includes two out of nine people who had been treated in a hospital and then returned to the community. The same is true of the one Eskimo individual with a psychotic pattern. Where Stirling County is concerned the one individual discovered in the community sample had not been hospitalized. This suggests that the difference cannot be dismissed on account of the hospital question. I am, therefore, inclined to believe that there is something different about the psychiatric profile of the group of Yorubas we studied. Many of us look upon the psychotic pattern as more noxious than the psychoneurotic and psychophysiologic. It is worth noting that the Yorubas had the lowest rates in the more benign categories as opposed to the highest in the psychotic pattern. The Yorubas were, on the whole, the healthiest of the three populations and the least prone to mild disorders. When a Yoruba becomes ill, apparently, he exhibits serious symptoms.

The greatest obstacle to exploring the meaning of this difference is, of course, the smallness of numbers. Of the 677 individuals in this study, only 11 are involved in the psychotic pattern differences (one Eskimo woman, one Nova Scotian man, six Yoruba men, and three Yoruba women). The Eskimo woman was evaluated as having a schizophrenic pattern, the Nova Scotian man an affective pattern, four of the Yorubas as "psychotic other," one as puerperal, two as schizophrenic, and two as schizophrenic with paranoid symptoms.[10] This degree of heterogeneity within a small number of people gives very little to go on in establishing what kind of a difference exists among the Yorubas. And the role of culture is an open question. We could not go very far in suggesting, for example, that Yoruba culture engenders or tolerates psychotic thinking by virtue of widely held magical beliefs. Magical beliefs are equally common among the Eskimos.

The cultural approach that seems to have the greatest probability of being useful is a stress model. It appeared to us that sociocultural stress was a factor in the Yoruba group due to rapid cultural change and modernization. Furthermore, it impinged to a greater degree on men than on women. Another form of stress, also more pronounced for males than females, stemmed from the cultural commitment to seniority in that it deprived many men, especially young and middle-aged men, of social prestige and power. This was especially the case for those who had acquired education or modern skills.

It is worth noting that there was a slightly higher prevalence of psychiatric disorders of all kinds (not just definite cases as given here) among the Yoruba men sampled as compared to Yoruba women. In addition, certain indicators of cultural change were significant regarding prevalence among men (Murphy, forthcoming). Looking solely at the psychotic pattern among the Yorubas, the male-female difference is much more pronounced. Twice as many men as women are in this group. It would seem worthwhile, therefore, to consider sociocultural stresses of the kinds suggested above as potentially involved in why the Yorubas, especially the men, have a high rate of the psychotic pattern.

The mental deficiency differences are significant at the .05 level with the Stirling population having the greatest amount (4 percent), the Eskimos next (2 percent), and the Yorubas least (.5 percent). Just as it was important to consider hospitals in interpreting the psychotic pattern, it is necessary to assess educational institutions here. We used performance in school and social roles as the main criterion for the mental deficiency pattern. We did not use I.Q. testing. It is not surprising, therefore, that the findings about the mental deficiency pattern parallel exactly the average level of educational achievement in the three cultural groups. In Stirling County, it is eighth grade; among these Eskimos, fourth grade; and among these Yorubas, it was less than two years in school for the men and virtually no schooling for the women. Attendance at school was compulsory at the time of investigation of the Stirling and Eskimo groups, though this did not necessarily apply to the older members of the study populations.

In view of the reliance on school performance and the differences in educational norms, I believe the mental deficiency differences to be in the method rather than in the populations. It seems evident that in a cultural group where education is widespread or compulsory, clear-cut cases of mental deficiency are more visible than elsewhere.

Turning to the sociopathic pattern, we have the only instance in which the Eskimos had a higher rate than the other two groups (Eskimo, 4 percent; Stirling, 2 percent; and Yoruba, .5 percent). Although this is not statistically significant if we use the .05 level, it is the next most prominent difference after the psychotic and mental deficiency patterns.

In view of the control of data for confidence of psychiatric judgment and seriousness of the disorder, this category concerns mainly frank abuse of alcohol, flagrant promiscuity, and deviant behaviors that warrant legal action. It raises the issue of cultural differences in the availability and use of penal institutions, a matter somewhat comparable to what was said before regarding hospitals or schools.

Each of the groups is served by a legal system that practices incarceration. Among the three study populations, 2 of the 14 individuals evaluated as sociopathic had been in jail, and both of them were Eskimo. As far as we are able to assess, there were no differential or prejudicial practices which exposed one of these groups more than the others to legal sanctions. In the two Eskimo cases, it was not a matter of the long arm of the law reaching out to take in offenders against the larger and more powerful Western society. It was a matter of the offenders' fellow Eskimos calling for help and protection. I was told by Eskimos that in the olden days when one displayed bad character, as they thought was involved in these cases, one would have been quietly pushed off the ice.

Since alcohol plays a role in the sociopathic differences, we should also look at cultural patterns regarding drinking. Among these rural Yorubas, palm wine is undoubtedly the most common form of alcohol taken; there are no governmental regulations regarding either its production or use; and there is minimal cost connected with making it. The two Yorubas who were evaluated as having a sociopathic pattern were men for whom palm wine was a factor.

In Nova Scotia, liquor is sold through provincially regulated stores.

However, access to these stores is fairly easy, and all types of liquor are consumed. Three men and three women in the Nova Scotia sample were evaluated as having the sociopathic pattern. With each of the men and one of the women, alcohol misuse was the main feature.

A self-imposed prohibition against the importation and use of alcohol had been instituted for the Eskimos on the island at the turn of the century. Alcohol was not therefore legally available, but some Eskimos bought or were given spirits (especially beer) by soldiers from a nearby installation. Three men and four women in the Eskimo group were found to have a sociopathic pattern; but alcohol figured in only two cases, and they were women who were friendly with the soldiers.

The prohibition against alcohol has undoubtedly made the recent history of these Eskimos quite unlike many Indian and Eskimo groups among whom drinking is a serious problem. It seems likely that the socio-cultural stress of entering the mainstream of American lifeways, including the fact of entering the larger society at the lowest levels of economic security, has something to do with the overuse of alcohol among native groups (Jessor et al., 1968). The control of alcohol among the St. Lawrence Island Eskimos was beginning to break down at the time of this study. Perhaps also the tightness of control was one reason for sociopathic patterns to be somewhat more common among the Eskimos than the other groups compared here. In the Eskimo case, the stresses of cultural change, the contrast with the dominant society, the deterioration of the traditional Eskimo values, and the disintegration of community processes, all did seem related to why there was an outcropping of behavior directed against social norms and in disregard of customary patterns.

Conclusion

In terminating this paper, I would like to refer to the fields of culture and personality and of psychiatric epidemiology, both of which are involved in the kind of problem and analysis I have discussed.

The main point of the culture-personality idea has been that the culture in which an individual grows up has pertinence for personality functioning, that is, for the basic, normal patterns of personality development and expression characteristic of that cultural group. By extension, it has come to be thought that culture would also have relevance for personality malfunction as exhibited in psychiatric symptomatology. The first of these has not been touched upon in this paper. We are not here concerned with depth psychology nor depth cultural interpretation but with manifest behaviors of psychiatric interest. Cultural difference has not stood up as a major factor at this level.

Implicit in a cross-cultural presentation of epidemiological findings are the questions, "Does culture cause psychiatric disorder?" and "Does a particular culture cause a particular psychiatric disorder?" Firm answers are clearly still unknown. If asked for my most carefully thought-out response (insofar as evidence from these studies pertains), I would say this. Culture probably does play a role in the causing of psychiatric disorder, but it is not one specific culture as opposed to another that attracts attention as a causative factor but human culture everywhere having a rather remarkably similar influence on the amount and kinds of disorder. Universal cultural processes of change and disintegration produce stress which is linked, in turn, to some disorders found in all groups.

Culture certainly cannot be ignored as context for understanding individual psychiatric cases or psychiatric prevalence rates. That one culture protects the members of its groups from psychiatric disorders while another culture causes its members to have disorder is the kind of interpretation that is called in question. Thus, to suggest that a particular culture causes a particular disorder is speculation far beyond the data. Nonetheless, it remains an intriguing question worthy of further work as to why, in this large arena of similarity, one group such as the Yorubas has a greater amount of the psychotic pattern and another group such as the Eskimos has a greater amount of the sociopathic pattern when, in many regards, both groups are experiencing the sociocultural stresses of modernization.

METHODOLOGICAL NOTE

The emphasis of the Harvard Program in Social Psychiatry has been on estimating true rather than treated prevalence of psychiatric disorder. We have made use of hospital and public records wherever possible. Our approach, however, has been to interview and observe representative samples of subjects from the communities and to gather systematic data from other persons selected for their knowledge about the subjects' social adjustment as well as their physical and psychiatric history.

In order to obtain the same information on each subject, we developed a structured interview schedule that can be administered by nonpsychiatrists. It consists of questions about symptoms of psychiatric interest. The information gathered is processed by what we term a "psychiatric evaluation." In such an evaluation, two psychiatrists first independently and later jointly organize the data and make a series of judgments. At the first level, these judgments concern the presence or absence of "detailed symptom patterns" that are later grouped into "major symptom patterns." For example, the psychiatrist decides whether the subject ever had cardiovascular or gastrointestinal symptoms (as detailed patterns) under the major heading of a psychophysiologic symptom pattern and whether the subject ever had symptoms of anxiety or depression (again as detailed patterns) under the major heading of psychoneurotic. For the detailed patterns assessed to be present, the psychiatrist then makes four other judgments: (1) whether the symptom pattern is currently experienced or was experienced only in the past; (2) the duration of its being experienced (3) the amount of impairment attributable to it; and (4) the psychiatrist's confidence that the pattern is indeed present and the symptoms appropriately categorized.

Up to this point, the psychiatrists have evaluated symptom patterns separately. As a final operation, he offers two overall judgments that concern the person as a whole. One is his answer to the question, "Is this person a psychiatric case?" His response is a measure of confidence in his judgment and is recorded as: "A" meaning definitely a psychiatric case, "B" meaning probably a psychiatric case, "C" meaning doubtful, and "D" meaning definitely not a case. The second is his estimate of the amount of impairment the subject exhibits in familial, occupational, and social functioning. This estimation is recorded as: "none" meaning no impairment, "minimal" meaning some but not significant impairment, "mild" meaning 20 percent to 30 percent, "moderate" meaning 30 percent to 50 percent, and "severe" meaning over 50 percent of the subject's total life space impaired due to psychiatric symptoms. For many purposes, it is useful to combine the two judgments concerning the person as a whole in order to show in one measure confidence of caseness, impairment, and the implication of certain symptom patterns.

For this, we developed a "Typology of Need for Psychiatric Attention." The typology consists of five categories: I, Most abnormal. "A" cases, i.e., definitely psychiatric cases with either (a) psychosis, brain syndrome, epilepsy, or mental deficiency as major symptom patterns or (b) a rating of moderate or more overall impairment irrespective of which kind of major symptom pattern is involved. II, Psychiatric disorder with significant impairment. "A" cases with mild overall impairment, mild being considered significant but not included in Type I. III, Probable psychiatric disorder. "A" cases with minimal impairment and "B" cases, i.e., probable psychiatric cases. IV, Doubtful. "C" cases. V, Probably well. "D" cases, i.e., cases in which the psychiatrist is confident that the subject is not a psychiatric case.

For the presentation of cross-cultural findings reported here, I have used this typology, because it gives a grouping of subjects so that all the main psychiatric judgments are engaged in one summary. In order to draw out definite and noteworthy cases, I have only those individuals designated as Type I or Type II.

ACKNOWLEDGMENTS

The work reported here has been conducted as part of the Harvard Program (formerly Cornell Program) in Social Psychiatry and has been supported through funds provided by the Milbank Memorial Fund, the Carnegie Corporation of New York, the Ford Foundation, the National Institute of Mental Health, the Dominion Provincial Mental Health Grants of Canada, the Social Science Research Council, and the Agency for International Development. The foundations are not, of course, the authors, publishers, or proprietors of this report and are not to be understood as approving by virtue of their grants any of the statements made or views expressed herein.

NOTES

1. The outline is a paraphrase of that in Leighton and Hughes (Murphy), 1961:343–58.
2. Numerous people have contributed to the work of the Harvard Program. Those mainly involved in the studies reported here are authors of the publications cited below.
3. See Leighton, 1959; Hughes et al., 1960; Leighton, D. C. et al., 1963.
4. See Murphy, 1960; Murphy and Leighton, 1965; Hughes et al., 1960; Murphy, 1964.
5. See Leighton, A. H. et al., 1963; Leighton and Murphy, 1963; Leighton and Murphy, 1955.
6. The results of the 1962 study in Stirling County have not previously been published. They are used here rather than the 1952 study (as reported in the three volumes listed above) because the sample of Stirling Communities in 1962 was made in the same fashion as the sample of Yoruba villages in 1961. The similarity in sampling and the proximity in time of investigation make the use of these data appropriate for comparison.
7. See Srole et al., 1962; Hollingshead and Redlich, 1958; Taylor and Chave, 1964. An example of an epidemiologic study in which age is inversely related to prevalence is found in Parker and Kleiner, 1966.
8. The psychiatric terms used here follow those of American Psychiatric Association, 1952. An explanation of their adaptation for this research is given in Leighton, 1959:93–129.
9. Symptom patterns in which the psychiatrists had medium confidence are retained in this analysis. It is not infrequent for a psychiatrist to have high confidence that a person is a psychiatric case (Types I and II cases are such) but have only medium confidence in his evaluation of one or more of the symptom patterns.
10. The psychiatrists had high confidence in their evaluation of the Eskimo, medium confidence regarding the Nova Scotian, and high confidence regarding five of the Yorubas and medium confidence about the remaining four Yorubas.

REFERENCES

American Psychiatric Association. 1952. Diagnostic and statistical manual of mental disorders. Washington, D.C.

Hollingshead, A. B., and F. C. Redlich. 1958. Social class and mental illness: a community study. New York, John Wiley and Sons.

Hughes, C. C., with the collaboration of J. M. Murphy. 1960. An Eskimo village in the modern world. Ithaca, Cornell University Press.

Hughes, C. C. et al. 1960. People of Cove and Woodlot. New York, Basic Books, Inc.

Jessor, R., T. D. Graves, R. C. Hansom, and S. L. Jessor. 1968. Society, personality and deviant behavior: A study of a tri-ethnic community. New York, Holt, Rinehart and Winston, Inc.

Leighton, A. H. 1959. My name is legion. New York, Basic Books, Inc.

Leighton, A. H., and J. M. Murphy. 1963. Yoruba concepts of psychiatric disorder. *In* Causes of mental disorders: A review of epidemiological knowledge, 1959. New York, Milbank Memorial Fund.

Leighton, A. H., and J. M. Murphy. 1963. Yoruba concepts of psychiatric disorder. *In* First Pan-African Psychiatric Conference. T. A. Lambo, ed. Ibadan, Nigeria, Government Printer.

Leighton, A. H., and J. M. Murphy. 1965. The problem of cultural distortation. *In* Comparability in international epidemiology, studies and techniques. R. M. Archeson, ed. New York, Milbank Memorial Fund.

Leighton, A. H., et al. 1963. Psychiatric disorder among the Yoruba: A report of the Cornell-Aro Mental Health Research Project. Ithaca, Cornell University Press.

Leighton, D. C. et al. 1963. The character of danger. New York, Basic Books, Inc.

Lin, T. Y. 1953. A study of the incidence of mental disorder in Chinese and other cultures. Psychiatry 16:313–36.

Mishler, E. G., and N. A. Scotch. 1965. Sociocultural factors in the epidemiology of schizophrenia. International Journal of Psychiatry 1:258–305.

Murphy, J. M. 1960. An epidemiological study of psychopathology in an Eskimo village, Ph.D. dissertation, Cornell University.

———. 1964. Psychotherapeutic aspects of shamanism on St. Lawrence Island, Alaska. *In* Magic, faith, and healing: Cross-cultural studies in psychotherapy. A. Kiev, ed. New York, Glencoe Free Press.

———. (In Press). Sociocultural change and mental illness among rural Yorubas. Proceedings of the Second Pan-African Psychiatric Congress.

Murphy, J. M., and A. H. Leighton. 1965. Native conceptions of psychiatric disorder. *In* Approaches to cross-cultural psychiatry. J. M. Murphy and A. H. Leighton, eds. Ithaca, Cornell University Press.

Parker, S., and R. J. Kleiner. 1966. Mental illness in the urban negro community. New York, The Free Press.

Srole, L., et al. 1962. Mental health in the metropolis: the Midtown Manhattan study vol. I. New York, McGraw-Hill Book Company, Inc.

Taylor, L., and S. Chave. 1964. Mental health and environment. London, Longmans, Green and Co., Ltd.

15. Variations in the Motivational Antecedents of Achievement among Hawaii's Ethnic Groups

RONALD GALLIMORE, Ph.D.

Department of Psychology and
Social Science Research Institute
University of Hawaii
Honolulu, Hawaii

IT IS BY NO MEANS novel to suggest that n Achievement may be unrelated to achievement in some cultures. DeVos (1968) has written that it is ethnocentric to dismiss as irrelevant other motivational antecedents of achievement. To illustrate this point, he cites the importance of affiliative motives among achievers in Japan, where striving for success is motivated more often by a concern for the reaction of others than by the pursuit of what we would consider self-satisfaction. In short, the correlation between n Achievement, as defined by McClelland (1961), and achievement may hold only among those cultures that train children to seek self-rewards as opposed to familial and social rewards.

This distinction between types of rewards is an explicit component of the McClelland definition of n Achievement; that is, the inclination to evaluate one's performance against an "internalized" standard of excellence. The standard of excellence may be externally specified as well, but presumably for the n achiever, maximum achievement satisfactions occur when he personally judges his performance to be successful, independent of the reactions of those whose opinions he may nevertheless value. This characteristically Western view of psychological motivation and achievement is, from DeVos's perspective (1968; 363), "too much dependent on an individualistically motivated" conception of human nature to provide the basis for a transcultural theory. Among the Japanese, for example, the pursuit of purely personal satisfaction is likely to be viewed as a "sign of excessive immoral egoism" (DeVos, 1968; 359) whereas rewards that the society can bestow to foster achievement, the pursuit of excellence, and the dedication to duty are qualities that characterize nineteenth- and twentieth-century Japanese culture.

Evidence for the notion that achievement may be fostered by varying motives can be found in psychological as well as anthropological sources. For example, Crandall (1963) developed a scheme which divided achievers into (1) those with autonomous achievement standards and (2) those with reflective achievement standards. Children and adults with the former are internally motivated, and the latter are approval motivated. Similarly, Atkinson and O'Connor (1966) have reported that in the presence of a salient social incentive, and on certain tasks, high affiliation, low achievement motivated individuals can be induced to behave as high n achievers. These writers, of course, have confined their observations to North America, but there are striking parallels between their conclusions and those DeVos has offered.

The hypothesis that there are cultural variations in the motivational antecedents of achievement has to date generated limited systematic research. There are a variety of reasons for this investigatory lag, but one of the most significant has been the problem of developing a culturally unbiased definition of achievement. The distress many observers feel about the Western conceptions emerges in large measure from the explicitly narrow and culturally bound definitions of achievement and achievement motivation such schemes employ. No doubt, it may be eminently practical as well as interesting to study modernization or Western-type economic striving among non-Western peoples. However, the validation of a transcultural theory of psychological motivation almost certainly cannot rest on culturally biased definitions of achievement.

More relevant to the purpose of this presentation than psychological discussions on motivation are anthropological objections to the extension of largely North American derived conceptions of motive and motivational dispositions, such as n Achievement, to non-Western cultures in particular. Empirical analyses are clearly in order, but before introducing some recent investigations conducted among Hawaii's non-Western ethnic groups (Gallimore and Howard, 1969; Gallimore and Howard, 1968; Kubany, Gallimore, and Buell, 1969; Sloggett, Gallimore, and Kubany, 1969), it will be necessary to discuss some basic conceptions as applied in this paper.

The term n achievement is applied to scores derived by a method detailed by McClelland, Atkinson, Clark, and Lowell (1953) for classifying fantasy responses elicited in story form by the Thematic Apperception Test (Murray, 1938) and other so-called projective measures. Validation of n Achievement as an operational definition of achievement motivation rested initially on comparing stories written under achievement arousing condi-

tions with productions written under neutral conditions. Subsequent validation efforts included investigations of the relation of fantasy *n* Achievement
to nonfantasy achievement (Atkinson and Feather, 1966). Nonfantasy
measures, or operational definitions of *n* Achievement, have been developed
(Atkinson, 1958) but have been employed much less frequently than the
TAT. Although few constructs can match either the appeal or the empirical
support enjoyed by *n* Achievement, for many North American psychologists its status as a motive or a motivational disposition remains in dispute
(Brown, 1965; Klinger, 1966).

A motive is a hypothetical construct generated by an observer to
account for behavior directed toward a goal; on the other hand, motivational dispositions are defined either in terms of the frequency, or
intensity, or both, with which particular classes of motives are observed to be
operative or aroused. Klinger (1966, 292) said, "Motivational dispositions
are assumed to be reflected in behavior only when the corresponding motives
have been 'aroused' or 'engaged' by theoretically specifiable stimuli of either
external or internal origin. Once aroused, the motive is thought to energize
behavior, both overt motor and covert symbolic behavior, that has been
established in the reinforcement history of the organism as instrumental in
attaining a relevant goal object." Fantasy behavior is presumed to result from
motive arousal under conditions in which there is no opportunity to seek
and/or attain a relevant goal.

Variations on this view of motive and motivational dispositions are
widely held among North American psychologists specifically interested in
n Achievement, such as Atkinson (1954, 84), who echoes the McClelland
group. "The arousal of a motive is equivalent to the arousal of a family of
perceptual and instrumental response dispositions whose strength may be
accounted for in terms of the principles of associative learning. . . . The
arousal of a motive, then, mediates the arousal of perceptual and instrumental
response dispositions. . . ."

Motives are fictions created by observers as mediates between
instrumental behaviors of various frequencies and intensities and specified
cues and thus round out the motivation triumvirate. In the case of the
achievement motive, individual differences in the motivation to achieve
(motivational disposition) are assessed most often by determining the extent
to which a person's TAT fantasy productions fit the scoring categories outlined by McClelland, Atkinson, Clark, and Lowell (1953). The varieties of
cues that are presumed to arouse the achievement motive and thereby increase the amount of fantasy *n* Achievement an individual produces in the
typical TAT testing session are described by McClelland et al. as: (1) cues in
the everyday environment and cues in relatively autonomous thought
processes of the individual; (2) specific experimentally introduced cues; (3)
controllable cues in a particular picture.

Our research was based on the assumptions outlined in the above
paragraphs. As our investigations continued, however, we began to question

the usefulness of hypothetical motivational constructs in cross-cultural research. Our doubts concerning the usefulness of the motive concept were by no means original, and the sources which have influenced us will be clearly evident (Bandura and Walters, 1963; Dollard and Miller, 1950; Klinger, 1966; Staats, 1963; Sechrest and Wallace, 1967; Wallace, 1967; Walters and Parke, 1964).

Background of Research

In 1966 my colleague, Alan Howard, and I began a study of socialization and related behavioral development of an indigenous Hawaiian group in Hawaii. We centered our efforts on a single rural community with a large proportion of individuals of Hawaiian descent. We have described the community and the research samples in detail elsewhere (Gallimore and Howard, 1968, pp. 1–2).

Americans of Hawaiian descent are best considered part-Hawaiian. Virtually all have some Hawaiian ancestry but few can be considered "pure" Hawaiians. Most identify themselves as Hawaiian plus one or more other ethnic groups, the others usually being Chinese, Filipino, Japanese, Portuguese, Korean, Puerto Rican, or *haole* (i.e., Caucasian). They speak a colloquial dialect of English, often described as "pidgin," which includes some words from Hawaiian as well as a few from other languages. Hawaiian is spoken by a minority, most of whom are elderly; in general, there is little familiarity with the old culture.

In 1960, 100,000 persons with Hawaiian blood (10,000 Hawaiians [a recent study indicates this to be a vastly inflated estimate of the number of pure Hawaiians (Schmitt, 1967)] and 90,000 part-Hawaiians) comprised 17 % of the State population and were the third ranking ethnic group. Their number would have been larger if 20,000 had not left the state in the previous ten years.

They are a very young group with an equal distribution of men and women. The median age for Hawaiian and part-Hawaiian males was 16 years, the lowest of all the major races.

Seventy per cent of the Hawaiian and part-Hawaiian group were estimated to be living in the city of Honolulu, where, by residence, they were the most widely and evenly distributed of all racial groups. "Full" Hawaiians were concentrated in such economically undeveloped areas as Kohala and Kona on the island of Hawaii, Hana on Maui, Koolauloa on Oahu, the island of Niihau, and parts of Molokai. More than ten per cent reside on Hawaiian homestead lands and in public housing projects throughout the state. Fifty per cent or more Hawaiian blood is required in order to qualify for Hawaiian homestead lands. The 1960 total population on Hawaiian homesteads was 8,420. Of the 4,018 families living in public housing projects in 1960, 1,481, or 34%, were Hawaiian and part-Hawaiian.

Although the major purpose of our over-all research is a general study of Hawaiian culture, community, and behavior, our data were collected in a single community. The reason behind this choice was simple: when we began there was little published material on the Hawaiian population and we had no reasonable basis for deciding who was culturally a Hawaiian. As a consequence, we chose a community in which there is a large proportion of individuals with Hawaiian ancestry, many of whom are living on land set aside for persons who could demonstrate to the Department of Hawaiian Home Lands that they are 50 % or more Hawaiian. Thus, if an individual was the lessee of a homestead lot in 'Aina Pumehana,[1] he was considered by our working definition to be Hawaiian. It is clear that this is not the only possible definition, given the diverse circumstances under which the Hawaiian population lives.

On a variety of indices the people of 'Aina Pumehana as well as the entire Hawaiian population of the state are overrepresented: among the indices are rates of deviance, school failure, unemployment, health problems, and most of the other characteristics generally used to describe an impoverished group in the United States. These kinds of data almost exhaust what had been reported at the time we initiated our research; for a variety of reasons, we chose to avoid a problem oriented investigation and, instead, simply studied Hawaiians.

The project was begun in proper anthropological style with a full year of participant observation; although this method was practiced throughout the research, at the beginning of the second year we initiated a hypothesis-testing phase which continues to the present. A major strategy has been the use of a wide variety of methods both in the generation and testing of hypotheses.

The Distribution of *n* Achievement among Ethnic Groups in Hawaii

As we planned our research in 'Aina Pumehana, it seemed almost mandatory that *n* Achievement be included as a variable of interest not only because of its currency, but also because Hawaiians are characteristically regarded as low achievers in all spheres of life, save perhaps rates of deviance. Thus, the hypothesis that poor achievement, for example in the schools, could be accounted for in the Hawaiian case by low levels of *n* Achievement was almost inevitable. Certainly nothing in the ethnographic phase of the project suggested otherwise, and with something less than firm conviction that the obvious required testing, we set out to carefully evaluate the relative status of Hawaiians on a fair measure of *n* Achievement.

Awareness that the explicit facial cues in the TAT cards employed by McClelland and his associates were inappropriate for cross-racial and cultural comparisons of *n* Achievement had already stimulated the development of a less obviously biased measure (Merbaum, 1961; Minigione, 1965), thus granting us two advantages; first, a saving of valuable time and second, a set of norms for a less racially biased measure of *n* Achievement than the TAT against which to compare the Hawaiian samples. Minigione, following an exacting psychometric procedure, developed a set of twelve pictures; these stimuli were line drawings of scenes such as a boy sitting at a desk, a boy standing on a street corner, etc. From the set, six were selected for the Hawaii study on the basis of the absence of cues not common to the local environment, e.g., a man on a farm tractor. Otherwise, such cues as skin color, facial features, clothing styles, and so forth were effectively eliminated; copies of these six pictures have been reported by Ruth Finney to be satisfactory stimuli in the eastern highlands of New Guinea.

Although data were obtained on the Minigione pictures from a variety of age groups and for both males and females, attention will be confined here to high school males, as this is the group for whom some have suggested a fantasy measure of *n* Achievement is most appropriate (Klinger, 1966). For these high school boys, the TAT-like device was administered in a group setting at their respective schools; the instructions presented to the samples were copies from those reported by Minigione (1965). Each of the six pictures for which stories were written was reproduced on a separate page and accompanied by the four questions ordinarily used by *n* Achievement researchers including Minigione. Method of scoring conformed to the standard procedure, and the reliability of scoring was assessed by comparison of scores assigned by an experienced graduate student to stories scored by expert scorers as reported in Atkinson (1958). The degree of reliability was highly satisfactory, ranging from .80 to .94.

As Sloggett, Gallimore, and Kubany (1969) have reported, the Hawaiian groups scored lower on fantasy *n* Achievement for each of the four groups of high school boys; the data was ranked in order of magnitude and grouped to illustrate significant statistical differences. Thus, Table 1 shows the Hawaiian groups to be significantly lower in *n* Achievement than the remaining comparison groups, the Japanese and Filipinos.

Of particular interest is the absence of *n* Achievement within the urban Hawaiian sample; this group was obtained from a private school estab-

Table 1:   Mean Score Showing *n* Achievement in Four
Groups of Boys

Group	n	M	SD*
Rural Japanese	13	4.77	3.92
Rural Filipino	15	4.13	4.12
Urban Hawaiians	48	2.86	
Rural Hawaiians	32	1.72	2.23
('Aina Pumehana)			

$p < .001$

* No significant difference

Table 2:   Percentage of Boys Writing
at least One Story with *n*
Achievement Theme

Group	Percentage
Rural Japanese	69
Rural Filipino	67
Urban Hawaiian	46
Rural Hawaiian ('Aina Pumehana)	44

lished in the last century specifically for children of Hawaiian descent. The school currently selects for admission only those youngsters who meet high academic standards. It is evident that the picture of stimuli elicits little *n* Achievement fantasy from Hawaiian high school boys, good students or not. An even more striking illustration of the differences among the samples is presented in Table 2 which contains the percentage of boys within each ethnic group who wrote at least one story containing at least one achievement theme.

This method of arranging the data produces a rank order identical to that reflected in the mean scores reported in Table 1. These percentages illustrate clearly that the differences between ethnic groups in mean *n* Achievement shown in Table 1 are not statistical artifacts as might be suspected from the gross differences in variability reflected by the standard deviations also presented in Table 1. Recorded in Table 3 are the percentages of boys, within each ethnic group, who wrote 1, 2, 3, 4, 5, 6, or no stories with an *n* Achievement theme. Again the data indicate that fewer Hawaiian boys write fewer stories with *n* Achievement themes.

These data made explanation of the indifferent academic behavior of the 'Aina Pumehana Hawaiian youths a relatively simple matter. The boys are regarded by the schools not only as notoriously poor scholars (more than 75 percent of the population scored below the 25 percentile on a commonly used test of academic achievement) but unmotivated as well. Indeed, our ethnographic analysis of child rearing and socialization corroborated the results of the *n* Achievement study. Hawaiian youngsters have little *n* Achievement due to particular child-rearing practices of Hawaiian parents. This is a neat and tidy explanation if one is willing to ignore the question of what does motivate the youngsters of 'Aina Pumehana other than *n* Achievement. After all, they obviously are motivated to do some things, and among the group, there are some youngsters who do well in school.

Table 3: Percentage of Boys Writing Various Numbers of *n* Achievement Themes

Group	Number of Themes						
	0	1	2	3	4	5	6
Rural Japanese	31	15	54	0	0	0	0
Rural Filipino	33	33	20	13	0	0	0
Urban Hawaiian	54	31	13	2	0	0	0
Rural Hawaiian	56	41	3	0	0	0	0

We had accepted unwittingly a deficiency explanation of behavior. That is, we had concluded that Hawaiians fail in school because they lack *n* Achievement. As we have noted elsewhere (Gallimore and Howard, 1968, 5), such a conceptualization does not explain why Hawaiians behave as they do; at best, it may merely explain why they do not behave like middle-class Caucasians, the population within which the *n* Achievement construct has been most thoroughly validated. Thus, it is not a question of doubting the findings that Hawaiians do not write *n* Achievement themes, although the validity of our method can be challenged, but rather it is the issue of whether a simple intergroup comparison is a sufficient base upon which to build a theory of achievement behavior for a particular ethnic group. Thus, we set out to determine what motive, if not *n* Achievement, was important among Hawaiians, independent of the other groups.

Also at issue is the handicap imposed by the use of a purely verbal measure. Inspection of the *n* Achievement test protocols reveals that Hawaiians, particularly those in 'Aina Pumehana, wrote shorter stories than the other groups in the Hawaii sample. Although we have not made the test, it is likely that there is a correlation between story length and *n* Achievement for the Hawaii samples as has been found among other groups (Minigione, 1965). Thus, with this verbal handicap issue in mind, we elected to follow up the projective test study with an investigation that would allow not only an intragroup analysis of the relevance of *n* Achievement among Hawaiians but also permit a cross-cultural or intergroup comparison on a more behavioral and less verbal measure.

The first problem we addressed was the question of what motives are important to Hawaiians. Once we stumbled onto this issue of what motives other than *n* Achievement might potentially be used to account for variations in achievement within the Hawaiian group, the problem was readily solved. Both the ethnographic evidence and the studies of early socialization (Gallimore and Howard, 1968, 1969; Gallimore, Howard, and Jordan, 1969; Jordan, 1967) had clearly indicated that affiliative concerns are focal to any description of Hawaiian behavior and behavioral development.

Curiously, a study by Atkinson and O'Connor (1966) using North American college students contributed to our hypothesis about Hawaiians. In their study, and to their evident surprise, a high *n* Affiliation existed— low achievement motivated individuals were induced to behave in an achievement oriented fashion when social approval was available. As they concluded, "This hypothesis means that a person in whom the achievement motive is very weak (i.e., a person who produces very little imagery having to do with excellence of performance in thematic apperceptive stories under neutral conditions) might display all of the behavioral symptoms of 'an entrepreneurial risk-taker' if some extrinsic reward like love or money, for which he does have a strong motive, were offered as a general inducement for performance" (Atkinson and Feather, 1966, 317–18). It appeared that for some persons what matters is social approval and not competition with a standard of excellence; such persons would presumably be more concerned with what others thought of their performance than what they thought themselves. The parallel with DeVos's argument is striking. We, thus, undertook a test of the notion that affiliative motivation, and not achievement motivation, represents a more significant factor in accounting for achievement among Hawaiians.

It will be necessary to review first the elaboration of the theory of achievement motivation outlined by Atkinson and Feather (1966). Although it is the earlier work of McClelland on fantasy n Achievement that is best known outside of psychology, it has been Atkinson and his associates (e.g., Atkinson, 1957; Atkinson and Feather, 1966; Atkinson and Litwin, 1960; Atkinson and Reitman, 1960) who have addressed themselves most consistently to the study of nonfantasy achievement motivation. In the Atkinson-Feather theory of achievement motivation, n Achievement is only one element. In addition to n Achievement, which they generally term the need to achieve success (M_s), there is fear of failure or the motive to avoid failure (M_{af}). By subtracting an individual's score on a measure of fear of failure (usually a test anxiety questionnaire) from his n Achievement score (derived from the TAT), one obtains an index of resultant achievement motivation. Thus, Atkinson and Feather view achievement motivation as the joint function of an individual's motive to achieve success and avoid failure.

The present issue requires only a review of the conceptual reasons for the relation between resultant achievement motivation (RAM) and the commonly employed operational definition of achievement oriented behavior as the preference for tasks in which the probability of success is near 50 percent. Correlated with preference for intermediate risks (likelihood of success near 50 percent) is the inclination to seek accurate feedback on performance and to set goals in terms of past performance. Although the theoretical terms which the theory employs are somewhat abstract, the intuitive appeal of the assumption of a correlation between intermediate risk-taking and achievement motivation is rather strong. In effect, the Atkinson and Feather scheme implies that an achievement motivated individual, i.e., one high in RAM, prefers tasks which test his skill; when the chances of success are near 50 percent, he should experience the highest level of satisfaction since he will be more challenged by the task. More difficult tasks reduce the chances of success to a lucky break and, thus, offer no test for the achievement motivated person. Similarly, very easy tasks are of no interest since success provides little in the way of achievement gratification. Part of the theory obviously is an inverse relation between task difficulty and incentive value. The individual low in RAM, the failure avoidant individual whose fear of failure is greater than his n Achievement, is predicted by the theory to prefer extreme risks—either very easy ones which assure success and minimize failure or very difficult ones, failure in which can be attributed to the impossibility of the task ("How can you blame a fellow for failure when the task was so hard!").

For Hawaiians we predicted that n Affiliation, not resultant achievement motivation, would correlate with preference for intermediate risks. For the study, we constructed a mock airplane cockpit, consisting of a panel about two feet high and five feet long with an array of lights and controls obtained from aircraft surplus houses similar to that used in a previous study (Kensinger, 1967). In the center of the apparatus was a glass-covered aperture through which could be seen three small airplanes moving in a continuous circular manner. Situated in front of the apparatus was a joy stick taken from a fighter aircraft. On the panel a knob was prominently displayed with five gradations of difficulty clearly marked, "easy," "medium," and "hard," with the remaining two notches (between easy and medium, and medium and hard) unlabeled but arranged to make their intermediate status unambiguous. In order to enhance the credibility of the apparatus, it was labeled "property of USAF." It was anticipated that such a device would have as much appeal to the relatively nonverbal Hawaiian youths who were the focus of the study as a set of TAT pictures might for their more verbal comrades.

The participants (thirty-two Hawaiian high school males randomly selected from the 'Aina Pumehana school) were told that the purpose of the task was to manipulate the joy stick and the range finder in order to shoot down the airplanes viewed through the glass aperture. Located on the joy stick was a trigger which, when pulled, activated a bright red signal lamp beneath the circling airplanes; the subjects were told this red light simulated the firing of a projectile. If they had aligned their controls properly, a loud buzzer would sound, indicating a hit. If the red light was seen but no buzzer sounded, that was to be regarded as a miss.

The task was described as a test of ability to be an Air Force pilot and was used officially for such purposes. Pretesting with college students had indicated that the mock device was sufficiently impressive to make such an assertion credible. Accordingly, it was emphasized that hits or misses were due to the ability to align the controls properly and, therefore, represented a test of skill. In reality, hits and misses were controlled by the experimenter.

The sessions were run individually and in a uniform manner for all participants. Each individual was allowed 12 practice shots, 4 at each of the 3 levels of difficulty—easy, medium, and hard. In all cases, the practice trials began with the hard level for which no hits were obtained (light but no buzzer); then 4 shots at easy on which 4 hits were obtained (light plus buzzer); and finally 4 shots at the medium level on which hits were obtained for the first and last shots. These 12 shots permitted the boys to gain familiarity with the controls and the task in general as well as to establish the validity of the various levels of difficulty.

After the 12 practice shots, the real test began and each individual received 10 shots. It was explained that preceding each shot the subject was to select the difficulty level he wished to attain and then give his subjective probability of success. On a 5 x 8 card, the word probability was written, and the 11 choices running from 0 out of 10 through 10 out of 10 were explained and each boy tested for comprehension. Thus, for each of the 10 shots, the preferred difficulty level and the subjective probability for each boy was obtained. The boys themselves were asked to give what they thought were their chances of a hit; they were not asked to give their probabilities.

Since we were also interested in the effects of failure, no hits were given for the first five trials, thus making the subjective probability obtained on trial one the most unbiased estimate of preference for intermediate risks, operationally defined in terms of subjective probability. That is, given only the experience of the 12 practice shots and with the opportunity to select any of the five difficulty levels, the question was whether high affiliation motivated or high achievement motivated individuals would select inter- mediate risks (chance of success near 50 percent). Of course, it would be possible to examine preference for intermediate risks across the entire series of trials, but it was anticipated that Hawaiians, with repeated failure, would show a decreasing preference for probabilities near .50. The data on effects of failure are not discussed in the present paper (Gallimore and Howard, 1969). Following the five consecutive misses, all subjects were allowed five consecutive hits in order to eliminate any imputation of incompetence.

Administration of the Minigione picture stimuli and a measure of fear of failure had been completed previous to the experimental task, and the boys were not aware of the connection between the two. Scoring the protocols for *n* Achievement and *n* Affiliation (Atkinson, 1958, 685–773) was done by the same graduate student who worked on the study of fantasy *n* Achievement (Sloggett et al., 1969). The simplest format for presenting the data is illustrated in Table 4. By reporting the percent choice of .4, .5, and .6 for the three ethnic groups tested, it is evident that the mock airplane task differentiates the groups as might be expected.

While there is no important difference between the Japanese and the Caucasian groups, both are significantly greater than the Hawaiian group. Given the results of the fantasy *n* Achievement study, this is not surprising since the airplane device, regardless of its inherent attractiveness, is neverthe- less the sort of achievement task for which Hawaiians might reasonably be expected to have little motivation to strive for success.

To illustrate the stability of choice of subjective probability, Table 5 contains the preference for .4, .5, and .6 for the three ethnic groups for all ten trials; these are, of course, compounded by the uncounter-balanced series of failures and success. These percentages are based on trials and not boys; thus, for example, the basis for calculating the percentage for the Hawaiian group is 330 trials (10 trials per boy, 33 boys), of which 91 choices were .4, .5, or .6. The data cast in this fashion are virtually identical to those

Table 4: Percentage of Boys Selecting Subjective Probabilities on Mock Airplane Risk-taking on Trial 1

Group	N	Probabilities of 0.4, 0.5, and 0.6
Hawaiians	33	27
Caucasians	12	58
Japanese	20	50

Table 5: Percentage of Boys' Probability Choices in Ten Trials on the Mock Airplane Task

Group	Choices of 0.4, 0.5, and 0.6
Hawaiians	28
Japanese	52
Caucasians	54

Table 6: Correlations between Preference for Intermediate Risks and *n* Achievement, RAM, and *n* Affiliation for Hawaiian High School Boys on Trial 1*

Type of Motivation	Correlation
n Achievement	0.19†
Resultant Achievement Motivation	0.009†
n Affiliation	0.39‡

* The measure used in the correlations was absolute deviation from 0.5; that is, the greater the deviation from 0.5, the less preference for intermediate risks. This measure, absolute deviation, correlates 0.93 with preference for 0.4, 0.5, and 0.6 and for convenience is expressed in reversed form (in order to obtain positive correlations). In other words, a score of 5 is assigned the probability of 0.5, 4 to 0.4 and 0.6, and so forth.

† Nonsignificant, one-tailed test for Pearson product moment correlation.

‡ $p < .01$, one-tailed test for Pearson product moment correlation.

presented in Table 4. Statistical analyses support the same conclusions: no differences between Japanese and Caucasians, with Hawaiians significantly less likely than either to select an intermediate probability.

However, examination of the correlations between *n* Achievement and resultant achievement motivation (*n* Achievement minus fear of failure) and intermediate risk preference does not produce the expected relationship, as interpreted in Table 6. As predicted, Hawaiian high school boys who are affiliatively motivated, as measured by a TAT-type test, are more likely to select a task in which their respective subjective probabilities are near .5. It appears that DeVos's observations may apply to Hawaiians.

However, to conclude that the correlation of *n* Affiliation with intermediate risk-taking demonstrates not only the viability of the general proposition that there are cultural variations in the motivational antecedents of achievement, but also supports the specific hypothesis related to Hawaiians, requires several assumptions. First, is intermediate risk-taking a reasonable facsimile of the real-life instrumental behaviors typically used to infer the operation of a motivational disposition? Reactions to that question no doubt will be correlated with disciplinary identification and, perhaps, with sympathy in general for laboratory procedures in social science. Perhaps, the more important issue is whether the Atkinson-Feather achievement motivation theory, and thus the appropriateness of intermediate risk-taking as an operational definition of achievement oriented behavior, can be generalized beyond the North American groups for which it has been validated. Another issue is the salience of Hawaiians to perform well on a mock achievement task. Indeed, relative to Japanese and Caucasians, the Hawaiians may have been at a disadvantage if this task was a culture-bound measure as was the case with the projective measure.

Neither of these issues can be dealt with definitively, because adequate data are not available. However, there is a certain appeal to the strategy of assuming that particular instrumental behaviors, such as intermediate risk-taking, facilitate achievement independent of the nature of the achievement goal or the presumed motivational antecedent. Whether it is high need affiliation Filipinos seeking maximum gains at cockfights (although in that situation an intermediate risk might entail different anchor points) or high *n* Achievement North American college students selecting academic courses, preference for intermediate risks, accurate feedback on performance, and cautious goal-setting all could reasonably be assumed to be characteristic of those most motivated to succeed within any group. The proposition that cross-cultural comparisons can be usefully made on instrumental behaviors, such as those which Atkinson and Feather have used to define achievement oriented behavior, is an intriguing one and worthy of serious investigation. For the present, however, our focus is on motivational antecedents of achievement and related instrumental behaviors (achievement oriented behavior).

Situational Factors versus Motivational Dispositions

Among the most interesting implications of the notion that achievement may be motivated by such factors as *n* Affiliation is the prospect that more attention must be paid to situational variables than has been typical of most studies of *n* Achievement and achievement. It is probably that for those cultures which train children to strive in order to obtain familial and social rewards, situational cues ought to be more important determinants of achievement and achievement oriented behavior than internalized motivational dispositions. This observation prompted us to test the following hypothesis: for members of a cultural group for which social approval is a salient environmental cue, increases in the amount of achievement oriented behavior (preference for intermediate risks) can be obtained by manipulating the availability of social evaluation and, by implication, social approval (Kubany, Gallimore, and Buell, 1969).

The population selected to test this proposition was Filipinos living in Hawaii. The genesis was a pilot study [2] concerned with the values, behavioral patterns, and child-rearing practices of Filipinos. The student observers who participated in the pilot project repeatedly commented on the importance attached by their informants to social approval, interpersonal harmony, and fulfillment of the perceived expectations and needs of others. Social scientists working in the Philippines have similarly described the behavior of Filipinos (Guthrie, 1968; Guthrie and Jacobs, 1966; Lynch, 1964; Whiting, 1963). For example, Whiting observed that Filipinos were socialized to be responsive to the expectations of others and, in particular, to members of their nuclear and extended families. The behavioral continuities between Filipinos in their home country and in our Hawaiian sample were probably due in large measure to the relative isolation of the latter in a plantation community. Although increasing numbers of Filipinos are moving to urban areas in Hawaii, their relatively recent arrival from the Philippines, largely in the 1930's and 1940's, has temporarily resulted in enclaves of high density Filipino population.

Given the projective *n* Achievement study (Sloggett et al., 1969), it is reasonable to suggest that achievement for Filipinos may not be significantly affected by internalized motives. Although the evidence is sparse, it also appears that *n* Achievement is relatively unimportant among Filipinos living in the Philippines (Bulatao, 1964). Among Filipinos, high achievement in school may be important, if the ethnographic data are accurate, not so much for the self-satisfaction that it may generate but because such success will please others, bring honor to the family, and assure one's safety from the shame of public failure. It may be that achievement and achievement oriented behavior among Filipinos is more affected by situational cues than by intrinsic ones, i.e., a motivational disposition such as *n* Achievement. If this analysis is accurate, Filipinos ought to exhibit more achievement oriented behavior in a public surveillance as opposed to a private anonymous condition. That is, the presence of a potential dispenser of social evaluation may elicit increased achievement oriented behavior among Filipino subjects, if the experimental instructions make it clear that such behavior is socially appropriate and desirable.

To this end, 20 Filipino high school boys were given an opportunity to choose between an easy, medium, or difficult task before attempting to shoot down airplanes, using the same apparatus employed by Kensinger (1967). In this case, however, hits and misses were randomized in likelihood according to the following arrangement: medium level (50 percent), easy (80 percent), and hard (20 percent). Thus, in this study, the dependent variable was the frequency with which an individual selects the medium level of difficulty on each of ten trials. By randomizing the probability of success, we artificially manipulated subjective probability or expectation of success.

Pre-task instructions explicitly stated that striving to do well was highly desirable. The experimenter observed and scored half the subjects (the public condition); for the remaining half (the private condition), the experimenter remained out of sight during the task leading the subject to believe that the experimenter would not obtain knowledge of their scores.

Subjects in the public condition selected the medium difficulty level on the average of 7.5 times per 10 trials compared to 4.6 times in the private condition ($t = 2.55$, 18 df, $p < .01$, one-tailed). The experimenter's presence was clearly significant. But what of the intragroup differences? In this instance, we administered the Marlowe-Crowne Social Desirability Scale (MC-SD) which has been advanced as a measure of need for social approval and fear of disapproval (Crowne and Marlowe, 1964); for North American college students, scores on this scale have been reported to be significantly correlated with fantasy n Affiliation ($r = .55$). Assuming the MC-SD to be a measure of a transsituational motivational disposition to seek affiliative reinforcers, we asked which is more important for predicting preference for intermediate risks—affiliative motivation or situational factors? In fact, there was no correlation between the MC-SD in the private condition ($r = + .05$) and a slight, but nonsignificant, relation in the public condition ($r = + .28$). Thus, there was a minimal interaction between the presumed motivational disposition and the social cues in the sense that those individuals with greater need for approval were only slightly more likely to select the intermediate risk.

Implications and Conclusions

The data reported here underline several important issues. First, the evidence supports the long-standing anthropological view that there are many possible motives which explain why peoples of different cultures behave as they do. The results are by no means definitive, but they are of some use, because they reflect the complexity of the question.

The data also illustrate the potential danger of interpreting the meaning of intergroup psychometric comparisons in the absence of intra-group analyses. For the Hawaiians, the apparent correlation between their reputation for poor scholarship and the results of the projective *n* Achievement study led temporarily to what was an incomplete interpretation; the addition of the mock airplane task results, in spite of the probable character-istics of the measure, provided the intragroup correlations that altered rather dramatically our earlier conceptions of the motivational antecedents of achievement among Hawaiians. Perhaps the inter-/intragroup design should become a methodological rule in cross-cultural comparisons on personality measures.

Another possibility raised by the research reported here is the use of behavioral measures of achievement motivation in cross-cultural compari-sons. Preference for intermediate risks may represent a potentially useful variable in the study of achievement motivation in task or game behavior in various cultures. A recent study (Leffcourt, 1965) illustrates the point perhaps most clearly; he found that, on a gambling task, the usually obtained differences in preference for intermediate risks was reversed for Caucasians and Afro-Americans. Typically, blacks relative to whites have been shown to be nonachievement oriented or failure avoidant on risk-taking tasks in-volving skill (Altman, Ryssel, and Gallimore, 1966; Leffcourt and Ladwig, 1965). The results on the gambling task suggests a number of alternative explanations; blacks may have had more experience with gambling, blacks may have been less fearful of failure since success is a function of luck and not personal skill, etc. Whatever the explanation, the results support the notion that it may be possible to use intermediate risk preferences as a measure of interest in cross-cultural comparisons, provided one first assesses game and task preferences for each culture. As Premack (1965, 123–188) demonstrated in his studies of reinforcer effects on anatomically different responses, it is possible to develop a measure that is free of specific behavior bias. He used time to solve the problem. Perhaps Premack's work will serve as an analogue for developing preference for intermediate risk-taking as a measure in cross-cultural comparison.

Potentially more important is the implication that the long-standing emphasis in North American personality research on assessment of trans-situational dispositions may be inappropriate for those cultures in which extrinsic factors are regnant. If, for example, *n* Achievement and the associated assumptions about internalized motivation are irrelevant or are secondary factors in non-Western groups, as may be the case with Hawaiians, it will be necessary to attend more closely to situational variables such as the salience and availability of social rewards for achievement. Particularly relevant to the issue is Klinger's (1966) argument that situational determi-nants of achievement are at least as important, if not more so, than trans-situational dispositions. Although his analysis of the literature on achieve-ment and fantasy *n* Achievement is confined to studies of North Americans, the conclusions indirectly illustrate the importance of the relation between situational factors and achievement in non-*n* Achievement cultures.

In his review Klinger (1966) finds that the correlations between fantasy *n* Achievement (for North Americans) and molar, long-term performance, e.g., school grades, achievement test scores, etc., have been more often demonstrated and are a more reliable phenomenon than correlations between *n* Achievement and relatively brief task performance, e.g., verbal problem-solving tasks. For example, it appears that for college males who live at home, in contrast to those attending noncommuter schools, the relation between *n* Achievement and molar performance is greater. Further, in an experimental demonstration of the importance of situational determinants, Klinger (1967) found that simple visual exposure via closed circuit television to an experimenter giving *n* Achievement instructions was sufficient to increase the amount of fantasy *n* Achievement—that is, observing participants did not need to hear the presumably motive arousing instructions which McClelland et al. (1949) used in the original validation studies. Control groups which viewed a variety of instructions being given did not show increased TAT *n* Achievement. Klinger contends (1966, 304) that individuals who perform well have grown up in environments that encouraged good performance. Their environments have been rich in achievement cues, and they will have experienced more frequent achievement oriented perceptions, thoughts, and fantasies. Similarly, the social learning history of the individual will be closely connected with his performance in a variety of achievement areas; for example, those North American youngsters with successful parents, in terms of education and vocation, are themselves more likely to succeed.

Applied to cross-cultural questions, the Klinger position provides an appealing explanation for both the variations in what is regarded as worthy of achieving and the reasons which motivate individuals to achieve. The Hawaiian parent shapes his child to be responsive to the concerns and expectations of others; those children exposed to consistent training toward such an end will presumably be more responsive to affiliative and social rewards. If such consequences are made contingent on school performance, or intermediate risk-taking, or delinquency, then the individual will be motivated to achieve.

As psychologists have come to appreciate what their anthropologist colleagues may have always known, that situational determinants of behavior are at least as important as motivational dispositions, the search for alternative conceptions of motivation and personality has intensified. A recent and attractive view is the Wallace (1967, 56–64) conception of personality as a set of abilities including motivational components specifically. That is, in the course of socialization and maturation, the individual acquires a behavioral repertoire which equips him to operate with varying degrees of effectiveness in both familiar and novel settings. In Wallace's scheme, it is not assumed that an individual is predisposed to behave in a certain manner, say because he has a need to achieve, but rather the following questions are asked: (1)

is he able (i.e., has he learned how) to behave in an n Achievement fashion (tell n Achievement stories, pick intermediate risks) and (2) are the situational cues ones which elicit or suppress such behavior? Such a view avoids one of the major pitfalls of the transsituational disposition conception—once one has measured an individual's dispositional characteristics, a generalized predictive statement about future behavior relatively independent of specific situational factors presumably follows.

Wallace argues that the traditional approach tends to confuse the issue of an individual's ability with his volition to behave in a certain fashion; the distinction between ability and performance has been ignored. In the abilities conception, it is necessary to assess, first, in what ways the individual is capable of acting; then, one must determine the situations and conditions in which he will so behave. To illustrate, Wallace (1966) asked college students to write the sexiest TAT stories they could. Some produced puritanical and decidedly nonerotic tales, and others wrote smut, indicating that some college students have richer sex-related fantasy behavior in their repertoire than others. Presumably such behavior may be generalized to other settings, but as Wallace points out, until the situational factors governing the production of such behavior are specified, it would be impossible to predict the other situations. The situational factors Wallace sees as important include the patterning of reinforcement and punishment, the availability of models, the specific expectancies associated with the situation (whether the outcome is a matter of luck or skill), the formal properties of the situation (cultural and social demands), and so forth.

The second and, for the present discussion, the most relevant value of the Wallace view is the emphasis placed on assessment of situational determinants as well as behavioral repertoires. It should be emphasized that the abilities conception does not in any way diminish either the importance or necessity of assessing the behaviors of which an individual is capable nor does it decrease the difficulties.

Finally, the Wallace view, deriving from a distinctively different theoretical base, is similar to the analysis recently presented by DeVos who, in conceptual as well as methodological terms, set the challenge for psychologists interested in cross-cultural studies of achievement and achievement motivation (DeVos, 1968, 367). I hope that our Hawaii studies have made a contribution to the sharper conceptual focus that DeVos has articulated as well as to the need for transculturally appropriate methods.

ACKNOWLEDGMENT
This research was partially supported by National Institute of Mental Health Grant MH-15032 to the Bernice P. Bishop Museum.

NOTES

1.   'Aina Pumehana was chosen as a pseudonym to protect the members of the community in accord with standard research procedure.
2.   As part of a seminar at the University of Hawaii, graduate students spent time as participant observers in a Filipino community.

REFERENCES

Altman, B., L. Ryssel, and R. Gallimore. 1966. Race, class, and expectancy. Unpublished paper. Mimeographed.

Atkinson, J. W. 1954. Explorations using imaginative thought to assess the strength of human motives. *In* Nebraska symposium on motivation. M. R. Jones, ed. Lincoln, University of Nebraska Press.

———. 1957. Motivational determinants of risk-taking behavior. Psychological Review 64:359–72.

———. 1958. Motives in fantasy, action, and society. Princeton, Van Nostrand.

Atkinson, J. W., and N. T. Feather, eds. 1966. A theory of achievement motivation. New York, John Wiley and Sons.

Atkinson, J. W., and G. H. Litwin. 1960. Achievement motive and test anxiety conceived as motive to approach success and motive to avoid failure. Journal of Abnormal and Social Psychology 60:52–63.

Atkinson, J. W., and P. O'Connor. 1966. Effects of ability grouping in schools related to individual differences in achievement-related motivation. *In* A theory of achievement motivation. J. W. Atkinson and N. T. Feather, eds. New York, John Wiley and Sons.

Atkinson, J. W., and W. R. Reitman. 1960. Performance as a function of motive strength and expectancy of goal attainment. Journal of Abnormal and Social Psychology 60:27–36.

Bandura, A., and R. H. Walters. 1963. Social learning and personality development. New York, Holt, Rinehart, and Winston.

Brown, R. 1965. Social psychology. New York, The Free Press.

Bulatao, J. 1964. Hiya. Philippine Studies 12:424–38.

Crandall, V. J. 1963. Achievement. *In* Sixty-second yearbook of the national society for the study of education. H. Stevenson, J. Kagan, and C. Spiker, eds. Chicago, University of Chicago Press.

Crowne, D. F., and D. Marlowe. 1964. The approval motive. New York, John Wiley and Sons.

DeVos, G. A. 1968. Achievement and innovation in culture and personality. *In* Personality and interdisciplinary approach. E. Norbeck, D. Price-Williams, and W. M. McCord, eds. New York, Holt, Rinehart, and Winston.

Dollard, J., and E. Miller. 1950. Personality and psychotherapy, an analysis in terms of learning, thinking, and culture. New York, McGraw-Hill.

Gallimore, R., and A. Howard. 1968. Studies in a Hawaiian Community: Na Makamaka O Nanakuli. Pacific Anthropological Records No. 1.

———. 1969. The development of Hawaiian behavior: an experimental approach to culture/personality. Unpublished manuscript.

Gallimore, R., A. Howard, and C. Jordan. Independence training among Hawaiians. *In* Contemporary research in social psychology. H. C. Lindgren, ed. New York, John Wiley and Sons.

Guthrie, G. M., ed. 1968. Six perspectives on the Philippines. Manila, The Bookmark.

Guthrie, G. M., and P. J. Jacobs. 1966. Child rearing and personality development in the Philippines. University Park, The Pennsylvania State University Press.

Jordan, C. 1967. Dependency and dependency training in a Hawaiian community. Master's thesis, University of Hawaii.

Kensinger, L. L. 1967. A relationship between affiliation and achievement-oriented behavior. Master's thesis, University of Hawaii.

Klinger, E. 1966. Fantasy need achievement as a motivational construct. Psychological Bulletin 66:291–308.

——. 1967. Modeling effects on achievement imagery. Journal of Personality and Social Psychology 7:49–62.

Kubany, E. S., R. Gallimore, and J. Buell. 1969. Achievement-oriented behavior among Filipinos living in Hawaii. Unpublished manuscript.

Leffcourt, H. M. 1965. Risk taking in Negro and White adults. Journal of Personality and Social Psychology 2:765–70.

Leffcourt, H. M., and G. W. Ladwig. 1965. The American Negro: a problem in expectancies. Journal of Personality and Social Psychology 1:377–80.

Lynch, F. 1964. Social acceptance. Four readings on Philippine values. Institute of Philippine Culture Papers, No. 2. F. Lynch, ed. Manila, Ateneo de Manila University Press.

McClelland, D. C., 1961. The achieving society. Princeton, Van Nostrand.

McClelland, D. C., et al. 1953. The achievement motive. New York, Appleton-Century-Crofts.

Merbaum, A. D. 1961. Need for achievement in Negro and White children. Ph.D. dissertation, University of North Carolina. University of Michigan Microfilms, No. 62-3140.

Minigione, A. D. 1965. Need for achievement in Negro and White children, Journal of Consulting Psychology 29:108–111.

Mischel, W. 1968. Personality and assessment. New York, John Wiley and Sons.

Murray, H. A. 1938. Explorations in personality. New York, Oxford University Press.

Premack, D. 1965. Reinforcement theory. *In* Nebraska symposium on motivation. D. Levine, ed. Lincoln, University of Nebraska Press.

Schmitt, R. C. 1967. How many Hawaiians? Journal of the Polynesian Society 76:467–76.

Sechrest, L., and J. Wallace, Jr. 1967. Psychology and human problems. Columbus, Charles E. Merrill Books.

Sloggett, B. B., R. Gallimore, and E. S. Kubany. 1969. A comparative analysis of projective need achievement among Caucasians, Filipino-Americans, Hawaiians, Japanese-Americans, and Afro-Americans. Unpublished manuscript.

Staats, A. W., and C. K. Staats. 1963. Complex human behavior. New York, Holt, Rinehart, and Winston.

Wallace, J. 1966. An abilities conception of personality: some implication for personality measurement. American Psychologist 21:132–38.

————. 1967. What units shall we employ? Journal of Consulting Psychology 31:56–64.

Walters, R. H., and R. D. Parke. 1964. Social motivation, dependency, and susceptibility to social influence. *In* Advances in experimental social psychology, I. L. Berkowitz, ed. New York, John Wiley and Sons.

Whiting, B. B. 1963. Six cultures. Studies of child rearing. New York, John Wiley and Sons.

16.   An Approach to the Analysis of Subjective Culture

HARRY C. TRIANDIS, Ph.D.

Department of Psychology
University of Illinois
Urbana, Illinois

MY REMARKS TODAY will analyze an aspect of situations in which two persons with different cultural backgrounds have to work together for some particular purpose. The dyads might consist, for example, of a psychiatrist and a patient or two government officials.

The assumptions behind our project must be stated. First, we assume that it is possible to get a useful map of the cognitive structure of individuals by using psychophysical procedures. Second, we assume that if data are obtained from representative samples of cultural populations, there will be sufficient consistency across sex, age, and social class groups to permit a discussion of cognitive structures that are characteristic of certain cultural or at least subcultural groups. Third, we assume that the differences in these cognitive structures are critical for human interaction and relevant to our understanding of the interpersonal relation in culturally heterogeneous dyads. Fourth, we assume that these differences can be measured, understood, and communicated so that a person's interaction with members of another culture can be improved.

Accordingly, we have developed a research program with three steps: (1) cultural analysis, (2) training in cultural similarities and differences, and (3) validation of the training, by establishing that trained individuals behave more effectively than untrained ones in social situations involving members of other cultures. Our research program has so far given us encouraging results. Time permits the discussion of only the first phase, cultural analysis.

For purposes of communication, we employ the concept of subjective culture. This is a cultural group's characteristic way of perceiving and thinking about its social environment.

In what way does the cultural analysis that we do differ from that done by a traditional anthropologist? It seems to me that the traditional anthropologist is concerned with the best possible descriptions of individual cultures, while our concern is the best possible description of the similarities and differences between two or more cultures. The anthropologist is also concerned with the broader problem of the effects of all aspects of culture on the individual, while we are looking only for the effects of subjective culture on behavior. Furthermore, our focus is psychological, since we are interested in human perception and cognition and attempt to look at the fine grain, so to speak, of those processes, while the anthropologist cannot take the time to look at cognition in such detail. So rather than being antagonistic, the two approaches are complementary. The anthropologist provides the broad context, and we provide the fine detail on perception and cognition.

In summary, our approach is different in three ways: (1) we focus on cognition; (2) we employ large samples of informants—typically several hundred people from each subculture; and (3) we analyze our data with multidimensional procedures, such as facet analysis, factor analysis, multidimensional scaling, or analysis of variance.

In this paper, I will attempt to do the following: first, I will describe a conceptual framework which I think is useful in analyses of subjective culture; second, I will suggest how each of the concepts of this framework might be studied; and, third, I will briefly mention some empirical findings which suggest something about the utility of this approach.

Before I discuss the theoretical constructs, however, I would like to state my views concerning some methodological issues. The focus of this analysis is comparison. In order to compare two things, it is necessary to determine: (1) some common dimensions, (2) whatever unique dimensions there are, and (3) the positions of the objects to be described on the common dimensions. Perhaps the orange-apple comparison will illustrate this issue. First, you state some dimensions shared by these two entities. For example, weight, size, thickness of skin, acidity, etc. Second, you state dimensions that are unique to apples or to oranges, like apple-flavor, or orange-flavor. Third, you determine where apples and oranges fall on the common dimensions. You might find, for example, that there are large overlaps in the weight distributions with a slight tendency for the mean of the apples to be higher than that of the oranges but with very little overlap on the thickness-of-skin dimension or on acidity. Obviously, this information does not tell you all there is to know about apples and oranges. You must also compare each apple on the apple-flavor dimension and other apple-specific dimensions and, similarly, each orange on the orange-specific dimensions. But note that the comparison, as such, can only be done on what is common. It may be that the most important aspect of apples is their apple-flavor not their size. If that is the case, the comparison with oranges is misleading. On the other hand, if you are a human who only knows oranges, and you have not the slightest idea about apples, the concept of apple-flavor will be meaningless, but the concept of size will be accessible to you. We are forced by the focus of our problem to be satisfied with the more limited goal of comparison of the common dimensions, although we fully realize that we may miss important aspects of culture. We hope that such comparisons will give enough information to improve cross-cultural interaction.

We turn now to our conceptual framework. Both anthropologists and psychologists agree that categorization is a ubiquitous human activity. By categorization, we mean that humans give the same response to discriminably different stimuli. For example, although the human eye is capable of discriminating about 7.5 million colors, we typically employ less than a dozen color names in describing our color environment. Cultures differ in the number of categories they employ within a particular domain of meaning —the well-known example is of snow and ice which have many names among the Eskimos and few among the Aztecs. Cultures also differ in the criterial attributes they employ for categorization. When we examine the similarities and differences in categorization, what we really want to do is to examine attributes that are used as clues to the categorization process. This is information that can be obtained by using standard cognitive tasks.

It is obvious that language is intimately implicated in the categorization process. We can learn much about categorization by learning about the language of a particular group. But this is only the beginning in our reconstruction of their cognitive maps.

Categories differ from each other in a number of ways. Some categories are very concrete, like Mr. Smith, my neighbor, and some are abstract, like man. Some are very central, such as the belief that my name is Triandis, and some, for example, that pulsars represent dead stars, are quite peripheral. You can change my peripheral beliefs very easily, but not my central beliefs. It seems quite probable that cultures differ in the degree of centrality of various types of categories. In psychiatric work, it would seem invaluable to know this type of information because much of the time, the psychiatrist is trying to change some belief or, in other words, some connections among categories.

Let us trace, now, some of the constructs of our theoretical scheme from the most concrete to the most abstract. At the most concrete level, we have discriminable stimuli. At the next level, we have elementary categories, which can be visual, auditory, aptic, behavioral, etc. The phoneme is a good example of an auditory elementary category. At the next level we have meaning categories, which are elemental categories that are associated with other categories including affective states. The morpheme is a good example of an auditory meaning category. Meaning categories combine to form concepts, and concepts combine to form beliefs. Beliefs combine to form cognitive structures, such as stereotypes, attitudes, behavioral intentions, norms, roles, ideals, tasks, etc. When abstract categories are combined and affect is attached to them, we have values. For example, the abstract category "man" and the abstract category "nature" may be combined with some other categories to form the belief that "Man should be the master of nature." If affect is attached to this belief, you have one of Kluckhohn's value orientations. (Kluckhohn, 1959; Kluckhohn and Strodtbeck, 1961.)

Now this is a strong dose of concepts, but subjective culture has many elements. If we are to understand it, we must analyze categories, beliefs, norms, roles, stereotypes, and behavioral intentions as well as values. From each of these constructs it is possible to develop appropriate cognitive tasks to allow cross-cultural comparisons. Time allows for only a few illustrations.

At the most detailed and specific level, we can ask what is categorized in each culture. Lenneberg and Roberts (1956) and Landar et al. (1960) have developed excellent procedures for the study of color categorization. We can extend this approach by asking questions such as: "Is A the same as B?" "Is A included in B?" "Is it possible for both A and B to be true at the same time?" There are many questions of this sort that can be asked.

In determining the criterial attributes which define each domain of meaning, we can employ a variety of procedures. Promising approaches have been suggested by anthropologists for the analysis of kinship structures, e.g., componential analysis (a good review in Wallace, 1962); by sociologists, e.g., facet analysis (Guttman, 1959; Foa, 1965); by psychologists, e.g., multidimensional scaling (Torgerson, 1958); and by psycholinguists, e.g., feature analysis (Osgood, 1968). Each of these approaches has particular strengths and particular weaknesses, but time does not allow for elaboration. The only point I wish to make is that there are several models available for an analysis of data obtained from cognitive tasks which results in the determination of the criterial attributes used by a group of people.

The exact attributes obtained by any approach depend on the sampling of the categories to be analyzed. For example, if you select a set of extremely heterogeneous concepts, such as man, God, stone, tooth, and fire, then you typically, in all parts of the world, obtain three criterial attributes. Let me describe the so-called semantic differential method further. It was developed by my colleague, Charles Osgood (Osgood, Suci, and Tannenbaum, 1957) at the University of Illinois. Osgood and his associates begin with a heterogeneous sample of 100 concepts. In each of the 25 language-culture-communities where this work has been done to date, samples of high school students are asked to fill sentences of the type, "The HOUSE is . . ." or "The . . . HOUSE." From this step, one obtains qualifiers such as red, white, empty, good, etc. He then asks a different sample of subjects to rate 100 concepts on scales that have each of the most frequent qualifiers and their opposites as descriptions of the end-poles. For example, HOUSE may be judged on the scale good-bad. The correlations among the ratings of the 100 concepts on 50 scales provide a correlation matrix of size 50 x 50, based on 100 observations for each correlation. This matrix is then factor analyzed, and typically, one obtains three factors—evaluation (good, clean, beautiful), potency (strong, powerful, heavy), and activity (active, fast, hot). Now the interesting thing about Osgood's approach is that once the original 100 concepts have been double translated (from English to X and back to English to make sure the original concepts emerge again), the data are collected entirely independently in each culture and the analyses are done on different data.

What comes out from these analyses is a set of three factors that are equivalent but not identical. For example, in English, evaluation might involve the scales good, desirable, and moral, while, in some other language, the concepts might be clean, beautiful, and true. Obviously, the words do not mean the same thing across the two cultures, but what is common to good, desirable, and moral is something vaguely affective and evaluative; what is common to clean, beautiful, and true is again something affective and evaluative. Thus, cross-cultural equivalence has been established.

Now notice that, by this method, Osgood obtains criterial attributes that are very abstract. The reason for this is that the sample of concepts which he employs is very heterogeneous. If a homogeneous sample is employed, then dimensions that are appropriate for that particular domain of meaning will emerge. For example, I studied (Triandis, 1960) a sample of job concepts and found dimensions such as job complexity, white vs. blue collar, etc.

The advantage of going to the highest level of abstraction, as far as particular criterial attributes are concerned, is that the dimensions or factors that are extracted are cross-culturally equivalent. For example, Osgood has equivalent instruments from Japan, Thailand, and several of the languages of India. He has found most interesting cultural differences (for example, in the concept "myself" and the concept "mother") between such languages and American English.

While these most abstract dimensions of evaluation, potency, and activity give some interesting facts, there is obviously a need to probe even deeper. In some countries, the concepts "God" and "Coca Cola" have similar profiles on evaluation, potency, and activity. In other words, while Osgood's procedure explores the broad outlines, and finds the most general criterial attributes, there is a need for more refinement.

Refinement in this approach can be obtained by several methods. I have often used the restriction of the domain approach. For example, in several studies (Triandis, 1964, 1967), I used various descriptions of people as concepts. It is possible to construct such stimuli quite systematically and to obtain the behavioral intentions of samples of subjects toward them.

Here, instead of rating a concept such as HOUSE on a good-bad scale, the subjects are asked to indicate how they would behave toward the stimulus persons. The scales are bound by the words "would" and "would not." A typical item looks like this:

A 60 year-old male Japanese physician
Would ___'___'___'___'___'___'___'___'___ would not ask
the advice of this person.

The data are again subjected to factor analysis, much as was done by Osgood, but the factors now consist of clusters of behaviors. Let us look at the results of one study (Triandis, Tanaka, and Shanmugam, 1966) done with Southern Indian, Japanese, and American college students. All three cultures defined three factors of interpersonal relations—respect, friendship, and marital acceptance. However, the specific behaviors that went into each factor were not the same. Let us look, for an example, at the factor loadings of the respect factor. The American males have loadings over .90 on "admire the character of this person," "be commanded by this person," "obey," "admire the ideas," and "not treat as a subordinate." The Japanese, while having high loadings on "be commanded by" and "obey," have a loading of only .63 on "admire the character of this person" and a loading of only .07 for "admire the ideas of this person." In other words, for the American males, subordination is fused with admiration; for the Japanese males, there is a distinction between the two. The Indians are intermediate, but closer to the Americans than to the Japanese. Let us, also, look at the friendship factor. The Americans define it with the behaviors "be partners in athletic game with," "permit to do me a favor," "teach," and "gossip with." The Japanese define it with "admire the ideas of," "gossip with," "admire the character of," "be partners in athletic game," "permit to do me a favor," etc. Now the two factors are similar, except for a .85 loading on "admire ideas of" for the Japanese, while the Americans have only a loading of .35. So we establish here a similarity in the dimension, but some differences, also, in the way the dimension is defined.

This last example concerns the study of behavioral intentions. Let us consider another example from an analysis of role perceptions (Triandis, Vassiliou, and Nassiakou, 1968). Here, the concepts that were investigated were 100 roles, such as father-son, son-father, psychologist-client, prostitute-client, etc. The scales were again descriptions of behavior, and the subjects indicated how appropriate they considered what the first member of the role did toward the second as described by the scale. For example, if the role was father-son and the scale was would-would not hit, the subjects indicated whether in their culture it is frequently or infrequently appropriate for a father to hit his son.

In the same study, we asked subjects to provide us with behaviors that they thought appropriate for each of the 100 roles. We then selected frequently-mentioned behaviors and constructed a questionnaire with 100 roles and 60 scales defined by behaviors. We correlated the scales and obtained the 60 x 60 matrix of correlations in each culture. I will not go into the methodological niceties here, such as several parallel factor analyses with different samples of different behaviors. Such checks on the reliability of the data are essential. Our analyses revealed four culture-common factors as well as half-a-dozen culture-specific factors.

Let me show some of the results of one study (Triandis et al., 1969) by examining one role, the father-son role in Illinois, Northern India, and Taiwan. First, there are three common dimensions—hostility, respect, and superordination. In all three cultures, it is wrong to be hostile, and one must show some respect and much superordination in this role. But on these common dimensions, we find differences. For example, take the taboo on the hostility factor which is defined by the behaviors "not to throw rocks at," "not be enemy of," "not fear," "not laugh at," and "not fight with" in Illinois; "not throw rocks at," "not be enemy of," "not ignore," and "not be indignant with" in India; and "not fear," "not laugh at," and "not hate" in Taiwan. First, note the slight difference in connotation where the Indian factor does not explicitly prohibit "laughing at" or "fearing." Then, we find the Indian and Taiwan samples are statistically significantly more extreme on this taboo than are the Americans. Hostility is, so to speak, more unheard of in the father-son role in the two Asian countries than it is in America.

Second, note some dimensions that emerge in one culture but not in the others. There is a dimension of plain love, with high loadings on "love," "appoint," and "have fun with," which emerges in India but not in the other cultures in which there is apparently more distance between father and son. The two Asian cultures use a dimension which might be called nurturance which is not used by the Illinois males. Nurturance is defined in India by "advise," "take care of," "admire," and "pet"; in Taiwan by "help," "love," "cooperate with," "forgive," and "protect." In vain do I look for the love scale to have a high loading on any American factor. Somehow American males see love as inappropriate in the father-son relation. Or, perhaps, love is an embarrassing matter in that relation (suggestions of the Oedipus complex?) and leads to random responses which produce no substantial correlations with other behavior scales. At any rate, the difference in the factor structures suggests to me, and here I will make a value judgment, that the father-son relation is better on the love dimension in the two Asian countries than it is in Illinois. On the other hand, there is more respect for the son in America than in the two Asian countries. There is more willingness "to admire his ideas," "respect him," "depend upon him," "learn with his help," and plain "ask for his help." In India, this factor did not even emerge.

India shows a strong control factor, defined by the behaviors "to scold," "castigate," and "quarrel with," which seems harsh and extreme, while the Americans define their control factor with less extreme behaviors such as "command," "teach," and "inspect work of," and the Taiwan sample defined it with "command" and "punish" which are also forms of control.

In summary, the Indians appear more involved in the relation—there is love and fighting, too; the Americans stand a bit more aloof—there is respect but not clearly love. What are the implications of such findings for psychiatric work in the two cultures? I leave this to the experts on this matter.

So far, I have discussed various ways in which categories can be studied, compared cross-culturally, and their criterial attributes determined. Let me turn to a study in which the relations among the categories were explored.

In this study, we (Triandis et al., 1968) used a different kind of questionnaire with American, Greek, Indian, and Japanese students. In phase I, we asked the students to complete sentences of the form: "If you have . . . , then you have justice," or "If you have justice, then you have . . . ." The concepts used to fill sentences of the first kind were called antecedents, and the concepts used to fill sentences of the second kind were called consequents. The most frequently obtained antecedents and conse-quents were then presented to subjects, in phase II, in a structured format. The subjects were required to choose out of a list of five antecedents, or five consequents, the one "that best completes the particular sentence." The five antecedents or consequents were selected from among the most fre-quently obtained antecedents and consequents in phase I in such a way that, in each case, there was one antecedent or consequent that was frequently given in America, one in Greece, one in India, and one in Japan. The fifth response alternative was culture-common. The subjects responded to phase II predominately by choosing either the culture-common response or the response generated, during phase I, by subjects from their own culture.

The frequency distributions of the choices of the subjects were compared by chi-square, and it was possible to show that there are a large number of cultural differences in the perception of antecedents and conse-quents. Nevertheless, the similarities in responding are more overwhelming than the differences, thus encouraging us to believe that we were, indeed, tapping the meaning of the particular concepts.

We have studied 20 concepts in four cultures, but space allows discussion of the findings for only one concept. I have selected the concept "fear" as one which attracts interest because of its psychopathological con-notations.

First, let us consider the correlations among the four cultures. These correlations are based on the frequencies of choice of particular antecedents or particular consequents out of a list of 30 antecedents or consequents. In other words, the N is 30. The Americans and the Japanese correlated .64, significant at the .001 level on the antecedent frequencies, and .62 on the consequent frequencies. In other words, there is a substantial similarity in the meaning of this concept in America and Japan. By contrast, America and Southern India gives a $-$ .03 on the antecedent side and a .34 on the consequent; obviously, neither of them are significant. Thus, it appears that the American and Indian meanings of this concept are different. There is a wide similarity in the meaning of this concept across cultures, because the Greeks agree with the Americans and the Japanese, but the Indians appear idiosyncratic. We also have Osgood semantic differential information on the concepts we have studied, and we note that fear has similar connotative meaning in all four cultures—it is very bad, relatively weak, and passive; except in India where it is bad, strong, and passive. If fear is strong in India, it may be, as suggested by Hebb, that industrialization, by providing a more structured planned environment, suppresses it.

Now, all cultures see danger and lack of confidence as leading to fear, but America and Japan also see ignorance and the unknown as leading to fear, while the Indians are significantly low in seeing a connection between ignorance or the unknown and fear. It would appear that in the more industrialized societies there is predictability, planning, and the use of knowledge to organize affairs, and when these conditions are not present, there may be fear. In India, one gets used to uncertainty and, therefore, the connection between uncertainty and fear appears less appropriate. In the two industrialized countries, one also finds strong connections between loneliness and uneasiness and fear, while in India these connections appear inappropriate. Could it be that the extended family makes loneliness less of a problem and hence, is less likely to occur in association with fear responses?

I just mentioned a number of bonds that are strong between certain concepts and fear in America and Japan. Now I turn to bonds that are strong in India but not in America or Japan. Four links are particularly strong in India: demon, excess wealth, lack of manliness, and fantasy. Demon and fantasy appear related to spooky stories, and their connection with fear is understandable. Excess wealth may be connected with fear arising from the possibility that the government will confiscate gold, a rumor that was particularly strong in India in 1967 when the data were collected. However, the connection between lack of manliness and fear is interesting. The method permits detailed examination of any bond. Thus, we find that the Americans chose this option only 24 times and the Japanese only 17 times, but the Indians chose it 77 times. The American and Japanese choices of this option are significantly fewer than what one might expect by chance; the Indian choices of this bond are significantly more frequent than one might expect by chance. All statistical findings are reliable beyond the .01 level. Thus, since the Americans and Japanese are significantly low and the Indians significantly high on this item, there is unquestionably a cultural difference.

Now, let us look at the consequences of fear. In all cultures, fear leads to flight, panic, and uneasiness, but the Americans and Japanese also mention a freezing response, such as hesitation, which the Indians choose significantly less frequently than one might expect by chance. The Americans also mentioned weakness and nervousness as consequents of fear; the Japanese emphasized shaking. The Indians stressed bad dreams.

The total pattern suggests that industrialization changes the perceived causes of fear from fantasies and sexual inadequacies to interpersonal crises and lack of certainty; appropriately, the consequences of fear seem more in the realm of fantasy in India and more physiological (freezing, shaking) in the two industrialized countries. What it all means exactly, I do not yet know, and I think it is appropriate to employ such findings purely as sources of hypotheses, and very tentatively, until they are corroborated by other evidence. But the advantage of the method I have just described is that it is possible to give the members of each culture the opportunity to choose responses appropriate for members of that culture, while making the task equivalent for all the samples in all the cultures. It permits a careful look at controlled associations and allows the development of norms, so that the responses of a particular subject might be compared with international norms. For example, an Indian psychiatrist who wishes to explore associations could discover that, although a particular patient gives unusual associations, they are not so unusual when compared with the responses of the Japanese, and this may start an exploration of what might cause such communalities between his patient and a Japanese patient.

This presentation has covered much ground. I have intentionally omitted much of the validation work, since my feeling was that it would be more profitable if I attempted to interest you in this approach rather than to convince you of the validity of some small aspect of it. We have done some validation studies in which, for example, we attempted to predict specific behaviors of the subjects from the knowledge of their subjective cultures (Davis and Triandis, 1965; Triandis and Vassiliou, 1968). Much still needs to be done, and we hope that others will also begin exploring the subjective cultures of their subjects.

ACKNOWLEDGMENTS

The work reported was supported by a contract to study "Communication, Cooperation and Negotiation in Culturally Heterogeneous Groups" between the Advanced Research Projects Agency (ARPA Order No. 454) and the Office of Naval Research (NR 177–472, Nonr 1834(36)) and the University of Illinois. Fred E. Fiedler and Harry C. Triandis are the Principal Investigators.

REFERENCES

Davis, E. E., and H. C. Triandis. 1965. An exploratory study of intercultural negotiations. Urbana, Ill., Group Effectiveness Research Laboratory.

Foa, U. 1965. New developments in facet design and analysis. Psychological Review 72:262–74.

Guttman, L. 1959. A structural theory of intergroup beliefs and action. American Sociological Review 24:318–28.

Kluckhohn, C. 1959. The scientific study of values. *In* Three lectures. Toronto, University of Toronto Press.

Kluckhohn, F., and F. L. Strodtbeck. 1961. Variations in value orientations. Evanston, Row, Peterson.

Landar, H. J., S. M. Ervin, and A. E. Horowitz. 1960. Navaho color categories. Language 36:368–82.

Lenneberg, E. H., and J. M. Roberts. 1956. The language of experience: a study in methodology. International Journal of American Linguistics 22 (supplement): No. 2:1–33.

Osgood, C. E. 1968. Interpersonal verbs and interpersonal behavior. Mimeo.

Osgood, C. E., G. J. Suci, and P. H. Tannenbaum. 1957. The measurement of meaning. Urbana, University of Illinois Press.

Torgerson, W. S. 1958. Theory and methods of scaling. New York, John Wiley and Sons.

Triandis, H. C. 1960. A comparative factorial analysis of job semantic structures of managers and workers. Journal of Applied Psychology 44:297–302.

———. 1964. Exploratory factor analyses of the behavioral component of social attitudes. Journal of Abnormal and Social Psychology 68:420–30.

———. 1967. Toward an analysis of the components of interpersonal attitudes. *In* Attitude, ego-involvement, and change. C. W. Sherif and M. Sherif, eds. New York, John Wiley and Sons.

Triandis, H. C., and V. Vassiliou. 1968. Interpersonal influence and employee selection in two cultures. Urbana, Ill., Group Effectiveness Research Laboratory.

Triandis, H. C., Y. Tanaka, and A. V. Shanmugan. 1966. Interpersonal attitudes among American, Indian and Japanese students. International Journal of Psychology 1:177–206.

Triandis, H. C., V. Vassiliou, and M. Nassiakou. 1968. Three cross-cultural studies of subjective culture. Journal of Personality and Social Psychology Monograph Supplement 8:No. 4, 1–42.

Triandis, H. C., et al. 1968. Cultural influences upon the perception of implicative relationships among concepts and the analysis of values. Urbana, Ill., Group Effectiveness Research Laboratory.

———. 1969. A cross-cultural study of role perceptions. Urbana, Ill., Group Effectiveness Research Laboratory.

Wallace, A. F. C. 1962. Culture and cognition. Science 135:351–57.

RELIGIOUS FACTORS IN MENTAL HEALTH

17. Some Psychiatric Problems at the Buddhist Priest's Hospital in Thailand

SUNDARANU DUSIT, M.D.

Psychiatric Department
Priest's Hospital
Bangkok, Thailand

THE BUDDHIST PRIEST'S HOSPITAL in Bangkok is a special hospital exclusively for the use of Buddhist priests and novices. It is a general hospital with a capacity of 300 beds including all departments except the obstetric and gynecological departments. The reasons for establishing this special hospital for priests and novices were several. About 95 percent of the Thai population is Buddhist, and priests are highly respected. It is considered improper for priests and laymen to mix in general hospitals. Moreover, one of the rules for priests is that they cannot touch or be touched by women which creates a special problem when they are ill and are admitted to hospitals where female nurses provide all nursing care. Finally, the sheer numbers of Buddhist priests and novices, about 300,000 throughout the country, necessitated special consideration.

For these reasons, the Priest's Hospital was established in 1951. Male practical nurses perform all nursing duties under the supervision of female graduate nurses. All services for the priests are free of charge, and the Hospital provides free lunch for the priests utilizing the Out-Patient Clinic. Although the Hospital is government-operated, a large proportion of the budget comes from the donations of the devout Buddhist laymen.

The Out-Patient Department can handle approximately 200 to 300 priests daily. The most common diseases found among them are pulmonary tuberculosis and psychiatric problems. With regard to the latter, psychosomatic diseases are most prevalent; the rest are cases of psychoneuroses, psychosis, and drug addiction.

Most of the psychotic patients are schizophrenic, but the psychotic priests' history is very difficult to obtain. Most of them have lived away from their families and relatives for at least several years and often have not been in contact with their families for a long time. The only persons who can provide any information about them are usually priest-friends and abbots, and the latter usually know them only superficially.

The number of the psychotic priests is not high, and undoubtedly some of them had these symptoms before becoming priests. Others may have vowed to become priests as a means of getting rid of their psychotic symptoms. Psychotics are relatively numerous among those priests who practice metaphysics. In the course of their practice, they must remain alone in a quiet place with their eyes closed while concentrating on some bodily exercise, such as inhaling and exhaling, in order to keep their minds clear. During the process, some unconscious events may occur in various forms of hallucination which may be auditory or visual. After such happenings, the priest may become extremely frightened. The practice itself may be the cause of their psychosis, but, in actuality, we need more studies to link these together.

In drug addiction cases, the patients are usually addicted to bromide which they take to relieve their psychosomatic symptoms. They can easily buy various brands of this drug without a prescription. Two commercial brands, whose names sound attractive, seem to be popular among them: "neurotone" and "nerve cure." Both contain potassium bromide.

The common symptoms in psychosomatic cases are headache, chest pain, back pain, insomnia, and burning sensation. The site of a headache varies: frontal, bitemporal, or all over the head. Most of the headache cases are afraid of some organic lesion including hypertension in their brains. The chest pain is either at the sides or in the middle. These patients are afraid of pulmonary tuberculosis and heart diseases. The group with back pains is afraid of kidney diseases. Most of the psychoneurotic patients have anxiety neurosis with some conversion reaction.

In the treatment of psychosomatic and psychoneurotic diseases, both psychotherapy and drug therapy are employed. The major problems encountered in the process of treatment are that, first, these patients do not want to talk about their own problems because they are not supposed to have any. If they do have problems they are supposed to be able to solve them by themselves. Secondly, the priests are accustomed to receiving high respect, so the doctors must be extremely cautious in questioning them, especially about sex. Most of the priest-patients deny having problems or really do not know that they have problems. Even after the examination, when the doctors have concluded that their symptoms are related to some psychic problems, the patients still think that their problems concern their studies. It is commonly held by the priests that psychosomatic disorders are the diseases of learned men; consequently, the treatment of psychosomatic cases depends mostly on drug therapy.

My research at the Buddhist Priest's Hospital discloses several possible factors which create a high incidence of psychosomatic disorders. These factors are: (1) their motivation for becoming priests, (2) their living conditions, (3) sexual inhibition, and (4) difficulties in pursuing their studies.

(1) *Motivation for becoming priests.* There are four common reasons for becoming priests.

a) Most Thai men become priests for a temporary period, because it is an established tradition. Each year about 60,000–70,000 men join the priesthood for this reason and remain as priests for the three months of Buddhist Lent. These priests normally do not have psychosomatic problems.

b) Some men become priests to escape from misery and personal problems. Generally, the men in this category have some psychic trauma or problems and desire to run away for a while. They believe that if they become priests, religious insight will help relieve their anxiety. However, they frequently end up seeking counsel and medical treatment at the Priest's Hospital.

c) Men who have suffered from a severe physical illness, to the extent that they expect to die, frequently pledge to be priests. As their last recourse, they vow to become priests if their health will be restored. In such cases, they may even be ordained on their sick beds, believing that priesthood will more readily cure their illnesses.

d) Others become priests to have the opportunity to study more. The priests in this group have been increasing in numbers since the end of World War II. Most of them come from the northeast of Thailand and from a low economic status. These men cannot afford to pursue higher education, primarily because of lack of funds. The priesthood, therefore, provides an opportunity for them to continue their education. Because most of the higher educational institutions for priests are located in Bangkok, many living in the provinces try to move to Bangkok. In the last decade, the number of priests in Bangkok and its neighboring areas has increased so tremendously that the temples in these cities are exceptionally crowded. Many of the priests cannot obtain permission from their abbots to stay in Bangkok because of crowded conditions. As a result, they are denied the opportunity for advanced studies, and the best they can do is to wait and hope to find a place to stay. This is one of the causes of their anxiety symptoms.

(2) *Living conditions.* As a general rule, priests must obtain their

food as an offering from the merit-making people during their routine morning walk. The priests in Bangkok generally do not receive a sufficient quantity of food, because:

a) As previously noted, there are too many priests residing in Bangkok.

b) Relatively speaking, fewer Bangkok residents perform the merit-making act of presenting food to the priests in the morning than do the country people. As a result of the typically hurried and busy life in a large urban capital, the majority of the people do not have time to prepare food to offer to the priests. Instead, they are rushing to their offices or getting their children ready for school. Therefore, many priests are simply worried about how to obtain sufficient food to maintain their life. There is a high incidence of psychosomatic disorders in this group. On the other hand, those priests who enjoy good living conditions are the ones in the temples providing services such as cremation. Belonging to this group are the priests who have knowledge of astrology and fortunetelling; they determine the auspicious moments and dates for various social activities. Those who have a knowledge of folk medicine very often gain a reputation for successfully curing certain illnesses. The priests who can provide such services usually receive abundant compensation from the people, and consequently their standard of living is high. The incidence of psychosomatic disorders in this group of priests is very low.

(3) *Sexual problems.* Since priests are required to observe total sexual abstinence, this inhibition undoubtedly creates some amount of anxiety and frustration.

(4) *Study problems.* Higher education is difficult for most priests. Most of them have completed only the basic education of Prathom 4 (equivalent to Grade 4). As priests, they are required to study Pali which is more difficult for them than studying Latin would be for a Westerner. The higher the level of study, the more complex and difficult admission and graduation become. In Bangkok, there are two Buddhist priest universities which admit only 150–200 students each year and approximately twenty to thirty are graduated each year.

Conclusion

Psychiatric problems among the Buddhist priests in Thailand have required special facilities for their treatment. Psychosomatic disorders show the highest incidence, and these appear to derive from a variety of factors, some specially attendant on the nature of monastic life. Urgently required are more detailed studies to shed further light on this subject.

18. Javanese Mystical Groups

BONOKAMSI DIPOJONO, M.D.

Department of Psychiatry
University of Indonesia
Djakarta, Indonesia

Javanese Beliefs and Values

Indonesia consists of more than 3,000 islands and has a population in excess of 110 million including a great variety of ethnic groups, each with a distinctive culture. Of the five main islands, Java is the smallest but the most populated. The Javanese, who, as the major ethnic group, form about 60 percent of the whole Indonesian population, live mainly in the central and eastern part of the island.

Javanese mystical beliefs have been influenced mainly by animism, Hinduism-Buddhism, and Islam. Depending on the local circumstances, one of these influences may predominate over others. Prior to the time of Hindu influence in Java, the people seem to have believed that all beings and non-living matter possessed a spirit and were imbued with a magical life-power. Influence from this period can still be seen in widespread evidences of ancestor worship manifested in the shadow or puppet play where the puppets are symbols of ancestors, the worship of non-living matter such as stones and weapons, belief in the existence of good and bad spirits who are able to assume human form and belief in possession of human bodies by those spirits, belief in men's latent supernatural powers which when cultivated in various ways can be used for good or evil purposes and also in sacred weapons which can be strengthened by those powers. The influence of

Hinduism and Buddhism, evidenced by large and small temples scattered throughout Java, became even more widespread through the popular puppet plays, depicting stories from the Mahabharata and Ramajana epics among others. The supernatural world became more structured and systematized under the Hindu influence; thus, there are supposed to be several strata of heavens and hells, each with its inhabitants. Supernatural beings are also distributed according to a kind of hierarchical system. The belief in reincarnation and various ways of meditation are also of Hindu-Buddhist origin.

According to many scholars, the first Moslem settlers on Java possibly came from Iran and India. They were not orthodox Moslems but members of the so-called Sufii sect (Islam with preponderant mystical aspects). These first Moslems may have strengthened the existing mystical beliefs. Some of the so-called nine wali's (*Wali Sanga*) were teachers in mysticism before becoming teachers and propagators of Islam. The orthodox Moslems from Saudi Arabia came later. Islam added several angels to the supernatural pantheon, while Islamic chants and prayers and short passages of the Koran were used to prevent disaster or as a defense against evil spirits and magic. Christianity has not had much influence on Javanese mystical beliefs.

Because of the constant threat of evil spirits, the burning of incense, offering of ritual feast (*selamatan*) and flowers (*sesadji*), and the use of a complicated numerological system are common protective measures to satisfy those spirits and/or prevent encounter with them. It is not surprising then that evil spirits, human magical power, magic power of sacred weapons, inadequate prayers and offerings, and inadequate knowledge of the numerological system may cause suffering and illnesses, physical as well as mental. Although 90 percent of the Javanese are Moslems, most of them are strongly influenced by these cultural beliefs of which spirit worship is the most important.

The Javanese philosophy of life seems to be based on certain principles, usually taught and integrated in family education, of which the *narima* (acceptance), the *sabar* (patience), the *waspada* (alertness), the *eling* (being conscious of), the *tatakrama* (etiquette), *kapradjan* (dignity), *andap asor* and *prasadja* (simplicity and modesty) principles and the submissive attitude are the most important.

The *narima* principle is the attitude of resignation: to accept one's fate however unpleasant it may be. It is usually accompanied by a kind of rationalization to enhance the tolerance of frustration. If, for instance, a Javanese is facing difficulties in finding a job, he usually will make comments such as: *"durung pestine"* ("it is not yet his fate"), *"idep-idep nglakoni"* ("he has to experience"), *"durung kepareng"* ("it is not yet His will"), *"wus kersane sing kuasa"* (it is God's will"), etc. With this outlook, the Javanese does not easily blame others for his failures. For example, if a business run by a lazy son is not functioning well, the father will say: "Well, why did I choose such a lazy boy to run my business? If he were more active, I still doubt whether it would run better if it is not yet God's will."

The *sabar* principle is the attitude of patience, to be patient in any kind of situation. A Javanese usually will not attempt to fulfill his drives and needs by dramatic overacting but rather will wait for the right moment, in the belief that he has plenty of time. Emotionally, he will not react spontaneously by bursting into great laughter or tears or by becoming angry. Control of the emotions also may be attributed to principles of etiquette (*tatakrama*). The Javanese are usually slow workers, never hurrying or rushing through their daily activities. Their motto is: *"alon-alon waton kelakon"* ("slowly but surely"). The occasional conscious control of certain basic human needs, such as abstinence from certain foods and drinks, sleep, and sexual relations, may be seen as an exercise of the patience principle.

The *waspada* principle is the attitude of alertness, to be alert to bad influences from the outside world. The Javanese are usually very reticent in giving information about personal matters and are reserved and cautious in interpersonal relations. They would rather wait than actively approach someone they do not know. In gatherings they always try to avoid becoming the center of attention, so as not to expose themselves and be placed in a vulnerable position.

The *eling* principle is the attitude of awareness or being conscious of inner drives and emotions so as to be able to control these at all times. Aggressive drives, anger, hostility feelings, and sadness especially are to be controlled to prevent extroverted behavior. It is not surprising that Javanese usually do not like alcoholic drinks as alcohol may stimulate uncontrollable behavior.

The *tatakrama* principle is the Javanese etiquette, although the word "etiquette" is only an approximation. The attitude, posture, facial and verbal expressions, and behavior in general are usually controlled by this principle. Traditionally, *tatakrama* was most highly cultivated in aristocratic circles and least cultivated by the rural dwellers. The higher their status in society the more *tatakrama* was cultivated in the family. Today, the inculcation *tatakrama* in most family circles may be a kind of preservation of old family traditions. The former stratified society greatly stimulated the cultivation of this principle. To point with the thumb rather than with the index finger, how to dress properly, how to walk, how to wear the dagger, are but a few examples of the *tatakrama* principle.

The *kapradjan* principle is the preservation of dignity. Javanese have accepted certain standards of behavior for given situations. Behavior that goes beyond the standards is regarded as unworthy. To show off in a gathering, to stumble at every trifle when making a contract, to debate fiercely in public, are but a few examples of unworthy behavior. The Javanese tend to preserve their dignity according to their status in society.

The *andap asor* and *prasadja* principles are the attitudes of simplicity and modesty, although, again, these are only approximate translations. In a social gathering the Javanese will usually compete to see who will be the most modest and take a seat in the hindmost row, permitting others to occupy the front seats. In walking through a door, he will let his guest pass through the door before himself. He will always give deference to others, especially older people. Clothes are to be kept simple and not striking. These are but a few examples of these principles.

The principle of maintaining a submissive attitude enables the Javanese to accept authority very easily. This may be reinforced by an authoritative father figure in childhood, the highly stratified society, and 300 years of colonial rule. The consequences of this attitude are inferiority feelings and the creation of the so-called *bapak*-ism attitude (devotion to the father-symbol or leader of the group).

It is not known with certainty which of the aforementioned principles were original Javanese principles predating the colonial period and which were created as a kind of defense against the authoritative colonial power. At the very least, these characteristics were stimulated, exploited, and cultivated with great skill by the colonial rulers.

In childhood a Javanese faces an omnipotent father figure and protective (perhaps overprotective) mother figure. The father figure usually keeps some distance from the child in order to facilitate the child's early understanding of the *tatakrama* principle. Family education will be rather a one-way procedure; the child has to obey and accept his parent's advice and corrections. In later life this may result in credulity or suggestibility and hamper the ability to criticize. The so-called "yes" attitude (always answering with "yes" when he sometimes may mean "no") may create some further difficulties. If, for instance, an employee is suddenly asked to do something for his supervisor, he will say "yes" but may not fulfill his task.

The father figure preserves the family's dignity and social status and is usually the main provider. In this respect he will be accepted as the protector by the child and will be respected (by the *tatakrama* education), though also feared (as being omnipotent). There usually will be a lack of emotional love toward the father figure. All this tends to create an ambivalent attitude toward him.

The extended period of motherly protection until adulthood facilitates strong dependency feelings in the child, and, in turn, the mother feels strongly dependent on her children.

Spirit worship is greatly emphasized and creates some fear, but it is also an acquired means of protection and projection. The offering of meals (*selamatan*) and flowers (*sesadji*), burning of incense, visits to graves of ancestors, and the cult of sacred family weapons are but a few examples of spirit worship in the child's environment, the purpose of which is to ask the protection of the various spirits and especially to placate the evil spirits.

Education at home may be a mixture of *isin* (shyness and embarrassment) and *wedi* (fear). The parents may feel that in order to preserve the dignity of the family it is better that a child undergo *isin* rather than not conform to the *tatakrama* principle. Reward and punishment are not emphasized. To receive greater love and attention from the parents may be a major reward, but punishment is seldom carried out. The child will be taught especially to fear strange people, his father, and supernatural beings. "I will ask that man to take you away," "A soldier will come if you don't stop crying," "A spirit will take you away," "We shall leave you alone," "I will tell your father that you are naughty" are but a few examples. This type of threatening may create an attitude of alertness, especially in interpersonal relations. The type of parent-child relation and general family education described above may result in a tendency toward a shy, submissive, reserved, and overcontrolled individual.

The influence of society may strengthen or weaken these personality characteristics. Among the upper classes with comfortable houses and large gardens, children are kept at home, and socialization in the community will be minimal. For the lower classes in urban and rural areas, there is more interaction with the community and, therefore, a greater possibility of counterbalancing personality traits emphasized in the home. Nowadays, educational institutes are less authoritative and family education is becoming more flexible in accepting modern ways of child education.

A small Javanese community will function like a big family, where conformity to *tatakrama* rules, strong social control, and the *gotong rojong* and *rukun* principles are stressed. *Rukun* (harmony, being in peace) in the family, in the community, and in the country is the ideal state of interpersonal relations between Javanese individuals which, of course, in actuality is very difficult to accomplish. But in order to conform to the expectations of the community, a family will pretend to be *rukun*. This *rukun* principle later on became the motive power of *musjawarah* (gatherings, meetings, official conferences) where decisions are accepted by acclamation rather than by vote. *Gotong rojong* (neighborhood solidarity) is an ideal state of group solidarity, where individuals are expected to give spontaneous support to their neighbors when they need help and to join every effort concerning the welfare of the community. This *gotong rojong* is felt as a moral and social obligation toward the community—in order to conform to the expectations of this community—although it seldom entails strong emotional involvement. Neighborhood solidarity also stimulates and facilitates an attitude of hospitality and more intimate interpersonal relations, especially with the members of the same sex. The ideals of *rukun* and *gotong rojong* superficially give the impression that the Javanese individual is a strong socializing individual with a real feeling of belonging to his community. But in actuality the strong social control, the expectation of conformity to the *tatakrama* principle, and the too demanding idealism of *rukun* and *gotong rojong* may be felt rather as a burden and as too traumatic for the individual, the consequence of which is retreat to the more secure family environment.

The demands of society, however, may still be felt even with a *masa bodowa* attitude (do not care or apathetic attitude) toward events beyond the family circles.

The Javanese family system is usually a paternal extended family where two or more generations live together. The oldest male member has the highest authority. In case of polygamy (Islam allows four wives), the wives may stay in the same house or in separate houses. Breast-feeding continues sometimes until the age of three. The mother and all other female members of the family take care of the children and of the household in general. The emphasis on autonomy for the child is not very great and comes at a late age. Members of the family may change home environments by moving in with relatives rather easily. In this respect there is a great hospitality not only for relatives, but for friends as well, and members of the household may go so far as to move into a small room while permitting their guests to use the largest room. The mother usually prefers a daughter who can help with housekeeping. If a married couple has no children after being married several years, they try to adopt a child, preferably from a close relative, usually a brother or sister, in the belief that this will stimulate the wife to have a child of her own (Islam does not recognize adopted children in connection with inheritance).

In marriage, the parents usually choose the partner for their children, preferably a relative, in order to *ngupulake balung apisah* (to put separate bones together). The wedding ceremony will be held in the bride's house. In seven to forty days the bride and groom will establish permanent residence with either parents or separately.

Family ties are very strong and extend far beyond the usual family boundaries. Distant relatives such as nephews and cousins are recognized sometimes until the seventh generation or more. Family groups (*kumpulan trah*) are created based on kinship to a common ancestor. These social organizations, whose members are all related, are usually named after the common ancestor. The main purpose of the formation of such groups is usually *ngupulake balung apisah* (bring relatives together) to recognize each other as relatives, to help each other, and to stimulate the *gotong rojong* spirit among members. In case of marriage, the husband and wife automatically become members of each other's family group.

Javanese society is a stratified society with a division into *prijaji* and non-*prijaji*. The meaning of *prijaji* has never been formulated in a clear way. In former times only the family of a king (*sultan/sunan*) could be called *prijaji;* later this grouping was extended to include all government officials. For the peasants in the small villages all people from the city were called *prijaji kuta* (*prijaji* from the city). The divisions have now faded away. According to Islam, there is an unofficial division into *putihan* or *santri* (Moslems who live strictly to the religious rules) and the *abangan* (Moslems who are greatly influenced by the Javanese cultural beliefs).

Nowadays, many aspects of life in Java have been modified as people become adjusted to life as citizens of an independent country. Through the leveling process, the stratified society has faded away, and as a consequence of modern education, family education has had to accept some changes. Certain principles of life which were imposed by the colonial administration have been abandoned. Nevertheless, old beliefs, especially spirit worship, have not changed appreciably among the present generation. Many artistic expressions, particularly the puppet play, which is still popular, remind the Javanese of old beliefs. Some psychological factors also support the continuing acceptance of old cultural beliefs.

Javanese Mystical Groups

Mystical movements have always been very active, especially on Java where they can be found everywhere throughout the island. In Djakarta alone, more than one hundred groups are in existence. Most of these groups have branches throughout the country and some have branches in foreign countries. In the pre-World War II period, such movements were more or less suppressed but after the war, during the period of great turmoil and heightened social tension, they greatly accelerated their activities. The number of members varies from 100 in the smaller groups to tens of thousands in the larger groups.

Mystical groups tend to be well-organized; some have formal rules and bylaws. Although there may be a clear division into organizational and spiritual sections, the spiritual leader (usually male) is the accepted leader of the group and is assisted by teachers and guides. The organization is usually controlled by the more sophisticated members of the group, who may become so powerful that they greatly influence the movement's orientation, often not to the advantage of spiritual aspirations. The membership comes from all levels of society; usually only adult men and women are accepted as members. All groups use similar modes of devotion, worship by meditation, which may be called *sudjud, sembahjang,* or *samadi.*

Each group has its particular style of meditation. Meditation is cultivated by the worshiper through a learning process of diligent exercises in order to achieve perfection. The duration and level of worship by meditation greatly depends upon the individual member of the group. Many groups use offerings, abstinence, incense, visits to the graves of ancestors, and mantras and prayers as devotional adjuncts. The chief symbol of devotion is usually the one God, sometimes with subsymbols such as ancestors, angels, or other spirits.

The philosophical ideas of the group—its concepts of life, death, the spiritual world, and cosmic life—create its specific frame of orientation. Most groups claim their teachings and thought are traditional Javanese science (*ilmu kedjawen*). The teachings and thoughts of these groups are usually a mixture of Hindu-Buddhistic, Islamic, and old animistic beliefs, although several groups claim to be based on a specific religion (usually Islam).

The ultimate goal of these movements is often *Djumbuhing Kawula lan Gusti,* eternal unity with the One God. There tends to be a great diversity of opinion concerning this ultimate goal, its conceptualization as well as the method of attaining it through meditation. Several groups may share the same concept, but not the same method of its attainment. There is also a social goal which has been conceptualized by the Congress of the Indonesian Kebatinan (mysticism) as follows: to work as much as possible for the sake of the world without any other intentions (such as personal profit). The minor goals of a movement may include: the worship of ancestors, perfection of the human soul, purification of the self, reaching a higher heaven after death, preservation of Javanese science, and the cultivation of supernatural power (occult power, healing power, communication with the various spirits).

For most Javanese, human life is seen as part of an endless cosmic life cycle. There is a strong belief in the existence of a structured supernatural world inhabited by spirits and souls which is reinforced by a gratifying belief in spirit protection. From childhood, the Javanese is accustomed to spirit worship. Spirits in general are usually feared, but certain spirits are also seen as protectors. Spirit worship is an acquired way of asking for spirit protection, blessing, and forgiveness. The belief in being protected or forgiven may reduce an individual's insecurity and guilt feelings in facing his emotional problems even though the problems are not resolved. Spirits also become objects of projection. To blame the spirit as the probable cause of emotional tension may transform anxieties and frustrations into irrational fears that can then be handled more easily by actions such as offerings and visits to the graves of ancestors. The worshiper may learn a proper form of projection and proper actions for protection in the group, or forms may be suggested on an ad hoc basis by the spiritual leader.

The belief in a supernatural world with its supernatural beings may stimulate the need for further knowledge of this world and its possible relationship to the natural world of human beings. The word *kebatinan (batin* means inner experience) implies not only the human inner life but also the exploration of the supernatural world and its relationship with the natural world. Mystical movements are called *aliran kebatinan* in Javanese (*aliran* means movement). The tendency of a Javanese, especially the elderly, to preoccupy themselves with problems of *kebatinan* may be related to childhood fantasies of wishing to communicate with spirits, to a wish for supernatural power, or to a desire for knowledge about life after death. Desire for *kebatinan* also may be stimulated when the individual faces insoluble emotional conflicts, especially feelings of insecurity about the future. The common sequence of probing further into problems of *kebatinan* is as follows: preoccupation, need of experience (meditation), need of expression, need of recognition, and a *kebatinan* frame of orientation accompanied by distortion of external reality. In stages of preoccupation, experience, and expression, one may feel that joining a mystical group of the same orientation may be beneficial. In the secure group environment, free expression of supernatural experience will be accepted, and the individual will receive protection, guidance, and control from the group and its spiritual leader. If the individual has a great need for recognition, he may seek to become a mystical leader. The maintenance of a clear boundary between these two worlds may be important in order to keep in touch with the world of reality. If the boundary fades away, a distortion of reality occurs with a strong *kebatinan* frame of orientation. Social functioning will then be disturbed.

Mystical movements may function as small religions with major emphasis on the concrete experience of meditation. Theoretical explanation of philosophical and religious doctrines is kept simple and easily comprehensible. The intellectual content is played down. The basic concepts are usually in accord with the Javanese philosophy of life in general, of which submission, dogmatism, acceptance, patience, alertness, dependency, etiquette, and spirit worship are the most important. Because mystical movements may function as religions, the process of the mystical experience may involve an alteration of previously held religious beliefs. The repetition of meditation and the purification process may arouse feelings of guilt, sin, and fear which the mystical group's rewards and punishments may stimulate. Some mystical movements are well aware of this change. Sometimes dramatic reactions during the so-called period of crisis (also called evolution or cleansing), which occasionally shows symptoms of acute psychotic reactions, may be seen as the climax in the process of change or as the manifestation of multiple conflicts—among others, a conflict between an individual's existing religious beliefs and his acceptance of the beliefs of the movement. With emotional support and kindly guidance from the teachers, the member may be able to overcome this change-induced crisis. It should be noted that the officially recognized religions greatly oppose the existence of the mystical groups. Members of some mystical groups may practice the art of healing which is a *dukun*-like practice (*dukun* is a native healer) with a more or less supernatural orientation, the description of which is beyond the scope of this paper. Other groups consider their meditation exercises to have sufficient healing power and do not seek additional practices.

A mystical group may be created by one or more people, usually under the same *dukun* teacher or mystical school. Another way of creating a mystical group is by a supernatural message; someone suddenly receives a message to give enlightenment to his fellow Javanese and to propagate the teachings given afterwards by a supernatural messenger. An individual native healer (*dukun*) may change his private healing practice into a mystical movement by accepting pupils in apprenticeship and becoming well known.

For the leader, the formation of a group around him may fulfill certain psychological and sociopsychological needs. He may enhance his social status in the community and at the same time have his economic needs cared for by the members. It may provide an expedient solution for his emotional conflicts by, for example, compensating for insecurity and inferiority feelings. By receiving devotion and affection from the membership, he may, in turn, become entirely dependent on them.

An important Javanese ideal, the so-called just king, greatly facilitates the creation of mystical groups, especially in periods of social turmoil. The emphasis on justice may have been stimulated by the past 300 years of colonial rule and Javanese dissatisfaction with social conditions in general, factors which could easily create the social insecurity and the constant feeling of the ordinary Javanese that he was being treated unjustly. The impressive performance of a spiritual leader and the devotion of his pupils appear to be modeled on the ideal of a just king.

The government will always be suspicious when new movements are created. This is especially true when these movements internalize the just king attitude which greatly enhances devotion to the spiritual leader and promotes the fighting spirit of the group. During the pre-World War II period, such movements were viewed as a prelude to possible uprising and nowadays are regarded as potential political movements. Therefore, they are usually checked by the government as early as possible. Unfortunately, it is not easy to readily determine whether new movements may have other aspirations beside their spiritual activities. Mystical movements in general are well tolerated by the government as long as their practices are not in conflict with law and regulations (especially political activities, amoral and asocial acts). The urban groups tend to operate in more secrecy and have less opportunity for extension than the rural groups which are more open and where whole villages may join the movement.

Urban mystical group leaders come from all levels of society, but least often from the upper classes. They may be full-time spiritual leaders, but there are also government officials, bankers, businessmen, teachers, medical doctors, engineers, etc. In addition, they may have a profitable (*dukun*) native healing practice, although most mystical movements regard healing for profit as a violation of *kebatinan* (rules). Despite the high respect given by the group to the leader, the role does not enhance status in the community or in their professions as government official, banker, doctor.

In rural areas, the spiritual leaders of mystical groups are usually peasants and are more active in propagating their teachings, e.g., by frequent visits to neighbors who may need some spiritual help. The peasant role is shared by almost all members of the village community, and in this rural setting the spiritual leader may enjoy high status. With high status for the leader, the prospects for enlarging the group increase, but the larger a mystical group, the greater need for organization. With greater need for organization and diversity of membership, a hierarchical system of leadership emerges. In a hierarchical system of leadership, when a spiritual leader passes away, the group may fall apart into smaller and opposing groups.

One of the most important aspects of a mystical group may be the free healing practices. Healing also may be interpreted as a way of not becoming too involved with *kebatinan* and as a means of maintaining social communication with the natural world. Some of these groups even have outpatient facilities. While not officially endorsed by the government, these facilities are not prohibited. Mystical groups also may be regarded as preservers of old Javanese principles of life, *narima, sabar, waspada, eling, tatakrama, andap asor,* and *prasadja.* Newer, more modern principles of life, although not resisted are not encouraged. Nowadays with the process of Indonesianization being encouraged, many (especially elderly) Javanese may try to preserve their Javanese identity by joining a mystical group.

GROUP ASPECTS

Members of a movement accept their spiritual leader as the worldly representation of a deity. Decisions concerning each individual member will be made by him. Without the members' devotion for the spiritual leader, the existence of the group would be impossible. The leader is actually the binding force of the group; the representation of the omnipotent father figure. The family motif is reinforced by the old rule that members of the same group have to regard each other as brothers and sisters of the same (father) teacher (*kadang* or *saderek tunggal guru*). The emotional ties between members may be even stronger than ties within the family.

We suggest that this member-movement relation is a reliving of childhood experiences in the extended family system. The spiritual leader is head of the family, the omnipotent father figure, while the teachers and guides are the uncles and aunts. The teacher of a class may be regarded as the direct father or mother figure. Members of the upper classes are seen as elder siblings while members of the lower classes are younger brothers and sisters. While, in childhood, superstitious beliefs may influence the fantasy world of the child, mystical teachings and experiences may fulfill childhood fantasies of obtaining supernatural power such as healing power, communication with spirits, etc. The intensive teacher-pupil relation facilitates continuous guidance and support for the member. The active interaction between the group members in a secure group environment may fulfill the member's need of belonging and dependency. This may be especially beneficial if the family environment of an unmarried individual is becoming unbearable and relations with relatives are becoming too traumatic. Active participation in group activities and diligent exercises may facilitate the member's efforts toward a possible way out of existing internal conflicts.

THE EXERCISE OF MEDITATION

The word meditation is used here to indicate every deliberate attempt by an individual to produce a special state of mind that is open to supernatural experience, with or without withdrawal of awareness of the environment. With a marked or total withdrawal of awareness of the environment, the meditation may become a trance state. The various groups use different names for their exercises, such as *sudjud, sembahjang, samadi,* or *wening.* Each group may have one or more kinds of meditation. Meditation itself is a learning process that passes through various stages. Many movements call meditation a process of purification or maturation. A member will start at the lowest level and, at a time decided by the spiritual leader, will proceed to the next higher level. The member is constantly guided and controlled by the leader's assistants. Certain rituals such as prayers, mantras, and burning of incense may be performed prior to the meditation proper. Abstinence from all or certain foods or drinks and from sexual relationship as well as deprivation of sleep, retreat into seclusiveness, and visits to graves of ancestors may be suggested occasionally. While rituals prior to meditation may be objects of concentration, abstinence from food and drinks and deprivation of sleep may fatigue the nervous system. The retreat into seclusiveness and visits to graves of ancestors may create a monotonous environment with a minimum of external stimuli. All these measures serve to facilitate a smoother meditation. The occasional inability to meditate may be seen as an indication of existing emotional conflicts that must be discussed with the teacher afterwards. In the more modern movements, the measures noted above, as well as much of the spirit beliefs, are abandoned and regarded as primitive.

THE EXERCISE OF MEDITATION IN THE SUMARAH MOVEMENT

Some mystical groups have tried to interpret the process of meditation by giving a theoretical explanation of a hypothetical mental structure and the possible relation of its components during the various stages of meditation. One of these groups is the Sumarah movement which was created in 1935 when the spiritual leader received a supernatural message to propagate the knowledge of Sumarah. An attempt will be made to give one of the many possible psychological interpretations of the process of meditation in this movement and, at the same time, to keep this interpretation as close as possible to the group's theoretical explanation. *Sumarah* means *sudjud-marang-Allah* (meditation to Allah). It is well organized with branches in many parts of the country. The members are distributed in five classes; each class has a teacher. The movement may be regarded as one of the modern groups. It has abandoned spirit worship, and members are not allowed to communicate with spirits whom they possibly may encounter during the meditation. In the first stage of meditation, the member is not allowed to meditate except in the presence of a teacher, because there is a risk of becoming possessed by these spirits. The exercise of meditation is called *sudjud.*

At the lowest level of *sudjud,* the member meditates in a standing position and is asked to close his eyes, to stop thinking, and not to pay any attention to external stimuli or to counteract body movements. The member usually will fall down on the floor and start showing automatic motor behavior. Certain of these acts are easily recognized as praying, fighting, imitating sexual acts, running around, or speaking in tongues. A member is supposed to develop a greater sensitivity to danger during the *sudjud* than in non-*sudjud* states; thus, he will easily find his way without colliding with other members or obstacles. If suddenly attacked by another member, he will automatically avoid or foil the attack. When the exercise is over, the member will have some recollection of inner experiences (certain sensations and hallucinations), but other happenings during the *sudjud* will be totally forgotten. According to the group's theories, at this level of *sudjud,* the *angen-angen,* the preserver of knowledge and experience (memory), separates from the *pamikir* (thought). A possible explanation may be that, by a minimum of cortical arousal and a lower level of information input, dissociation (here a trance state) occurs with an abreaction of stored significant experiences (a discharge of energy through more or less meaningful motor behavior). The ability to develop a greater sensitivity to certain stimuli indicates that a functioning component of the personality is still in contact with the environment.

On a higher level of *sudjud,* automatic motor behavior becomes less pronounced and finally ceases. The *sudjud* may be felt as something in the middle of the breast as big as a tennis ball that becomes smaller with diligent exercises. At this stage, the member may receive messages from voices suddenly speaking through his mouth or from the middle of his breast. According to Sumarah theories, the *angen-angen* unite with the *rasa sutji* (holy feeling) located in the middle of the breast and the *sudjud* is felt. After the *sudjud,* both components separate again. All happenings during the *sudjud* may be partially or fully remembered. The middle of the breast may be a suggested point of concentration and consequently of a certain feeling which arises in this area. With more skill strong concentration will be unnecessary, and the feeling of the ball will be less pronounced. The sudden voices through the mouth may be remnants of automatic motor behavior, while voices from the middle of the breast may be a hallucinatory kind of experience, when stored portions of information emerge into awareness and are experienced as incoming conscious information.

When, according to Sumarah theories, the *angen-angen* and *rasa* unite permanently—twenty-four hours a day—the messages will be heard at any time or place. The member is fully aware of his surroundings and can communicate with, and is responsive to, his environment. Automatic motor behavior may sometimes occur. A member on his way to a meeting may suddenly feel that his legs are carrying him to the house of a sick member. The message is interpreted by the member as his not being allowed by the deity to go to the meeting but, instead, as being required to take care of the sick member. The feeling of constantly being under control of the deity is the ultimate objective of the Sumarah movement which has three basic principles. A human being can do nothing (unless with God's will), he has nothing (his worldly possessions are borrowed), and he should surrender his body and soul to the deity.

Since memory is not impaired, the concept *angen-angen* may not mean the memory of past experiences itself but rather the emotional components of it. The permanent separation of the *angen-angen* from the *pamikir* and unity with the *rasa* may thus involve a constant effort to separate past experiences from their emotional components. The *rasa* acts as a kind of screening mechanism for these emotional components and enables one to constantly dispose of them. The main aim on this level of *sudjud* may be the constant suppression of emotional feelings in daily life by the technique of meditation with the constant possibility for discharge. Members who have reached the level of *sudjud* described above may be somewhat apathetic and detached. They may show some flatness of facial expression, poverty of emotions, and indifferent attitudes. In interpersonal relations, they exhibit some indifference, even toward relatives. Orientation and memory are not impaired, while thinking is less critical, and general response toward external stimuli is somewhat slow.

The highest level of *sudjud* has been attained solely by the spiritual leader when the *sudjud* is suddenly felt in his heart area, instead of the middle of the breast, and then disappears. It is said that unity with the deity, the ultimate goal of the movement, has been accomplished, and this individual has become the transmitter of God's words. The spiritual leader strongly identifies himself with the deity; a kind of transformation of personality has been accomplished. With a great skill in *sudjud,* a point of concentration is no longer necessary.

This movement considers its meditation exercises to have significant healing power, and the patient requesting help will usually be asked to join the movement. The creation of healing facilities is prohibited, but occasional healing practice by a member is allowed as long as he does not receive gifts in any form. If because of his illness a patient is not able to *sudjud* himself, a teacher in the movement may *sudjud* for his well-being. Later on, he must *sudjud* himself and join the movement. The teacher is only a mediator, and the deity alone decides whether a patient is cured or not.

During a meditation exercise, the teacher is supposed to be able to feel his pupil's meditation and to be able to correct it by giving advice. This ability is called *njemak* (to feel another's feeling) and is supposed to be accomplished with the support of his *rasa sutji* during the *sudjud. Njemak* does not enable a teacher to know what other people think, but only what they feel at a given moment, such as feelings of pain, anxiety, distress, fever, hostility, or depression as well as feelings during meditation. If he is meditating for a patient's well-being, the teacher will experience the symptoms of the illness and suffering himself. It is not surprising, therefore, that the treatment of a mentally ill patient (psychotic disturbance), where the *pamong* has to *sudjud* for the well-being of the patient since the patient is unable to *sudjud* himself, is supposed to be the most difficult, because the teacher will experience the mental disturbance.

Conclusion

It seems that the main function of the Javanese mystical groups is to provide a secure environment for the individual when he is suffering from emotional conflicts which he is not able to solve even with the help of the native healer. The group aspects of the mystical groups may be beneficial for the member as long as he does not estrange himself from his family relationships and as long as he is able to fulfill his social obligations in the family setting. Former childhood education with strong emphasis on spirit worship and other old Javanese beliefs may greatly influence a member's decision to join a mystical group in adulthood.

The suppression of emotional feelings is a learned attitude and is in accord with the principles of the Javanese etiquette and preservation of dignity. This suppression of emotional feelings may create many insoluble emotional conflicts in the individual. The reinforcement of this suppression by the exercises of meditation, with possible discharge of energy-loaded emotions, may be a possible way out of dealing with emotional conflicts. On the higher levels of meditation, which potentially can engender an indifferent attitude in interpersonal relations, many social complications may occur, especially in family and marital relations.

The joining of mystical groups may be most beneficial for the elderly Javanese. Although they are tolerated and taken care of by younger family members, elderly Javanese may have feelings of isolation or rejection. As a result they may tend to preoccupy themselves with problems of *kebatinan* and even try to exercise meditation with a possible retreat into seclusiveness. The secure environment of a mystical group can provide these older citizens with some guidance and control.

Several members of mystical groups who have exhibited symptoms of psychotic reactions have been seen by psychiatric practitioners. Existing religious beliefs may come in conflict with the philosophical doctrines of the movement, experiences during meditation may create intensive fears, or the member may be so preoccupied with supernatural thought that it may interfere with his dealing with external reality.

19.   Religious Conversion and Elimination of the Sick Role:
A Japanese Sect in Hawaii

TAKIE SUGIYAMA LEBRA, Ph.D.

Department of Anthropology and
Social Science Research Institute
University of Hawaii
Honolulu, Hawaii

IT SEEMS SAFE to assume that every society has its definition of illness as a social role. The sick person as a role occupant can claim certain rights, such as the right to be exempted from work and other normal obligations and to be treated with "compassion, support, and help" (Parsons, 1964, 113). Precisely because illness is a social role, the contents of privilege vested in illness are likely to vary from one social system to another such that they are fitted into a particular system as a whole, of which the sick role is a part. When a new social system emerges, a new definition is likely to be given of the sick role. An emerging religious sect is most likely to carry its own definition of health and illness, as well as death, as an essential component of its culture. If healing takes place as a sectarian performance, it can be understood, I assume, in the light of the sectarian definition of the sick role.

I would like to explore possible relations between religious commitment and healing phenomena, with special attention to the redefined sick role. Religious commitment here specifically refers to conversion to a new sect which involves intense interaction between the candidate and proselytizer for conversion, exclusive membership in the sect, sustained participation in the sect's collective action, and rigorous conformity to the sectarian norms.

The sect studied is formally called Tenshō Kōtai Jingū Kyō, more commonly known as the Dancing Religion because of the outdoor collective dance, a part of its regular ritual which is most visible to the outside public. Here I shall abbreviate it as Tenshō. Tenshō emerged in postwar Japan under the leadership of a middle-aged farmer's wife, Sayo Kitamura, who came to be addressed as Ōgamisama, great deity. In 1952, the first overseas division of the sect was established in Hawaii, and its membership is roughly estimated to have reached 500 as of 1965. The following analysis is based on a year-long field research (Lebra, 1967) on Tenshō converts in Hawaii. The data were collected through interviews with 55 Honolulu members over 30 years old and through observation of collective activities at local branch meetings. Most interviewees had had direct contact with Ōgamisama, the self-appointed messiah, at one phase of conversion or another, which was made possible by her occasional visits to Hawaii or by the follower's pilgrimage to the sect's headquarters in Japan. Being either *issei* (Japan-born immigrants) or *nisei* (*issei*'s American-born children) including *kibei* (American-born returnees from Japan after growing up there), the informants all understood Japanese with varying degrees of literacy and binguality. As for class background, they were found distinctly lower in education and occupation than members of a Buddhist church in Honolulu. Among various reported evidences of salvation, healing was mentioned most frequently. Sixty percent of the informants who had been ill or whose family members had been ill or both, (N = 40) declared that complete healing had taken place due to conversion; 20 percent claimed definite improvement. Post-conversion experience of healing was reported even more frequently in both interviews and weekly congregations. Whether one should accept such information as reliable or reject it as a wishful distortion, or whether conversion did not bring the opposite outcome (aggravation of illness or death) as well, does not affect our analysis. Our interpretation of the sectarian redefinition of the sick role should account for both the reported successful curing and unreported aggravation of illness.

As in many other religions, Tenshō ideology identifies illness as a sign of supernatural potency. Therefore, a brief review of Tenshō concepts of the supernatural is necessary. In my informants' vocabulary a variety of supernatural agents associated with illness were found. The supernatural being may be suprahuman, human, or infrahuman (e.g., dog spirit); it may be emitted from a dead person (a dead spirit) or a living person (a live spirit); and it may be familiar or strange to the person being possessed by it. It may be benevolent, malevolent, or neutral, and thus sickness may be taken as a sign of the disciplinarian intent of a fatherly supernatural, as an attack by a hostile spirit which is jealous or holding a grudge or as a gesture of a dead person's spirit trying to call attention and solicit help from the living person.

The central supernatural figure in Tenshō is the Kami, specifically identified as Tenshō Kōtai Jin (the heaven-illuminating, great-ruling deity), who is claimed to have descended into Sayo Kitamura's abdomen and transformed her from a simple farmer into a third messiah after Buddha and Christ. Tenshō Kōtai Jin has partial identity with the Shinto Sun-Goddess, Amaterasu—a point which cannot be overlooked in understanding the conversion of the people of Japanese ancestry, particularly of *issei* and *kibei*. This supreme Kami causes sickness to give divine tests. However, sickness is usually associated more with lesser spirits, or both the Kami and lesser supernatural agents are believed to be jointly responsible for sickness.

A word about a semi-supernatural agent called *innen*. *Innen* is understood as a Karma chain, fate or bondage that is transmitted from one individual to another through consanguineal links in most cases but not always. *Innen* is the most frequently mentioned symbol to explain sickness, although, here again, *innen* may join the spirit of one or another dead person in causing illness.

Given the above cognitive orientation toward sickness, it follows that the sick role must be redefined. The following analysis focuses upon the evaluative change of the sick role. Evaluation of the sick role refers to judgment of sick-role occupancy in terms of good or bad. It falls into two categories. One is evaluative judgment by a collectively shared and sanctioned standard involving moral principles; the other refers to judgment by the evaluator's own emotional acceptability. The former is objective; the latter, subjective. These two standards of judgment are identified here as legitimacy and desirability.

Change in Legitimacy

In Japan, where the individual is rigidly bound by role obligation as a member of a group, illness appears as a primary opportunity for release from obligation. Excessive legitimacy of the sick role seems to be necessitated to compensate for excessive demands for role conformity in daily life. This is shown by the overtolerance of the Japanese for the public figure who fails to fulfill his public responsibility because of illness as well as by the false pretense of being sick which the Japanese frequently resort to when they want to resign from a job. This tendency may be explained not only by the social function of sickness as suggested here but by the deep layer of personality system. The studies conducted by DeVos (1960) and DeVos and Wagatsuma (1959) delineated the Japanese conception of illness in connection with guilt. Illness is viewed as a sign of moral masochism which characterizes the behavior of Japanese women, particularly of the mother. The mother's illness as the physical expression of her self-sacrifice and self-blame for others' faults, the authors contended, induces guilt in the child, and the latter may also find in his own illness the desired expiation of his guilt. It may be said that the moral tone surrounding illness is so generalized that the sick person feels or appears righteous, and the people around him are compelled to feel guilty. Conversion to Tenshō brought about a radical change in this orientation. Illness, as such, has lost claim to legitimacy. It is not that what was described above as Japanese disappeared completely but that it was channeled in another direction.

In Tenshō, illness is looked upon as a signal of neglect of one's duty; it reflects or arouses guilt and shame in the sick person. This view is internalized in two ways: either through the relation between ego and the identified supernatural that is believed to be causing the sickness, through the relation between ego and Ōgamisama or fellow members or both.

Conversion reestablishes not only cognitive but also moral relation between the convert and the supernatural. Sickness is caused by a spirit, it is true, but the spirit's activation is partly contingent upon the sick person's action. The Kami, for example, gives more tests to those who neglect the duty to Him than to those who are faithful.[1] The convert suffers from muscular pain because, as Ōgamisama interprets, he is greatly indebted to a deceased kin. As long as the latter's spirit continues to visit him and cause pain, he will feel guilty for not repaying the debt. Even hostile spirits such as *jashin* (a false deity), *inugami* (a dog spirit), and *ikiryō* (a live spirit) are supposed to be activated, at least in part, in response to ego's disposition or behavior. "*Jashin* comes from *janen* (wicked intent) [of the possessed]"; "to be possessed [by a spirit] is just as shameful as to possess [someone]." If a person is attacked by *ikiryō*, he must reflect that he has done something which made the *ikiryō* originator jealous or caused him to hold a grudge. Such retributive significance is clearly associated with *innen* as well; here is involved the idea that a person receives a certain *innen* as a reward or punishment for what he did in his present or previous life.

Moral masochism of the mother and the child's guilt toward her are both effectively mobilized toward denial of the legitimacy of sickness. The convert is reminded to recall his deceased mother who suffered all her life for the sake of her drunken husband and unfilial son. His guilt sometimes reaches the point that he bursts into tears. The only way he can expiate his guilt is to save her spirit which is signified by his own recovery. Righteousness is associated with being healthy.

The convert's moral obligation to the supernatural is effectively supported and controlled by his social relation to Ōgamisama and fellow members. Obligation to the supernatural seems to overlap with obligation as a member of Tenshō sect, as Ōgamisama's disciple, and as a *dōshi* (comrade) to other members. To become sick and unable to attend regular meetings is taken as a consequence of violating the sectarian norms. Among the norms are: renunciation of external religious memberships, symbols, and paraphernalia; minimization of social affiliations; minimization of non-religious solution of problems such as medical treatment; and avoidance of worldly indulgence. These norms are difficult to follow. Particularly, renunciation of religious symbols such as ancestral altars, mortuary tablets, ashes and graveyards, and withdrawal from the family-inherited Buddhist and Shinto affiliation creates utmost conflict and, in some cases, results in family dissolution. Once the convert overcomes this conflict and becomes committed to the sectarian norms, he tends to dramatize his experience and to be intolerant of uncommitted fellow members whose sickness he sees as the Kami's punishment. It is interesting to note, in passing, that Tenshō emphasis upon guilt toward deceased kin and ancestors may be reinforced by the required destruction of their reminders such as tablets and altars.

To what extent sickness is associated with guilt depends upon internalization of sectarian norms. It is proposed here that the driving force for internalization of sectarian norms was provided by the deep sense of indebtedness to the proselytizers (Ōgamisama or members). The benefits ranged from tangible to interactional. Tangible benefits include provision of food, shelter, money, employment, professional services, and customers for traders. One informant was assigned a house by Ōgamisama's order which had belonged to her brother against the expressed wishes of her parents and siblings, not to mention the rule of patrilineal inheritance. Another claimed that Ōgamisama saved him from bankruptcy by giving advice on management of his business. Several informants benefited from the professional services of fellow members such as carpenters, painters, masseurs. By receiving such benefits, an initially uncommitted convert feels increasingly obligated to become a true Tenshō follower. Among other tangible benefits, the provision of marriage partners and children for adoption may be included. Locally, a number of new families emerged through Ōgamisama's matchmaking, in most cases between a local convert and a convert in Japan. The sense of indebtedness for tangible benefits is further strengthened by Ōgamisama's declaration that this religion demands no membership dues. This alleged pecuniary indifference on the part of the prophet seems an exceedingly important factor in generating the obligation of total compliance among the converts.

More important locally than tangible benefits are interactional benefits. The benefit here is derived from the behavioral capacity of the proselytizer, verbal and nonverbal, in public or private scenes, to initiate and maintain interaction. At the most physical level, it includes tactile interaction—patting or pressing parts of the candidate's body where a spirit is supposed to be located, such as shoulder, back, stomach; pulling the candidate by the hand to stand up; in execptional cases, eating and sleeping with Ōgamisama. It is not coincidental that masseurs have been effective proselytizers, as numerous local cases indicate. At another level, interaction consists of expressive communication. This includes facial movements (Ōgamisama's radiant face, compassionate smile, frightening gaze, frown, tearful eyes) hand movements (pointing at a person, beckoning to him to come forward) head movements (nodding, shaking) and combined movements (bowing with folded palms in a prayer form, showing a smile of welcome for any candidate).

Verbal interaction is through either direct speech or correspondence. The benefactor may play an active role as a speaker or a passive role as an eager sympathetic listener. Most early converts have the treasured memories of what Ōgamisama said to them in their first encounter with her. The meaning of the verbalized content does not necessarily seem to count. Many did not understand Ōgamisama's particular dialect and yet felt as if struck by a thunderbolt. The effect of exposure to vocal stimulation from the whole congregation chanting the meaningless phrase is another example.

Another dimension of interaction may be added. While the interaction described above refers to Ōgamisama's or a member's action directly oriented toward the convert, this involves the introduction of a third party, individual or collective, into the interaction situation. First, a transmitter's role or a go-between role is played by the third person, as when Ōgamisama's favorable comment on a new convert is transmitted to the latter through a leader close to her. As the access to Ōgamisama decreases, reliance upon such a go-between increases in order to maintain interaction. In fact, this form of communication can be even more effective than a direct one in that the third person, with better knowledge of the potential or new convert, can adjust or modify the information to be transmitted. Secondly, in a public scene where the candidate is introduced to Ōgamisama in front of a large audience, the audience's responses can be utilized effectively to gratify the candidate. Ōgamisama fully used this social resource to flatter, approve, upset, or shame the candidate.

Tangible and interactional benefits presented by Ōgamisama or members, however trivial they may look, tend to have a tremendous impact in obligating a new convert and urging him to do whatever the Kami (that is, Ōgamisama) tells him. The way he comes to feel deeply obligated, for a seemingly negligible benefit, may reflect the degree of deprivation, material and social, which made him inordinately appreciative of the slightest favor offered. The scarcity value of the benefit, in other words, must have been high. This was confirmed by the fact that livelihood had been a serious problem for many converts and by the fact that still more converts had been lonely as a result of family disharmony, especially of marital friction or of family dissolution. Thus, they were hungry for human warmth. The process of becoming obligated may have been accelerated also by the Japanese cultural idiom surrounding the concept of *on*.[2] Simply by labeling whatever is received an *on,* the convert may feel compelled to generalize it into an unpayable debt and to attempt to repay it at any cost.

When these benefits are accompanied, as they often are, by at least temporary relief from illness, the beneficiary becomes convinced that Ōgamisama is his lifesaver or, as informants put it, *inochi-no-onjin,* the *on*-person to whom he owes his life. To repay the *on,* he must become a further committed follower, and to be healthy is a sign of such commitment. As Ōgamisama says, "If you discipline yourself hard enough, you will enter the world where there is no need of doctors or drugs." Where there is any degree of ambivalence on the part of the convert, he is more likely to dramatize and publicly announce his experience of salvation, letting the audience know how deeply he is indebted to Ōgamisama for his life. Once committed to this extent, the convert must maintain his state of salvation (being healthy), not only as a moral obligation to the benefactor but to save face vis-à-vis fellow members. Thus, a deeply committed convert shows embarrassment and apologizes to Ōgamisama in his testimony when he falls ill.

As a human being subject to illness, Ōgamisama plays two roles. She takes a typically "exemplary" leadership role (Weber, 1963) by stressing that she has attained absolute salvation and by telling her followers to emulate her. She says, "Come up where I am. How good I feel!" At the same time, she lets them know that she constantly suffers from all sorts of illness. It is here that moral masochism is fully displayed. And yet masochism does not lie so much in being sick as in ignoring sickness and working regularly like a healthy person. Ōgamisama takes pride in the fact that she has never had a single day off from the duty of preaching even when she has been seriously ill. This form of masochism is demanded of the members. One of the local pilgrims to the headquarters testified that, while there, she had been scolded by Ōgamisama for using sickness as a reason for not attending the daily disciplinary meeting. She was told that she was indulging herself. Seventy-nine years old, this informant could not get out of bed because of pain and stiffness throughout her body. After learning of Ōgamisama's scoldings through a go-between, she made up her mind to attend the meeting and even participated in yard work to which all pilgrims were assigned.

It has been shown that the legitimacy of the sick role is denied to Tenshō members and that they are obligated, once ill, to recover as promptly as possible.

Change in Desirability

With regard to the Japanese attitude toward illness, Caudill (1962) singled out the characteristically gratifying aspect of the sick role. Specifically, he noted that in Japan sickness provides an important social occasion for the emotionally satisfying communication between the patient and the nursing person from which they are ordinarily inhibited. People in Japan, it was observed, like to go to bed with mild illnesses. Caudill related such expectation of communication through sickness to the Japanese tendency to live out emotions. Institutionalization of *tsukisoi* (subprofessional nurses attached to particular patients on a 24-hour basis), also studied by Caudill (1961), shows that such expectation of the sick role is not confined to home care but extended to the hospital situation. The desirability of the sick role described here is shared by the patient and the nursing person, and thus we can say that the function of sickness is socially integrative as well as ego integrative. If sickness justifies the wish to depend upon and be indulged by the attending person, it also legitimizes the wish to be depended upon and indulged upon by the patient. It may be recalled, in this connection, that many pure love stories widely read in Japan involve a love partner who is sick and sometimes fatally so. The socially integrative function of sickness can be seen not only in the form of reciprocity and communication between the patient and the attendant. Sickness further gratifies the wish for physical gregariousness with a larger group of people since relatives, friends, and other concerned people gravitate toward the patient to do *mimai* (inquiry after a sick person).

The general desirability of the sick role described here is also eliminated through Tenshō conversion. As the illegitimate aspect of the sick role is internalized by Tenshō converts, so is the undesirable expectation of it. Elimination of desirability can be analyzed from two points of view: change in expectation of dependency and gregariousness and vested interest in exemplary well-being.

Through conversion, sickness ceases to be an occasion for gratification of the wish for dependency and solidary gregariousness. Since sickness is believed to be caused supernaturally, recovery is expected to follow the ritual effort (prayer) of the sick person himself. The individuals around him, on the other hand, are supposed to stay away from him lest they should catch and carry with them the spirit causing the illness. This is one reason why Tenshō members are discouraged from attending secular funerals as well as visiting hospitals. Contact with a sick person is to be avoided, particularly by vulnerable members. Coupled with the realization of the supernatural causation, the conceptualization of sickness as illegitimate reduces sympathy for the sick. Such a cold attitude facilitates severing oneself from old secular obligations to sick people outside the sect, thus contributing to the autonomy of the sect. When a member becomes sick, he tends to express discontent with such forced isolation, as some informants indicated. However, this isolation seems only to reinforce the patient's wish to get well, to go back to the regular meeting, and to be approved by fellow members; the temporarily frustrated wish for solidary gathering is gratified through restored health. Ōgamisama strongly disapproves the desire for dependency and indulgence and stresses discipline and self-help even with sick followers, as we have observed before.

Desire to be sick is further inhibited by the fact that the convert has made a social investment in his well-being. First, commitment to sectarian norms involves self-sacrifice on the part of the convert in his secular interest which is likely to amount to an overpayment for whatever debt he owes to the sect. Not only does he cut himself off from secular ties, but he also positively contributes to the sect in money or kind on a voluntary basis. One important means to secure the payoff is to expand the sect and to make its prophecy—final salvation of the Kami's children and damnation of the rest of mankind on the coming day of judgment—come true. The convert has a vested interest in the successful recruitment of new converts. To demonstrate how the proselytizer himself has been saved is a most effective and generally used technique for persuasion. As living evidence of the experienced miracle, he must manage his front, as Goffman (1959) would phrase it, as a revitalized, young, healthy-looking man. His face is more persuasive than words. It is all too understandable that Tenshō emphasizes the importance of the facial look as the window of the soul. Such "face-work" (Goffman, 1955) is constantly required when potential converts are within one's family. It is also necessary for self-defense when one's conversion has created family conflict, since any symptom of sickness on the part of the convert will give a reason for the family members opposed to Tenshō to attack him.

Social investment in well-being has further implications. Payoff for sacrifice is partly derived from the status obtained by the convert within the members' community. Particularly for those who are frustrated with status aspirations in the outside world, it seems crucial to assume and maintain a leader's status in the local branch. Here again, leadership is mainly exemplary in that the leader himself must look saved. Physical vulnerability will cost him the exalted status as well as his face.

The desirability of the sick role, or rather its undesirability, has been discussed with reference to both emotional pleasurability and calculated interest. We can see how change in desirability and change in legitimacy reinforce each other until the point is reached where the sick role is eliminated. This may account not only for Tenshō members' willingness to get well and to exaggerate healing miracles but also for actual instances of cures. At the same time, elimination of the sick role may be responsible for aggravation of illness, including sudden death, whenever recovery would have required physical and psychological rest more than anything else. Aggravation and death did occur frequently, though they were not reported as such. When death occurs, the survivors explain it this way: the deceased person was completely cured before he died, when he was dying, or after he died. The evidence of such a cure is found in the following situations: Ōgamisama's declaration such as, "Don't worry, your husband has now attained Buddahood in heaven"; the corpse remaining soft and warm long after death occurred; the survivor's hallucination with the vision of the deceased appearing healthy; and the belief that all poisons were squeezed out of the body right before death occurred.

Qualifications

The preceding analysis was carried on with the assumption that Tenshō converts in Hawaii have redefined the sick role from a typically Japanese image into a less Japanese image. A close examination of interview materials, however, justifies this assumption only in part.

It is unlikely that Japanese culture, as the point of departure for redefinition of the sick role in legitimacy and desirability, applies to Hawaii's members of Tenshō completely. First, both legitimacy and desirability of the sick role in Japan are structurally supported by the availability of the nursing personnel as well as by economic security within a household. The multi-generational family system, together with solidary ties with collateral kin, will guarantee an attendant to a sick member and transference of economic responsibility in case the major breadwinner gets sick. Such security for emergency may be further provided by the mutual aid network in rural communities. In Hawaii, as far as my informants are concerned, the nuclear family, including single member households, was predominant [3] and the mutual aid, systems, e.g., association of immigrants from the same provinces, were breaking down. Thus, the sickness of one member tends to be disastrous. The working wife may share economic responsibility but then is not available as a nurse. No wonder that many informants, especially male converts, expressed deep attachment to their mothers from whom they had been long separated and that Ōgamisama struck the responsive cord in their hearts when she reminded them of the unpayable debt to their mothers. No more surprising is the fact that Ōgamisama was identified as "like my mother or grandmother" or "someone even more missed."

Secondly, probably conditioned by such structural change of the family system and also by social contact with other ethnic groups, Hawaii's Japanese seem to have internalized some of the American compulsion for independence and autonomy. The informants recalled their sickness having caused depression and even suicidal attempts because the physical incapacity and forced dependency were too painful to bear.

It is now necessary to modify our assumption as to legitimacy and desirability of the sick role. Hawaii's members of Tenshō may have internalized the Japanese expectation of the sick role but lacked a structural basis for realizing it, and they may have learned two types of value regarding dependency—Japanese and American. What Tenshō did was to get rid of frustrations arising from the discrepancy between expectation and gratification, and it expelled ambivalence stemming from bicultural learning by demoting the Japanese expectation pattern. With all these qualifications, it is still clear that Tenshō brought about a change in the sick role which encouraged its total elimination.

Conclusions

With the hope of delineating an explanatory variable for faith healing, I have analyzed redefinition of the sick role triggered by religious conversion. Two aspects of the sick role—legitimacy and desirability—were analyzed with reference to their change through sectarian commitment. It was noted that sickness lost its legitimacy by being identified as a sign of moral deficiency and lost its desirability because of the isolation forced upon the patient and because of the new investment in well-being. A number of problems were implied: the influence of religious commitment, in general, upon sickness; the Japanese background of the conversion phenomena in relation to sickness, because the sect studied was Japanese and its sampled members were of Japanese ancestry; and the variations in Hawaii's members of the sect who were specifically studied. Despite the complexity of issues involved, it may be concluded that redefinition of the sick role, learned through the particular sectarian conversion, amounted to its elimination and that this change may account, in part, for miraculous healing.

NOTES

1.   This view does not preclude the totally opposite view equally held by the converts that the Kami does not bother to test the hopeless but only tests his true children (Lebra, 1970).
2.   *On* refers to a relation between a benefit-giver and a benefit-recipient, implying the former's generosity and the latter's debt.
3.   This was partly necessitated by the migration. Many of the parent generation either never came to Hawaii or returned to Japan for good.

REFERENCES

Caudill, W. 1961. Around the clock patient care in Japanese psychiatric hospitals: the role of the *tsukisoi.* American Sociological Review 26:204–14.

———. 1962. Patterns of emotion in modern Japan. *In* Japanese culture: its development and characteristics. R. J. Smith and R. K. Beardsley, eds. Chicago, Aldine.

DeVos, G. 1960. The relation of guilt toward parents to achievement and arranged marriage among the Japanese. Psychiatry 23:287–301.

DeVos, G., and H. Wagatsuma. 1959. Psycho-cultural significance of concern over death and illness among rural Japanese. International Journal of Social Psychiatry 5:5–19.

Goffman, E. 1955. On face-work. Psychiatry 18:213–31.

———. 1959. The presentation of self in everyday life. Garden City, Doubleday.

Lebra, T. S. 1967. An interpretation of religious conversion: A millenial movement among Japanese-Americans in Hawaii. Ph.D. dissertation. University of Pittsburgh.

———. 1970. Logic of salvation: the case of a Japanese sect in Hawaii. International Journal of Social Psychiatry 16:45–53.

Parsons, T. 1964. Some reflections on the problem of psychosomatic relationships in health and illness. *In* Social structure and personality. London, The Free Press.

Weber, M. 1963. The sociology of religion. Boston, Beacon Press.

PROBLEMS OF TRANSCULTURAL ADAPTATION:
MIGRATION, STUDY ABROAD, EXPATRIATION, AND FUSION

20. Migration and Mental Disorders in Taiwan

HUNG-MING CHU, M.D.

Department of Neurology and Psychiatry
National Taiwan University Hospital
Taipei, Taiwan, Republic of China

MIGRATION is a complicated process involving social, economic, cultural, political, religious, and psychological factors. The characteristic of each migrant population varies, and so does the effect of migration on the mental health of the population concerned. Much of the current literature supports the association between migration and high rates of mental illness, but a reverse trend has been noted by some studies.[1] Studies of the relation between internal migration and mental illness have been rather inconsistent in their results.[2]

Two main hypotheses have been applied by investigators to explain the effect of migration on mental health. (1) The selective migration hypothesis holds that migrants (internal or foreign born) are sick or potentially ill before migration and, also, that a positive or negative screening effect may occur, not only for the potentially ill but also for those with a psychological and socioeconomic readiness to move.[3] (2) The stress hypothesis asserts that the process of migration, including culture shock, creates stress which precipitates mental disorder in susceptible individuals.[4] Generally speaking, these two effects often work together simultaneously, and they are not clearly separable.

These contradictory findings on migration and mental disorders possibly can be explained in several ways. (1) Most of the studies were based on hospital admission data which have serious limitations for generalizing the results.[5] (2) Various methods, such as health questionnaires, interviews, and clinical diagnoses by psychiatrists or general practitioners were employed to identify the ill population. The identified subgroups can display different patterns in reacting to migration, and most of the previous studies were confined to schizophrenia or psychosis. (3) The definition and duration of the migration were not the same, and these factors were significantly related to the prevalence of mental disorders.[6] (4) Because of the lack of detailed demographic data, both in migrants and nonmigrants, the effect of migration is often confused with the effect of other social factors such as age, sex, social class, or culture. Some statistical standardization methods are essential in the comparison of the different prevalences.[7]

A comprehensive survey of mental disorders in defined districts, as reported in this study, should provide the information needed to shed light on the relation between migration and mental disorders. The main objectives of this study were: (a) to obtain the prevalence rates of mental disorders of mainland Chinese immigrants in the sample communities, (b) to compare the prevalence of mental disorders between the natives (Taiwanese) and immigrants (Chinese mainlanders) with respect to various socioenvironmental factors, and (c) to identify the high risk groups in immigrant and native populations.

The present study has the following characteristics. (1) The data were collected by one research team by house-to-house visits using a uniform methodology; (2) subjects were the inhabitants of three defined communities —a rural and suburban area outside of Taipei, a small town, and a section of a large city—all sharing the same Chinese culture. (3) There were three distinct population groups: (a) native Taiwanese, born into families living in the above investigated communities before the end of World War II; (b) migrant Taiwanese, who moved from other parts of Taiwan with their families to the communities investigated above after World War II; and (c) the mainland Chinese, who came from mainland China to Taiwan after the war and settled in the investigated areas. (4) Systematic collection of demographic information of the communities was carried out in the survey together with a psychiatric investigation of the inhabitants. (5) Identification of a large number of psychoneurotics provided an opportunity to study the effect of migration upon neurotic disorders.

Geographical Sketch of Populations Investigated

A prevalence survey of mental disorders in the entire population of the Taiwanese in the three communities was conducted in 1946–48 (Lin, 1953). Fifteen years later a follow-up survey in the same three communities was carried out (Lin et al., 1969) with the total population consisting of: (a) original inhabitants and their children (native Taiwanese), (b) migrant Taiwanese who moved to these communities from other parts of Taiwan

Figure 1: Age and Sex Distribution of Three Investigated Populations

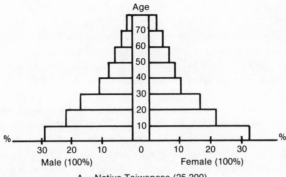

A. Native Taiwanese (25,200)
(M : F = 1.05)

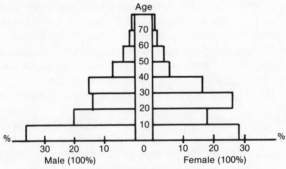

B. Migrant Taiwanese (3,984)
(M : F = 0.34)

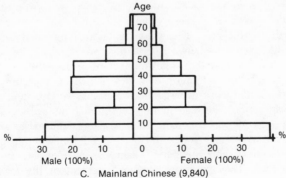

C. Mainland Chinese (9,840)
(M : F = 1.47)

during the last fifteen years, and (c) Chinese mainlanders who moved from mainland China after World War II. The mass migration of mainland Chinese took place in 1949–50. The proportion of registered mainland Chinese population to the total registered population in Taiwan was about 2 percent in 1948 and 6 percent in 1949. It increased steadily from 7 percent in 1950 to 12 percent in 1961 (Department of Civil Affairs, Taiwan Provincial Government, 1965), as migrants dispersed themselves all over the island. Overpopulation, especially in large cities, necessitated an expansion of various facilities.

Baksa, originally a rural community, underwent rapid social change to become a suburban district of Taipei City containing a number of government offices and schools. The population of the Baksa area tripled in fifteen years due mostly to migration, starting in 1949–50, of mainland Chinese, the majority of whom were civil workers and their families. The natural increase of the original inhabitants and a number of Taiwanese migrants also added to the population. In Simpo, a small town about fifteen miles north of Shin-Chou, which is still a market center mixed with a rural population, the proportion of migrant population was lower than the Baksa area. The district of Amping, located in the narrow strip between the sea and the center of Tainan, a large modern city in South Taiwan, was once a prosperous seaport of the old capital in Taiwan. Trade has been in continuous decline as a result of Tainan's urbanization. When a rubber factory manufacturing military articles was moved from mainland China to Amping after World War II, about 80 percent of the mainland Chinese in Amping migrated as employees of the factory.

At the time of our survey the population in the three areas totaled 25,200 native Taiwanese, 3,984 migrant Taiwanese, and 9,840 mainland Chinese. Demographically the three populations showed considerable differences: 1) As Figure 1 shows, the age and sex composition of the native Taiwanese exhibited a fairly normal distribution similar to the general population of Taiwan (Report of Department of Civil Affairs, Taiwan Provincial Government, 1965). The mainland Chinese showed a very irregular distribution. The age groups 30–40, 40–50, and 50–60 were disproportionately large, and the sex ratio of these groups was over 2.0. Members of these groups constituted the bulk of the population that migrated to Taiwan 15 years ago, when they were between 15 and 45 years old. On the other hand, there was a disproportionately small number of men in the age groups 10–19 and 20–29. The out-migration of males in these age groups to schools, military services, and work in large cities may account for their small numbers. The disproportionately small number of migrant Taiwanese males in the age group 20–29 was due to the same factors. The excess of mainland Chinese females in the age groups 10–19 and 20–29 may be attributed to the addition of a considerable number of Taiwanese women who were married to mainland men. They comprised about 5 percent of the total mainland population. 2) Household size was largest for native Taiwanese and smallest for mainland Chinese. Native Taiwanese had the highest proportion of three-generation families (45.5 percent), while the other two groups had a much higher proportion of two-generation families (over 70 percent). The mainland Chinese had a considerable number of single person households (8.9 percent). A larger proportion of mainland Chinese, 54.5 percent in males and 50.8 percent in females, were firstborn among the same sex siblings than native Taiwanese, 35.3 percent and 37.5 percent, respectively. It may be that large numbers of first born left mainland China because it was thought necessary for them to leave the troubled home for a safe place in order to perpetuate the family line. It may be related to the fact that more firstborn mainland Chinese entered the civil service and therefore migrated to Taiwan with the government. 3) Native Taiwanese and the mainland Chinese again showed striking differences in regard to education (Table 1), while the migrant Taiwanese fall between. The percentage of the population receiving primary education and no education at all was highest among the Taiwanese, while those receiving high school education and college education were highest for mainland Chinese. In occupation (Table 2) a striking difference between native Taiwanese and mainland Chinese was clearly observed. Laborers, the unemployed, and farmers were highest in number among native Taiwanese, while the professionals, salaried workers, and students were highest among the mainland Chinese. Again, the migrant Taiwanese fell between these two groups in almost all occupational groups.

A similar relationship of these three groups was observed (Table 3) with respect to the main family occupation. The unemployed percentage, which was extremely high when individuals were tabulated, almost completely disappeared when families were concerned in the native Taiwanese group and the migrant Taiwanese group, while the mainland Chinese still showed a considerable proportion (2.9 percent) as unemployed. This may speak for the capacity, or the strength, of the Taiwanese family to absorb those members who are less capable of looking after themselves. The occupational class distribution (Table 4) clearly reflects the educational backgrounds and occupations of the three.

Methods of Field Survey

The methods of case finding applied in field survey were described and discussed in detail by Lin (1953) and Lin et al. (1969). The investigation of each area lasted approximately a year and fell into three stages. In the first stage, information was collected in the following ways regarding members of the community suspected of mental abnormality. 1) Visits to community leaders were made—to the mayor, district chief or village chief, officials of the adminstrative offices, particularly those dealing with census, welfare, and health, members of the town council, elders, doctors, nurses, principals and teachers of the schools, and police. These visits were intended to explain the purpose of field investigation and to acquire firsthand and

Table 1:   Percentage of Individual Education of Three Population Groups

Individual Education (Age over 16)	Native Taiwanese	Migrant Taiwanese	Mainland Chinese
No formal education	26.1	23.7	10.4
Primary	60.8	57.2	34.4
Junior high	8.0	10.0	17.5
Senior high	4.2	6.5	21.6
College	0.9	2.6	16.1
Total	100.0	100.0	100.0

Table 2:   Percentage of Individual Occupation of Three Population Groups

Individual Occupation (Age over 16)	Native Taiwanese	Migrant Taiwanese	Mainland Chinese
Professionals	1.4	2.7	5.5
Salaried workers	4.7	7.9	32.0
Merchants	5.8	5.4	4.4
Farmers and fishermen	9.7	3.1	0.1
Laborers	26.5	25.9	20.2
Unemployed	21.0	10.3	7.8
Housewives	27.0	38.6	20.4
Students	3.4	5.6	8.8
Others	0.4	0.4	0.7
Total	100.0	100.0	100.0

Table 3: Percentage of Family Main Occupation of Three Population Groups

Family Main Occupation	Native Taiwanese	Migrant Taiwanese	Mainland Chinese
Professionals	2.5	6.0	7.6
Salaried workers	7.7	19.6	57.8
Merchants	15.7	13.8	6.4
Farmers and fishermen	24.8	7.8	0.2
Laborers	47.3	48.5	24.6
Unemployed	0.7	1.0	2.9
Others	1.2	3.2	0.5
Total	100.0	100.0	100.0

Table 4: Percentage of Family Occupational Class of Three Population Groups

Family Occupational Class	Native Taiwanese	Migrant Taiwanese	Mainland Chinese
Professional and semiprofessional	3.6	10.5	20.5
Skilled	5.8	15.9	40.0
Semiskilled	58.1	42.2	26.6
Unskilled	32.5	31.4	13.2
Total	100.0	100.0	100.0

intimate knowledge about the community and the major changes that had taken place during the fifteen years since the previous study. 2) Demographic data was collected through copying the population registration record. Taiwan uses a continuous registration system, i.e., the local registration office always keeps the very latest registration information of residents. Precoded schedules used in copying items from registration records were designed to contain information about each family as well as its individuals, i.e., name, sex, date of birth, education, occupation, size of household, social class, duration of residence, religion, and health. 3) Psychiatric information was collected. In addition to psychiatric information volunteered by the leaders of the community, an effort was made to obtain the names of possible psychiatric cases by asking a set of standard questions to a number of selected informants, such as doctors, teachers, policemen, and elders of the community, who were in possession of intimate knowledge about the inhabitants regarding their professional, business, and personal affairs. The items of the standard questionnaire include indications of gross signs of abnormal behavior: attempted suicide, poor work record, poor school record, police record, and drug addiction. The family record sheets copied from the registration records were most useful for this purpose, since they enabled the informants to go over each member of a family systematically and retrospectively. The first stage lasted about four to six months in each community.

The second stage lasted about two to three months and focused on collection of detailed personal histories of suspect cases from families or neighbors. An effort was made to discover any mental cases not previously reported by consulting records of public and private psychiatric hospitals, general hospitals, and health centers in nearby localities. This work was carried out by two psychiatrists and a psychiatric social worker or a psychiatric nurse.

The third stage of field work lasted about one month and consisted of household visits by small psychiatric teams (a psychiatrist and a social worker, a clinical psychologist, or a psychiatric nurse) who conducted interviews were carried out in a friendly atmosphere which was enhanced by the presence of a community leader. The latter would introduce the research team to the head of the family and explain the purpose of the visit as a health inquiry. It was prearranged so that all adult members of a household were present for the visit, and they talked to the research team first in a group. Conversation started usually by asking the main occupation of the family and the state of education and health of each member of the family. Every detail of personal data was checked while each member's behavior, attitude, and content of conversation were scrutinized systematically. If someone in a household was found to belong to one of the following categories, he was singled out then for an individual interview for intensive psychiatric examination: (1) those on record, through the first stage investigation, as suffering, or possibly suffering, from some kind of mental disorders; (2) those discovered as having a poor work record, a poor school record, a poor health record, a police record; and (3) those found to manifest abnormal behavior during the interview.

The intensive psychiatric screening took the form of general psychiatric examination including history-taking. Those who were judged to be sick in accordance with the prescribed criteria and were in need of some kind of psychiatric treatment were identified as cases and were referred to the principal investigator who gave clinical diagnosis after examination. When the diagnoses did not agree, a follow-up study for the final diagnosis was prescribed.

Results

The age-specific prevalence rates of the total mental disorders of the three groups are shown in Figure 2. The higher rates in age groups 30–39, 40–49, and 50–59 are noteworthy, particularly among mainland Chinese and migrant Taiwanese, and the psychoneurotic disorders (Figure 3) contributed greatly to the marked concentration of mental disorders in those age groups. In age group 30–39, the prevalence of psychoneuroses among mainland Chinese was higher than in migrant Taiwanese, but in age groups 40–49 and 50–59, the reverse obtained. In age-specific rates of psychoses (Figure 4), little difference was observed in the three groups up to age 40. The native Taiwanese showed a higher rate of total mental disorders after the age of 60, and the higher rates of psychoses, especially of senile psychoses and mental deficiency, of that age group were related to this finding. For prevalent differences between the two sexes among the different diagnostic and age groups (Tables 5 and 6), the tendency among the three populations was almost the same; females had higher rates in psychoneuroses and schizophrenia, and males had higher rates in mental deficiency and psycho- pathic personality.

The prevalence rates of different types of mental disorders adjusted to age in both sexes of the three groups (Table 7) showed the native Taiwanese with the highest rates in mental deficiency and the lowest in psychoneurosis which contrasted sharply with the mainland Chinese who showed highest rates in psychoneurosis and lowest in mental deficiency. These differences were most prominently observed in male Taiwanese and female mainland Chinese. There was an opposite trend between males and females in psychoses, i.e., among males, native Taiwanese had the highest rates, followed by native Taiwanese and migrant Taiwanese with no dif- ferences between the latter two. The male Taiwanese showed a significantly higher rate of manic-depressive psychosis, and the female mainland Chinese showed higher rates of schizophrenia.

After the prevalence rates of mental disorders in native and migrant populations were further adjusted to age and various social factors simulta- neously in both sexes (Table 8), no further significant prevalence difference in female schizophrenics could be observed among the three populations.

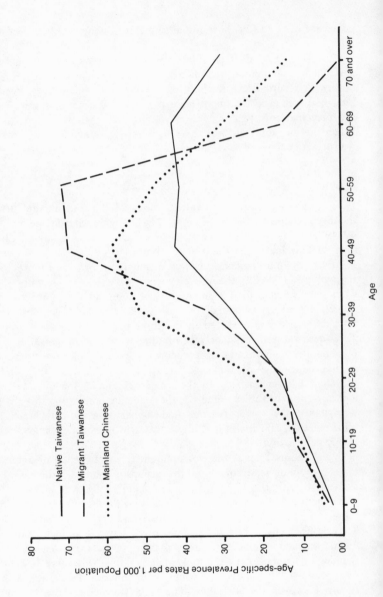

Figure 2: Prevalence Rates per 1,000 Population of Total Mental Disorders of Three Investigated Populations (Sex-adjusted)

Figure 3: Prevalence Rates per 1,000 Population of Psychoneuroses of Three Investigated Populations (Sex-adjusted)

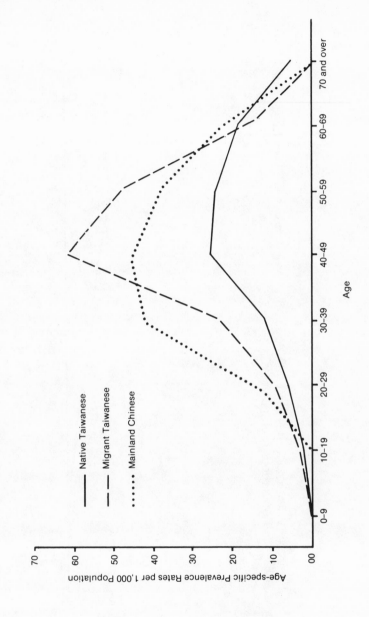

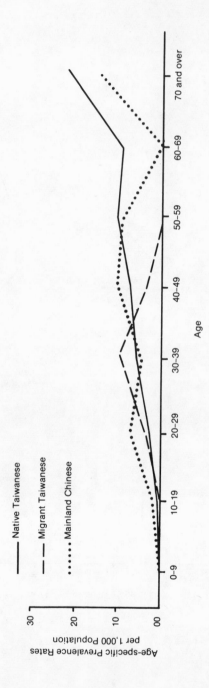

Figure 4: Prevalence Rates per 1,000 Population of Psychoses of Three Investigated Populations (Sex-adjusted)

Using the same procedure, the prevalence in both sexes was adjusted to age and one of the other nine social factors: (1) size of household (1, 2–5, 6–9, 10–13, 14 and over); (2) type of family (single, basic, extended, others); (3) ownership of house (private, supplied by employer, rent, others); (4) sibling position among same sex sibs (first, second, third, fourth, fifth, sixth and over); (5) marital status (single, married, separated, widowed, divorced, others); (6) individual education (Table 1); (7) individual occupation (Table 2); (8) family occupation (Table 3); (9) average years of education of family member over the age of 12 (0–3, 4–6, 7–9, 10 and over). The higher rate of schizophrenia in mainland females also disappeared after the adjustment to age and one of the other two social factors (Table 12): (1) ownership of house and (2) individual education. These findings suggest that the family socioeconomic status (family occupational class), individual education, and economic or psychological security (ownership of house) played an important role in the higher prevalence rate of schizophrenia in mainland females in the comparison of rate difference between migrant and nonmigrant populations as far as sex and age factors are concerned. In other words, the prevalence difference in schizophrenia between migrant and nonmigrant populations can be due to the different composition of the sample population in terms of socioeconomic factors.

In other diagnoses, the same adjustment to age and one of the ten social factors was applied in both sexes. The significant difference in prevalence of manic-depressive psychoses, all psychoses (females), mental deficiency, and psychopathic personality among the three populations was noted in less than half of the ten social factors (Tables 10 and 12 in summary form). The higher rate of all psychoses (Tables 9 and 12) in native Taiwanese males disappeared after the adjustment to age and one of the following four social factors: (1) ownership of house, (2) individual education, (3) individual occupation, and (4) average years of education of the family member over the age of 12. Again, these findings indicate that socioeconomic factors played an important role in the different prevalence rates of psychotic disorders between migrant and nonmigrant male populations.

In psychoneurotic disorders, the significant prevalence difference between migrant and nonmigrant populations was very consistent, in spite of the adjustment with age and one of the ten social factors in both sexes. The native Taiwanese had the lowest prevalence rate in psychoneurosis among the three populations (Tables 11 and 12). Results suggest that sex, age, and one of the ten social factors could not be the determinant factors related to the prevalence difference between migrants and nonmigrants; some other factors, selective and/or stress factors, may be the underlying causes for the disproportionally high rate of psychoneurotic disorders in migrant population. In each subgroup of the social factors, the prevalence differences of mental disorders among the three populations were consistent with the general trends after adjustment to age and sex. Only the significant level of difference decreased or became non-significant due to the decrease of

Table 5:   Frequency Distribution of Mental Disorders by Age, Sex, Diagnosis, and Investigated Populations

Diagnosis	Investigated Populations	Sex and Age Groups in Years					
		0–9		10–19		20–29	
		M	F	M	F	M	F
Schizophrenia	A	—	—	1	—	3	3
	B	—	—	—	—	1	—
	C	—	—	1	—	1	3
Manic-depressive psychoses	A	—	—	1	—	3	1
	B	—	—	—	—	—	—
	C	—	—	—	—	—	1
Senile psychoses	A	—	—	—	—	—	—
	B	—	—	—	—	—	—
	C	—	—	—	—	—	—
Other psychoses	A	—	—	2	2	2	—
	B	—	—	—	—	1	—
	C	—	—	1	—	—	1
Mental deficiency	A	12	8	18	15	16	7
	B	5	—	4	3	—	2
	C	8	6	5	8	1	—
Psychoneuroses	A	—	—	7	4	12	14
	B	—	—	1	1	—	11
	C	—	—	—	—	3	8
Psychopathic personality	A	—	—	2	1	8	—
	B	—	—	—	—	—	—
	C	—	—	1	—	1	—
Total mental disorders	A	12	8	31	22	44	25
	B	5	—	5	4	2	13
	C	8	6	8	8	6	13

A) Native Taiwanese
B) Migrant Taiwanese
C) Mainland Chinese

Table 5: (Continued)

	Sex and Age Groups in Years										
30–39		40–49		50–59		60–69		70 and over		All Ages	
M	F	M	F	M	F	M	F	M	F	M	F
6	3	3	2	2	6	1	4	—	2	16	20
—	3	1	—	—	—	—	—	—	—	2	3
1	2	1	6	1	2	—	—	—	1	5	14
1	—	3	3	1	1	1	—	—	—	10	5
—	1	—	—	—	—	—	—	—	—	—	1
—	—	—	—	—	—	—	—	—	—	—	1
—	—	—	—	—	—	—	2	4	5	4	7
--	—	—	—	—	—	—	—	—	—	—	—
—	—	—	—	—	—	—	—	—	—	—	—
1	3	2	1	5	1	1	—	—	1	13	8
1	1	—	—	—	—	—	—	—	—	2	1
1	3	—	2	1	—	—	—	—	—	3	6
21	4	3	8	5	2	7	—	1	—	83	44
—	1	—	—	1	—	—	—	—	—	10	6
—	—	1	—	—	—	—	—	—	—	15	14
9	22	10	42	11	25	5	12	—	3	54	122
3	12	5	10	—	7	—	1	—	—	9	42
32	34	30	26	15	7	—	3	—	—	80	78
4	—	8	1	2	1	7	1	—	2	31	6
—	—	1	—	2	—	—	—	—	—	3	—
7	2	2	2	2	—	2	—	—	—	15	4
42	32	29	57	26	36	22	19	5	13	211	212
4	18	7	10	3	7	—	1	—	—	26	53
41	41	34	36	19	9	2	3	—	1	118	117

Table 6:   Prevalence Rate per 1,000 Population of Mental Disorders by Age, Sex, Diagnosis, and Investigated Populations

Diagnosis	Investigated Populations	Sex and Age Groups in Years					
		0–9		10–19		20–29	
		M	F	M	F	M	F
Schizophrenia	A	—	—	0.3	—	1.3	1.5
	B	—	—	—	—	3.9	—
	C	—	—	1.3	—	2.8	6.2
Manic-depressive psychoses	A	—	—	0.3	—	1.3	0.5
	B	—	—	—	—	—	—
	C	—	—	—	—	—	2.1
Senile psychoses	A	—	—	—	—	—	—
	B	—	—	—	—	—	—
	C	—	—	—	—	—	—
Other psychoses	A	—	—	0.7	0.7	0.9	—
	B	—	—	—	—	3.9	—
	C	—	—	1.3	—	—	2.1
Mental deficiency	A	3.1	2.1	6.2	5.6	6.9	3.4
	B	7.4†	—	10.7	7.8	—	3.4
	C	4.8	3.7	6.7	10.8	2.8	—
Psychoneuroses	A	—	—	2.4	1.5	5.2	6.8
	B	—	—	2.7	2.6	—††	19.0
	C	—	—	—	—	8.5	16.6
Psychopathic personality	A	—	—	0.7	0.4	3.5††	—
	B	—	—	—	—	—	—
	C	—	—	1.3	—	2.8	—
Total mental disorders	A	3.1	2.1	10.7	8.3	19.0	12.3
	B	7.4†	—	13.3	10.5	7.8	22.5
	C	4.8	3.7	10.8	10.9	17.0	27.0

A) Native Taiwanese
B) Migrant Taiwanese
C) Mainland Chinese
Significant test between males and females: † $p < 0.05$, †† $p < 0.01$

Table 6: (Continued)

30–39		40–49		50–59		60–69		70 and over		All Ages	
M	F	M	F	M	F	M	F	M	F	M	F
4.4	2.4	3.1	1.9	2.7	7.8	2.1	8.3	—	6.0	1.2	1.6
—	8.6	7.3	—	—	—	—	—	—	—	1.1	1.4
0.9	3.2	0.9††	14.5	2.1	12.8	—	—	—	23.8	0.9††	3.4
0.7	—	3.1	2.9	1.3	1.3	2.1	—	—	—	0.8	0.4
—	2.9	—	—	—	—	—	—	—	—	—	0.5
—	—	—	—	—	—	—	—	—	—	—	0.2
—	—	—	—	—	—	—	4.1	16.9	15.0	0.3	0.6
—	—	—	—	—	—	—	—	—	—	—	—
—	—	—	—	—	—	—	—	—	—	—	—
0.7	2.4	2.0	1.0	6.7	1.3	2.1	—	—	3.0	1.0	0.6
3.5	2.9	—	—	—	—	—	—	—	—	1.1	0.5
0.9	4.9	—	4.8	2.1	—	—	—	—	—	0.5	1.4
15.5††	3.2	3.1	7.7	6.7	2.6	15.0††	—	4.2	—	6.4††	3.6
—	2.9	—	—	16.4	—	—	—	—	—	5.5	2.8
—	—	0.9	—	—	—	—	—	—	—	2.6	3.4
6.6††	17.7	10.2††	40.6	14.7†	32.5	10.7	24.8	—	9.0	4.2††	9.9
10.6†	34.5	36.8	87.0	—†	93.3	—	30.3	—	—	5.0††	19.4
27.6††	55.2	26.8	62.6	30.9	44.9	—	42.9	—	—	14.1	18.9
3.0	—	8.2†	1.0	2.7	1.3	15.0†	2.1	—	6.0	2.4††	0.5
—	—	7.3	—	32.8	—	—	—	—	—	1.7	—
6.0	3.2	1.8	4.8	4.1	—	17.1	—	—	—	2.6	1.0
31.1	25.7	29.6††	55.1	34.9	46.7	47.4	39.3	21.2	39.0	16.4	17.3
14.2†	51.7	51.5	87.0	49.2	93.3	—	30.3	—	—	14.4†	24.5
35.4††	66.6	30.4††	86.7	39.2	57.7	17.1	42.9	—	23.8	20.8†	28.3

sample size divisions into small subgroups. As a rule, the prevalence of psychoneuroses in native Taiwanese was significantly lower than those in total migrant populations (migrant Taiwanese and mainland Chinese). This was demonstrated in the social subgroups that exhibited high rates, i.e., (1) size of household: 2–5 and 6–9 persons, (2) type of family: basic, (3) sibling position: first and second, (4) marital status: married, (5) education: none and primary school, (6) occupation: laborer and housewife, (7) family occupation: laborer, (8) average years of education of family member: 0–3, 4–6, and 7 and over, (9) family occupational class: classes IV and V (the lower classes).

The gradient relationship of prevalences of the three populations was different in both sexes and diagnostic subgroups (Table 12). In males, the prevalence rates of psychotic and neurotic disorders of migrant Taiwanese were between those of native Taiwanese and mainland Chinese and rather close to those of native Taiwanese. In females, the prevalences of psychoses of migrant Taiwanese were the lowest among the three populations and still very close to those of mainland Chinese. The findings suggest that males and females had different reaction patterns to migration.

Some social subgroups in the migrant populations were identified as related to the high risk of mental disorders. Table 13 shows the exact opposite trend on the prevalence of psychoneurotic disorders in the three populations. The higher the socioeconomic class, the higher prevalence of psychoneuroses was noted in native Taiwanese, and the reverse was the case in mainland Chinese. In psychoses, a common trend was noted in the three populations, i.e., the lower the socioeconomic class, the higher the rates of psychoses. These findings suggest that the lower socioeconomic migrants had higher susceptibility to mental disorders, especially to psychoneurotic disorders. The other subgroups among migrant populations with a high tendency to mental disorders were those who (1) lived in a one-person family, (2) lived in a dormitory, (3) were separated from their spouses, or (4) were still single over the age of 30 (especially in males). The population size of the above four high-risk subgroups was relatively small, but the prevalence of mental disorders in migrant populations was still consistently higher than those of the native population in a very signficant level after adjustment to age and sex.

The duration of illness in psychotic cases showed a similar trend for both migrant Taiwanese and native Taiwanese. Only 21 percent of mainland Chinese schizophrenics had a duration of illness of more than 15 years, starting before their migration, as against 54 percent of Taiwanese ($p < 0.02$). The difference was more obvious in females ($p < 0.01$). The same trend was noted in all psychoses ($p < 0.08$). In psychoneuroses, the duration of illness was less than 15 years in most of the cases (about 90 percent), and the higher proportion of cases with more than a 15-year duration in Taiwanese was still noted ($p < 0.01$). No significant difference of

Table 7: Age-adjusted Prevalence Rate per 1,000 Population of Mental Disorders of Native Taiwanese, Migrant Taiwanese, and Mainland Chinese*

Diagnosis	Male			Female			Total		
	Native Taiwanese	Migrant Taiwanese	Mainland Chinese	Native Taiwanese	Migrant Taiwanese	Mainland Chinese	Native Taiwanese	Migrant Taiwanese	Mainland Chinese
Schizophrenia	1.2	1.2	1.1	1.6	1.0	4.0‡	1.4	1.1	2.5
Manic-depressive psychoses	0.8†	—	—	0.4	0.3	0.4	0.6†	0.2	0.2
Senile psychoses	0.3	—	—	0.5	—	—	0.4	—	—
Other psychoses	1.0	1.1	0.5	0.6	0.3	1.3	0.8	0.7	0.9
Subtotal	(3.3)§	(2.3)	(1.7)	(3.1)	(1.6)	(5.7)§	(3.2)	(2.0)	(3.6)
Mental deficiency	6.5‖	5.6	3.5	3.6	2.6	3.4	5.0‖	4.1	3.5
Psychoneuroses	4.1‖	4.6	8.3	9.7	21.3	18.2‖	6.9‖	12.8	13.2
Psychopathic personality	2.4	2.4	2.4	0.4	—	0.7	1.6	1.2	1.6
Subtotal	(6.5)‖	(7.0)	(10.7)	(10.1)	(21.3)	(18.9)‖	(8.5)‖	(14.0)	(14.8)
Total	16.3	14.9	15.9	16.8	25.5	28.0‖	16.7‖	20.1	21.9

* The combined population of native and migrant Taiwanese, as a standard population. Significant test (Chi square test) among investigated populations:

df=1   †p < 0.05,   ‡p < 0.01
df=2   §p < 0.05,   ‖p < 0.01

Table 8:   Observed and Expected Case Numbers of Schizophrenia by Migration Status in Both Sexes Adjusted by Age and Family Occupational Class

Population	Male		Female		Total	
	Observed	Expected	Observed	Expected	Observed	Expected
Native Taiwanese	16	15.6	20	23.1	36	38.7
Migrant Taiwanese	2	1.5	3	4.1	5	5.6
Mainland Chinese	5	6.0	14	9.8	19	15.8
Total	23	23.0	37	37.0	60	60.0
Chi square test	n.s.*		n.s.		n.s.	

* Not significant.

Table 9:   Observed and Expected Case Number of All Psychoses by Migration Status in Both Sexes Adjusted by Age and Family Occupational Class

Population	Male		Female		Total	
	Observed	Expected	Observed	Expected	Observed	Expected
Native Taiwanese	43	35.7	40	41.3	83	77.0
Migrant Taiwanese	4	3.8	5	7.0	9	10.8
Mainland Chinese	8*	15.6	21	17.7	29	33.3
Total	55	55.0	66	66.0	121	121.0
Chi square test	* df=1 $p < 0.05$		n.s.†		n.s.	

† Not significant.

Table 10: Observed and Expected Case Number of Mental Deficiency by Migration Status in Both Sexes Adjusted by Age and Family Occupational Class

Population	Male		Female		Total	
	Observed	Expected	Observed	Expected	Observed	Expected
Native Taiwanese	83	77.0	44	38.1	127	115.1
Migrant Taiwanese	10	9.6	6	7.3	16	16.9
Mainland Chinese	15	21.3	14	18.6	29	39.9
Total	108	108.0	64	64.0	172	172.0
Chi square test	n.s.*		n.s.		n.s.	

* Not significant.

Table 11: Observed and Expected Case Number of Psychoneuroses by Migration Status in Both Sexes Adjusted by Age and Family Occupational Class

Population	Male		Female		Total	
	Observed	Expected	Observed	Expected	Observed	Expected
Native Taiwanese	54	74.6	122	154.3	176	228.9
Migrant Taiwanese	9	11.2	42	26.9	51	38.1
Mainland Chinese	80	57.2	78	60.7	158	117.9
Total	143	143.0	242	242.0	385	385.0
Chi square test, df=2	$p < 0.01$		$p < 0.01$		$p < 0.01$	

Table 12: Ratios of Observed to Expected Case Number of Mental Disorders Adjusted by Age and Social Factors

Ratios of observed to expected case number adjusted by age and one of the factors below

Diagnoses	Investigated Populations	Observed Case Number M	F	Size of household M	F	Type of family M	F	Ownership of house M	F
Schizophrenia	A	16	20	1.2	0.8	1.2	0.8	1.1	1.0
	B	2	3	1.0	0.7	1.3	0.7	1.0	0.7
	C	5	14	0.6	1.6	0.6	1.7	0.8	1.1
	Signif. test	df p<		1	.05	1	.05		
All psychoses	A	43	40	1.2	0.9	1.2	0.9	1.1	1.0
	B	4	5	0.9	0.7	1.1	0.7	0.9	0.6
	C	8	21	0.5	1.4	0.5	1.5	0.6	1.1
	Signif. test	df p<		1	.05	1 .05	1 .05		
Mental deficiency	A	83	44	1.2	1.1	1.1	1.0	1.1	1.1
	B	10	6	1.0	0.7	1.1	0.8	1.0	0.8
	C	15	14	0.5	0.8	0.6	1.0	0.7	0.9
	Signif. test	df p<		2	.01	1	.05		
Psychoneuroses	A	54	122	0.8	0.8	0.8	0.8	0.9	0.9
	B	9	42	0.9	1.4	0.9	1.4	0.8	1.3
	C	80	78	1.1	1.2	1.2	1.3	1.1	1.1
	Signif. test	df p<			2 .01	1 .05	2 .01		1 .05
Total mental disorders	A	232	236	1.1	0.9	1.0	0.9	1.0	0.9
	B	28	56	0.9	1.1	1.0	1.1	0.9	1.1
	C	122	119	0.8	1.1	0.9	1.2	0.9	1.1
	Signif. test	df p<		1 .05	1 .05	2	.05		

A) Native Taiwanese
B) Migrant Taiwanese
C) Mainland Chinese

Table 12: (Continued)

Ratios of observed to expected case number adjusted by age and one of the factors below

Sibling position among same sex sib		Marital status		Individual education		Individual occupation		Family occupation		Average years of education of family member		Family occupational class	
M	M	M	F	M	F	M	F	M	F	M	F	M	F
1.3	0.8	1.2	0.8	1.1	0.8	1.2	0.7	1.2	0.8	1.0	0.8	1.0	0.9
1.0	0.7	1.3	0.8	1.0	0.8	1.0	0.7	1.1	0.7	1.1	0.7	1.3	0.7
0.6	1.9	0.6	1.8	0.7	1.5	0.7	2.1	0.7	1.6	0.8	1.9	0.8	1.4
			1		1				1	1		1	
			.01		.05				.01	.05		.01	
1.2	0.9	1.3	0.9	1.1	0.9	1.1	0.9	1.2	0.9	1.1	0.9	1.2	1.0
0.9	0.7	1.1	0.8	1.0	0.8	1.0	0.8	0.9	0.7	1.0	0.7	1.0	0.7
0.5	1.5	0.5	1.5	0.6	1.2	0.6	1.5	0.5	1.3	0.6	1.4	0.5	1.2
1	1	1	1						1	1			1
.05	.05	.05	.05						.05	.05			.05
1.2	1.0	1.2	1.0	1.0	0.9	1.1	1.0	1.1	1.0	1.1	0.9	1.1	1.1
1.0	0.8	1.1	0.8	1.0	0.7	1.0	0.8	1.0	0.8	0.9	0.8	1.0	0.8
0.5	1.0	0.5	1.1	0.8	1.5	0.7	1.0	0.8	1.2	0.8	1.4	0.7	0.7
2		2											
.05		.01											
0.7	0.7	0.7	0.8	0.7	0.8	0.7	0.8	0.8	0.8	0.7	0.8	0.7	0.8
0.9	1.5	0.9	1.4	0.9	1.6	0.8	1.5	0.8	1.5	0.8	1.5	0.8	1.6
1.4	1.4	1.3	1.4	1.3	1.3	1.3	1.3	1.3	1.2	1.4	1.3	1.4	1.3
2	2	2	2	2	2	2	2	2	2	2	2	2	2
.01	.01	.01	.01	.01	.01	.01	.01	.05	.01	.01	.01	.01	.01
1.0	0.8	1.0	0.8	1.0	0.8	1.0	0.9	1.0	0.9	1.0	0.9	1.0	0.9
0.9	1.2	1.0	1.2	0.9	1.2	0.9	1.2	0.9	1.2	0.9	1.2	0.9	1.2
1.0	1.3	0.9	1.3	1.1	1.3	1.0	1.3	1.0	1.2	1.1	1.3	1.1	1.1
	2		2		2		2		2		2		1
	.01		.01		.01		.01		.05		.01		.05

prevalence was noted among the populations with different duration of time of migration. The data only showed a mild trend that recently migrated population (5 years versus 6 to 15 years) may reflect a lower rate of psychoses and mental deficiency and a higher rate in psychoneuroses and psychopathic personality.

Discussion

Difficulty in comparison of the prevalence of mental disorders between two or more groups of population with various characteristics has been discussed in detail by Reid (1960), Dunham (1961), and Lin et al. (1969). Unfortunately most investigations of migration and mental disorders were based on probably biased hospital data and small samples. As Murphy (1961) pointed out: "The relationship between immigration and mental hospitalization has become quite doubtful, and its meaning equally so. If these (social class, type of residential milieu, years of schooling, and ratio of single to married) were controlled for, the immigrant/native difference in mental hospitalization rates would disappear completely." Our study provides strong support for Murphy's position in regard to psychotic disorders; however, this notion cannot be generalized for psychoneurotic disorders. Our research provides evidence that there was a strong association between the higher rates of psychoneurotic disorders and migration, and the effect of social factors upon the high rate of psychoneurosis was ruled out. The interaction among sex, age, readiness to move, socioeconomic status, and selec-

Table 13:   Observed and Expected Case Number of Psychoneuroses by Family Occupational Class in Three Population Groups Adjusted by Age and Sex

Family Occupational Class	Native Taiwanese		Migrant Taiwanese		Mainland Chinese	
	Observed	Expected	Observed	Expected	Observed	Expected
Professional and semiprofessional	10	4.7	3	4.1	22†	35.2
Skilled	18*	8.5	10	8.4	60	62.1
Semiskilled	89	100.7	22	22.6	44	38.9
Unskilled	59	62.1	16	15.9	32	21.8
Total	176	176.0	51	51.0	158	158.0

* df=1 $p < 0.01$
† df=2 $p < 0.01$

tive factors in terms of onset of illness and socioeconomic distribution of population has been demonstrated.

Two old Chinese sayings, *"An tu chung chien"* ("to dwell contentedly on one's native soil, unwilling to be moved from his native place") and *"Lo yen kuei ken"* ("the leaves fall and return to the root," i.e., people should return to their original place), express a basic Chinese attitude toward migration. This attitude can help us to understand the subculture of Chinese overseas. The migrant or immigrant Chinese are always longing and preparing to return to their native land. Very tight social groups such as Chinatown or an Association of Fellow Provincials are formed to help migrants alleviate homesickness. Even among the migrants within the same country, this basic psychology of sticking together can be clearly observed. Of course, the motivation and distance of migration have some influence on this attitude, but Chinese possess a strong cultural resistance to migration.

Murphy's study of Chinese in Singapore (1959) found inverse correlations between hospitalization rates and size of community group. Murphy also reported (1955) that the Chinese hospitalization rates in Chinatown in Canada were lowest of all ethnic minorities, but highest of all ethnic minorities in other provinces where the Chinese were scattered. Murphy's findings may, perhaps, show the different attitude to hospitalization in various Chinese subgroups rather than the different underlying effects of migration on those Chinese. My impression is that migration places a great mental stress on migrant Chinese.

Mainland Chinese migrants are refugees, whereas the migrant Taiwanese are voluntary internal migrants. However, according to the population composition and the reaction pattern to mental disorders, they shared many similarities. Both migrant populations showed strong positive selective characteristics in terms of higher individual and average family education, higher family occupational class, and more modern family units. Astrup and Ødegaard (1960) pointed out that the direction of migration (migration to the capital city of Oslo and to other parts of Norway) had different selective effects in terms of prevalence of mental disorders. Parker and Kleiner (1966) studied Negro residents in Philadelphia, using hospital and community samples, and they also showed the relationship of migration direction to mental illness (southern migrants were underrepresented, and native and northern migrants were overrepresented). The present study suggests that both migrant populations, migrant Taiwanese and mainland Chinese, moved in the same direction.

Murphy (1955) presented four factors that related to the increased susceptibility to mental disorders in refugee population: (1) loss of homeland, (2) experience of persecution, including physical injury and starvation, (3) cultural difficulty in adjusting to new conditions, and (4) general social isolation. Among these four factors, only the first one, loss of (or leaving) homeland, is an important factor in the increased rates of mental disorders among mainland Chinese migrants as well as among migrant Taiwanese in the present study of sample populations.

The distance of migration was another factor which produced different selective screening effects upon migrants; ill people could not travel long distances. The lower age-adjusted rates of psychoses and mental deficiency in mainland Chinese males may be due to this effect of screening. The relative rarity or low incidence of manic-depressive psychoses and senile psychoses in migrants may be due to the selective effect of migration. The male migrants displayed higher motivation for migration than female migrants who merely followed their families, so the selective effect played a less important role in female migrants. On the other hand, the female migrants were less prepared for migration and may have experienced more difficulty in adjusting to the new environment. The opposite trend of age-adjusted rates in male and female migrants in psychoses can be explained by the result of the interaction between the selective effect and the reaction to the stress of migration. Studies of Astrup and Ødegaard (1960), Lazarus et al. (1963), and Rin, Chu, and Lin (1966) showed a similar difference in tendency of prevalence of mental illness in migrant males and females.

Because of the small number of cases whose onset of illness preceded migration, the selective effect seems to play a less important role in psychoneuroses among migrants, although the selective effect cannot be excluded. The significant difference of prevalences in psychoneuroses between migrants (the prevalences in mainland Chinese and migrant Taiwanese were very close) and nonmigrants remained almost constant despite adjustment for age, sex, and each of the ten social factors. There was no social subgroup displaying significant opposite trends in the prevalence difference in psychoneuroses between migrants and nonmigrants. With very few exceptions, statistically significant difference in psychoneurotic prevalence between migrants and nonmigrants completely followed the chance rule—the larger the population, the higher the chance of obtaining a significant difference. The above strongly suggest that the stress of migration was a very influential factor in higher prevalence of psychoneuroses in migrants.

Lee (1963) reported that the adjustment to marital status, education, and occupation had no significant effect on the migrant rates of mental disorders in comparison with nonmigrants. Our study partially supports his findings. The adjustment with these three social factors did not have significant effects on the differences of total mental disorders among the three population groups, but some effect on the prevalence of psychoses by the adjustment with individual education and occupation was noted.

The tendency of recent migrants (within five years) to be associated with lower rates of psychoses and mental deficiency can be due to the screening effect of migration, and the higher rate of psychoneuroses in a recently migrated population may be due to the stress effect of migration being more important than the screening effect in psychoneurotic disorders.

The effect of duration of migration on the prevalence of mental disorders was demonstrated by Malzberg (1964, 1967) and Rin, Chu, and Lin (1966).

Among the ten social factors, "ownership of house" was noted as being insignificant to migrants' adjustment in the differences of mental disorders among the three populations. This tendency may imply that if the migrants owned a house they would be willing to settle down in the new environment, or the ownership of a house would give them a feeling of belonging to the new environment, so that they would be able to adjust to the new situation as well as the native who owned houses. On the other hand, it appears that people who did not own a house resisted settling down or had socioeconomic problems, so they experienced the equal stress, related to the higher prevalence of mental disorders, whether they were migrants or nonmigrants. It seems that efforts to aid the migrant Chinese in becoming homeowners can insure their better mental health.

The subgroups among migrants with a high tendency to mental disorders, such as those who were (1) living alone, (2) separated from their spouse, (3) single, especially males, and those over age 30, (4) living in a dormitory, and (5) in lower socioeconomic status, were identified in the present study. The factors were related to leaving their homeland and to lack of family support, and poor economic conditions made their adjustment even more difficult. Middle-aged female migrants were more affected by these factors than any other age group. The opposite trends in the association of social class and prevalence of psychoneuroses between migrant and non-migrant populations may be explained by Bremer's hypothesis (1951) that the secure population tended to suffer more psychoneurotic disorders in the upper class and the insecure population in the lower class.

In regard to marriage between Taiwanese females and mainland Chinese males, the prevalence of mental disorders for this subgroup did not show much difference from those of other migrant populations. In order to clarify the effect of intermarriage against the effect of migration, the mental cases of Taiwanese females who married mainland Chinese males were treated as migrated Taiwanese or native Taiwanese, according to the migration history.

This study indicated some of the social factors in the prevalence difference of mental disorders between migrant and nonmigrant populations and provided some evidence to support the selective or stress hypotheses. Almost all hypotheses derived from previous studies on the association of migration and mental disorders were based on clinical and retrospective data. More convincing facts are needed to support those hypotheses. A longitudinal study of a defined population, such as a group of postgraduate students who are going to a foreign country to study, can provide more elaborate information on the effect of migration on mental health than the studies undertaken thus far. Such a study is being conducted in Taiwan and the United States, but it will take time to obtain conclusive results.

Summary

As part of an extensive epidemiological investigation designed to explore the relation between mental illness and various demographic variables, a comprehensive household survey of three communities in Taiwan was conducted, including a native Taiwanese group, a migrant Taiwanese group, and a mainland Chinese group. The results indicate that psychotic and mental defective disorders were significantly related to migration but must be considererd within the context of age, sex, and various social factors; however, neurotic disorders were significantly related to migration regardless of these factors.

ACKNOWLEDGMENTS

This study has been aided by a grant from the Foundations' Fund for Research in Psychiatry (FFRP Grant 62-257). The author is greatly indebted to his teacher, Professor Tsung-yi Lin, for his encouragement and valuable guidance throughout this investigation. The author also wishes to take this opportunity to thank Drs. H. Rin, E. K. Yeh, C. C. Hsu, M. T. Tsuang, K. M. Chan, W. S. Tseng, and all those who took part in the field survey and data processing. Without their help, this study could not have been carried out.

NOTES

1.   The association between immigration and mental illness is supported in current literature by Malzberg, 1964, 1965; Locke et al., 1960; Cade and Krupinski, 1962; Lazarus et al., 1963; Lee, 1963; Tewfik and Okasha, 1965; Hoek et al., 1965; Shoham et al., 1966; Abramson, 1966. A reverse trend is noted by Locke and Duvall, 1964; Malzberg, 1965; Murphy, 1965.

2.   Higher rates for migrants were shown by Astrup and Ødegaard, 1960; Locke et al., 1960; Lazarus et al., 1963; Thomas and Locke, 1963; Lee, 1963; Malzberg, 1964, 1967; Locke and Duvall, 1964; Rin, Chu, and Lin, 1966. A negative or reverse association was shown by Jaco, 1960; Srole et al., 1962; Leighton et al., 1963; Fried, 1965; Price, 1965; Kantor, 1965; Parker and Kleiner, 1966.

3.   Keeler and Vitols, 1963.

4.   Last, 1960; Locke et al., 1960; Parker et al., 1960; Kleiner and Parker, 1965; Gordon, 1965; Parker and Kleiner, 1966.

5.   Reid, 1960; Leighton et al., 1963; Hoek, 1965; Murphy, 1965.

6.   Malzberg, 1964, 1967; Rin, Chu, and Lin, 1966.

7.   Murphy, 1961, 1965.

REFERENCES

Abramson, J. H. 1966. Emotional disorder, status inconsistency and migration: a health questionnaire survey in Jerusalem. Milbank Memorial Quarterly 44:23–48.

Astrup, C., and Ø. Ødegaard. 1960. Internal migration and mental disease in Norway. Psychiatric Quarterly Supplement 34:116–30.

Bremer, J. 1951. A social psychiatric investigation of a small community in Northern Norway. Acta Psychiatrica et Neurologica Scandinavica Supplement 62:1–166.

Cade, J. F. J., and J. Krupinski. 1962. Incidence of psychiatric disorders in Victoria in relation to country of birth. Medical Journal of Australia 1:400–404.

Department of Civil Affairs, Taiwan Provincial Government 1965. Household registration statistics of Taiwan, Republic of China, 1963–1964.

Dunham, H. W. 1961. Social structure and mental disorders: competing hypotheses of explanation. *In* Causes of mental disorders: a review of epidemiological knowledge. New York, Milbank Memorial Fund.

Fried, M. A. 1965. Transitional functions of working-class communities: implications for forced relocation. *In* Mobility and mental health. M. B. Kantor, ed. Springfield, Illinois, Charles C Thomas.

Gordon, E. B. 1965. Mentally ill West Indian immigrants. British Journal of Psychiatry 111:877–87.

Hoek, A., R. Moses, and L. Terrespolsky. 1965. Emotional disorder in an Israeli immigrant community. Israel Annuals of Psychiatry and Related Disciplines 3:213–28.

Jaco, E. G. 1960. The social epidemiology of mental disorder: a psychiatric survey of Texas. New York, Russell Sage Foundation.

Kantor, M. B., ed. 1965. Mobility and mental health. Springfield, Illinois, Charles C Thomas.

Keeler, M. H., and M. M. Vitols. 1963. Migration and schizophrenia in North Carolina Negroes. American Journal of Orthopsychiatry 33:554–57.

Kleiner, R. J., and S. Parker. 1965. Goal striving and psychosomatic symptoms in a migrant and non-migrant population. *In* Mobility and mental health. M. B. Kantor, ed. Springfield, Illinois, Charles C Thomas.

Last, J. M. 1960. The health of immigrants: some observations from general practice. Medical Journal of Australia 1:158–62.

Lazarus, J., B. Z. Locke, and D. S. Thomas. 1963. Migration differentials in mental disease: state patterns in first admissions to mental hospitals for all disorders and for schizophrenia, New York, Ohio, and California, as of 1950. Milbank Memorial Quarterly 41:25–42.

Lee, E. S. 1963. Socioeconomic and migration differentials in mental disease, New York State, 1949–1951. Milbank Memorial Quarterly 41:249–69.

Leighton, D. C., et al. 1963. Psychiatric findings of the Stirling County study. American Journal of Psychiatry. 119:1021–26.

————. 1963. The character of danger. New York, Basic Books, Inc.

Lin, T. 1953. A study of the incidence of mental disorder in Chinese and other cultures. Psychiatry 16:313–36.

Lin, T., et. al. 1969. Mental disorders in Taiwan, fifteen years later: a preliminary report. *In* Mental health research in Asia and the Pacific. W. Caudill and T. Lin, eds. Honolulu, East-West Center Press.

Locke, B. Z., and H. J. Duvall. 1964. Migration and mental illness. Eugenics Quarterly 11:216–21.

Locke, B. Z., M. Kramer, and B. Pasamanick. 1960. Immigration and insanity. Public Health Report 75:301–306.

Malzberg, B. 1964. Mental disease among foreign-born in Canada, 1950–1952, in relation to period of immigration. American Journal of Psychiatry 120:971–73.

———. 1965. Mental disease among the Puerto Rican population of New York State, 1960–1961. Albany, New York, Research Foundation of Mental Hygiene.

———. 1965. New data on mental disease among Negroes in New York State, 1960–1961. Albany, New York, Research Foundation for Mental Hygiene.

———. 1967. Internal migration and mental disorders among the white population of New York State, 1960–1961. International Journal of Social Psychiatry 30:184–91.

Mezey, A. G. 1960. Personal background, emigration and mental disorder in Hungarian refugees. Journal of Mental Science 106:618–27.

Murphy, H. B. M. 1955. Flight and resettlement. Paris, UNESCO.

———. 1959. Culture and mental disorder in Singapore. *In* Culture and mental health. Marvin K. Opler, ed. New York, The Macmillan Company.

———. 1961. Social change and mental health. *In* Cause of mental disorders: a review of epidemiological knowledge. New York, Milbank Memorial Fund.

———. 1965. Migration and the major mental disorders: a reappraisal. *In* Mobility and mental health. M. B. Kantor, ed. Springfield, Illinois, Charles C Thomas.

Parker, S., and R. J. Kleiner. 1966. Mental illness in the urban Negro community. New York, Free Press.

Parker, S., R. J. Kleiner, and H. G. Taylor. 1960. Level of aspiration and mental disorder: a research proposal. Annals of the New York Academy of Sciences 84:878–86.

Price, D. O. 1965. Next steps in studying mobility and mental health. *In* Mobility and mental health. M. B. Kantor, ed. Springfield, Illinois, Charles C Thomas.

Reid, D. D. 1960. Epidemiological methods in the study of mental disorder. Public Health Papers, No. 2. Geneva, World Health Organization.

Rin, H., H. M. Chu, and T. Lin. 1966. Psychophysiological reactions of a rural and suburban population in Taiwan. Acta Psychiatrica Scandinavica 42:410–73.

Shoham, S., N. Shoham, and A. Abd-El-Razek. 1966. Immigration, ethnicity, and ecology as related to juvenile delinquency in Israel. British Journal of Criminology 6:391–409.

Srole, L., et al. 1962. Mental health in the metropolis: the Midtown Manhattan study, volume I. New York, McGraw-Hill Book Company.

Tewfik, G. I., and A. Okasha. 1965. Psychosis and immigration. Postgraduate Medical Journal 41:603–12.

Thomas, D. S., and B. Z. Locke. 1963. Marital status, education and occupational differentials in mental disease: state patterns in first admissions to mental hospitals for all disorders and for schizophrenia, New York and Ohio, as of 1950. Milbank Memorial Quarterly 41:145–60.

21.　　Paranoid Manifestations among Chinese Students Studying Abroad: Some Preliminary Findings

ENG-KUNG YEH, M.D.

Department of Psychiatry
National Taiwan University
Taipei, Taiwan, Republic of China

THE WORLD has witnessed a tremendous increase in cultural interchange since World War II, creating transcultural experience common to many people, especially students studying in foreign countries. The increase in Chinese students studying abroad in recent years has made them the third largest group of foreign students in the United States today, next only to Canadians and Indians. The problems arising from transcultural adjustment have become topics of great concern to psychiatrists, social scientists, and educators. To date, however, there have been no psychiatric studies or reports on the adjustment problems of Chinese students studying abroad.

During the past fifteen years I have treated, in the Department of Neurology and Psychiatry, National Taiwan University Hospital, 40 cases of Chinese students who had had psychotic breakdowns during their study in foreign countries. Paranoid manifestations were observed in a majority of these cases. Based on clinical experiences with these cases, including some intensive individual case analyses, this paper reports the predominant psychiatric findings in relation to sociocultural factors which were thought to be significant in development of paranoid symptoms in these students. An attempt is made to discuss briefly, on a hypothetical formulation, paranoid formation in these cases, in light of the contemporary social conditions, orientations in child-rearing, interpersonal relations, and systems of behavior control among Chinese. Statistical data and detailed case reports are avoided; instead, an overall picture is presented. Further intensive studies in some specific areas are indicated in order to test the hypothesis formulated in this paper.

Findings

Out of 40 cases, 26 were males and 14 were females. Diagnostically, there were 29 cases of paranoid schizophrenia or paranoid psychoses, 7 cases of other types of schizophrenia out of which 5 cases manifested paranoid features, 3 cases of manic-depressive psychoses, and 1 postpartum psychosis. Twenty-nine were mainlanders, and the remaining 11 were Taiwanese.[1] There was no significant difference in the case-rate of paranoid manifestations between the two domicile and sex groups. Except for one case, who went to the United States early in 1949 from the China mainland and returned to Taiwan in 1956, the rest were seen in the Department of Neurology and Psychiatry at National Taiwan University during the past ten years. The increase of Chinese students studying abroad during this period accounts for the frequency and number of cases. Nearly all—37 out of 40—went to the United States to study, while the remaining three went to Canada, West Germany, and Japan.

CONTENTS OF DELUSIONS AND HALLUCINATIONS

A majority of the delusions and hallucinations manifested were predominantly persecutory in nature; they were verbalized as being investigated, being watched, being followed, being poisoned, and mind being read. Political coloration—such as being investigated by the F.B.I. in the United States or by Chinese government agents at home or being suspected by Americans as Communists—was common. These delusions were manifested predominantly among the male students. Similar findings have been observed in patients who had not been abroad. Among all paranoid outpatients at the Department of Psychiatry, National Taiwan University Hospital, mainland males have been found to have significantly more preoccupation with political affairs in the content of delusions (Rin et al., 1962; Rin et al., 1958). This may be explained on the basis of strict security control, prevailing social tensions, and the inhabitant's defensive attitude toward authority and political matters. Chinese students, under the circumstances, generally are not interested in talking about political matters, especially in an unfamiliar situation. Inhibited dissatisfaction toward reality or authority, thus, may be easily projected to the outside world and lead to persecutory delusions. One student, a former active Nationalist Party member at home, developed delusions of being investigated by Nationalist agents and F.B.I. agents a few months after his arrival in Canada. Just before his departure to Canada, his mother was fired during her sick leave by the new principal of the primary school where she had taught for ten years. Not only did she lose a job, but the whole family was forced to move, because the house belonged to the school. The father's repeated petitions to various levels of authority were all in vain. The crisis instilled tremendous anger and hostility to authority in this young man. In response to this episode, he did not report to the consulate which he was obliged to do on arrival in Canada. He isolated himself from the Chinese students on the campus and from social activities of the local Chinese. Strong feelings of antagonism to fellow Chinese students gradually changed to anxiety and fear of being criticized as a foreign body by the other Chinese students who supposedly were also speaking ill of him. He later changed to persecutory delusions of being investigated by F.B.I. and Chinese government agents, especially following his open criticism of the Vietnam War. The nature of his delusions further changed, and he ultimately believed that Communists were also investigating him as a double agent. After his return to Taiwan, however, he responded well to treatment. Within two months time, all paranoid symptoms disappeared completely, and he had gained reasonable insight into his illness.

For four months following his discharge from our department at National Taiwan University, he worked temporarily as a high school teacher. He then went back to Canada to continue graduate study for a Ph.D. and has been doing well. His return to the home country in this case not only provided him with an opportunity for psychiatric treatment but also for reality-testing and correction of his reality-distortion.

Suspicion of poison in tea or food as a method of persecution was manifested in ten cases. This may be rooted in the traditional Chinese belief in persecution by slow-acting poison. A case with this delusion recalled, after his recovery from psychosis, that his fantastic ideas about poisoning may have come from Chinese novels about ancient chivalry which he had read during his middle-school days.

Three female cases showed delusions of being cheated and mistreated by Americans following failures in obtaining jobs and schooling. They acquired strong feelings that Americans and school authorities were prejudiced against them, and they developed inferiority complexes. Manifestations of the idea that their minds were being read by telepathy were found in two cases.

Not infrequently the persecutors were fellow countrymen rather than the host-countrymen. Neurotic competition with fellow countrymen or frustrated dependency needs seemed to create anxiety and a sense of failure in the students, which in turn led to denial and the paranoid projection toward fellow countrymen. For example, student A., a major in physics, suddenly developed the idea that a slow-acting poison had been put into his soft drink after a ping-pong game with another Chinese student, B. He thought that the poison was put in by B. to dull his mind, disturb his memory, and paralyze him. A.'s persecution complex was supposedly initiated by another Chinese student, C., who hated A. Student C. had entered A.'s department two years ahead of him as a teaching assistant, and he had once given A. a lower examination score than A. thought was fair for a fellow country-man. A., in turn, put some provocative notes on the blackboard in C.'s laboratory. Just before this episode, C. had failed a subject in the Ph.D. qualification examination given by A.'s professor. Therefore, A. thought that C.'s action was a retaliation.

MARRIAGE AND SEX PROBLEMS

Among many factors that precipitate students' breakdowns, such as difficulties in academic achievement, finances, languages, and interpersonal relationships, marriage and sex problems deserve special mention.

Most of the Chinese students studying abroad, especially in the U.S., plan to stay a long time or not to return home at all because of better economic conditions and job opportunities. Finding an ideal partner for marriage is an important concern of these young people, especially the female students. With strong traditional prejudice against marriage to non-Chinese, the careful parents prefer to have their children engaged to the Chinese students who have already been or will be going abroad before their children's departure for overseas study. Those who go abroad alone have the freedom to choose their marriage partner, but it is not an easy task for them within the limited social circle in which Chinese students tend to confine themselves.

Not infrequently the psychotic breakdown was precipitated by failure in a love affair, real or imaginary, and by sexual frustration. A 26-year-old female student majoring in library science became acutely disturbed with crying spells and delusions of being poisoned, hearing voices accusing her of misconduct with boys and threatening to kill her, after receiving a threatening letter from another Chinese girlfriend of the Chinese doctor with whom she had been in love. An intelligent, highly sociable person and an active participant in various student activities (she had represented her school at an International Student Conference), she was a very popular campus figure in China. In spite of her extroverted, sociable, and forceful personality, she was kept at some distance by the Chinese students, especially those from Taiwan, in the local student community in the United States. After several unhappy episodes, with different Chinese students who left her and with an American student who was strongly disliked by her family, she became acquainted with a handsome Chinese doctor from Taiwan who was known to date many girls regardless of nationality. She recovered quickly from paranoid psychosis after she was sent back to Taiwan where she was treated for two months at our department. She continued to be well and taught English at a girls' high school in her hometown for nearly a year until her second psychotic breakdown which was precipitated by an unexpected tele-phone call from the same doctor who happened to be home for a short visit.

For Chinese students studying abroad, especially females, marriage or even steady dating with foreigners may create considerable anxiety and a sense of shame. The students may be disparaged by fellow countrymen and may even have to sacrifice their emotional ties with the other members of the group. Three female students developed delusions that their American professors were interested in them as prospective marriage partners. They became acutely disturbed when they were openly rejected. One of them had the delusion that the dean of the college, a man of German descent in his early fifties, was interested in her and was always watching her through a magic mirror. She believed that her blood was being exchanged with another's, two-thirds of her uterus was taken away, and also hallucinated that electrical charges were being made against her body by jealous male Chinese students. This young lady who was a shy, introverted, and modest person before going abroad became openly sexual in her behavior toward males and aggressive with female ward staff during her hospitalization. Another female student, following a courtship by an American whom she accepted, became ambivalent, depressed, and finally attempted suicide. Upon regaining consciousness from the head injury which she suffered in jumping from the second floor, she became acutely disturbed with delusions of being humiliated physically by Americans.

Two male students who had been preoccupied by sexual inadequacy at home developed the paranoia of being castrated by American girls when they were embarrassed by sexual impotence. A 33-year-old married Taiwanese male, the father of two children and a passive, dependent, submissive type of person, for a long time had suspected the infidelity of his active and domineering wife, whom he married through arrangements by his parents. He had, however, never expressed his suspicion at home. His going to the United States at the age of 32 against his wife's wishes was excusable on the grounds that further overseas study would result in better job opportunities in the future. Perhaps it was only the acting-out of his hostility toward his wife. In the United States, he became intimate with a female Chinese student, and when he received a letter from his wife accusing him of infidelity and desertion of the whole family, he became acutely disturbed and replied with a long letter full of anger and jealous delusions. Paranoid notions of being castrated followed this episode. Another male student, who had a strong attachment to his mother, became bothered by feelings that his penis was small in comparison to those of his American classmates at the student dormitory. He later developed ideas of being looked down upon and cheated by American students, and he became very hostile and antagonistic to them. Intensive study revealed, in nearly all of these cases, disturbed early parent-child relations and inadequate psychosexual development.

PERSONALITY PROBLEMS
AND ADJUSTMENT DIFFICULTIES AT HOME

Eight out of the 34 paranoid cases, 6 males and 2 females, had experienced paranoid breakdowns resulting in hospitalization before their departure for study abroad. Nine other cases, 6 males and 3 females, had manifested a series of behavior problems that were suggestive of either paranoid disorders or personality pattern disturbances. Among those who had the first paranoid breakdown during study abroad, two groups of personality problems were noted. One group can be described as having been rigid, self-assertive, stubborn, aggressive, suspicious, aloof, introverted, and as having a tendency to isolate themselves from others. The other group can be described as having been emotionally immature and unstable. These characteristics were found to be predominant among the female students. They were reported to be sensitive to criticism, with strong inferiority complexes especially related to their physical and external appearance, and to be competitive, with low thresholds of frustration.

A rather high rate of previous breakdowns in these samples deserves our attention. Some explanations may be relevant to this finding. Paranoid symptoms are mental disturbances that usually show little personality disintegration or emotional deterioration. These cases may have been in their remission states at the time of departure, or their mental conditions may have been such that, unless disturbed, they were easily overlooked within the context of their surroundings. That the paranoid behavior pattern is easily overlooked in present Chinese society can be understood on the basis of traditional Chinese culture in terms of psychological orientation in interpersonal relations, psychological mechanisms in behavior control, present-day social conditions, and the prevailing attitudes of the Chinese toward this behavior. This will be discussed later. Although the cases are rather extreme, I have recently seen two Chinese students whose motivation for going abroad for study was to escape from a situation in which they believed they had been persecuted for years.

For those students with previous adjustment problems, though not necessarily psychotic, it was found that going abroad was motivated by neurotic competition with others or by the parents who attempted to satisfy their neurotic needs vicariously, regardless of their children's psychological readiness for overseas study. Occasionally, students just wanted to run away from the difficult situation at home, or they were making a blind effort to redeem failure at home by seeking better opportunities abroad. In any case, these students went abroad without insight into their own problems and without adequate preparation for the difficulties of study abroad. This is certainly a serious problem from the mental health and educational point of view.

From our experience with these cases, I am convinced that one or two psychiatric interviews with students before departure, including careful inquiry into their health history, ability to adjust, and their life experiences will not only serve to detect some easily overlooked psychiatric conditions but will also serve to predict the risk of future maladjustment or psychiatric disorders. More systematic studies in this area with international collaboration are needed for confirmation.

FAMILY BACKGROUND AND PARENT-CHILD RELATIONSHIPS

Emotional deprivation or disturbed family relations were found in 21 out of 34 paranoid cases. This includes early death of one or both of the parents and separation of the parents or parents and children in childhood. In nearly all the cases where there was an early death of a parent, the father was the one who had died, and the mother became a neurotic, overprotective, controlling figure in the family with high expectations for the children's achievements. In the cases involving separation from parents, the Sino-Japanese War was the most frequent cause. Some cases were the result of disturbed marital relations between the parents, such as the father's living away from home with a concubine. During the Sino-Japanese War, many mainland students experienced childhood separation from their parents. It might be speculated, however, that the children were well taken care of by parent-substitutes under the extended family system, and thus emotional deprivation caused by this separation could have been diminished or avoided. In the present cases, this unfortunately was not the case. The existence of concubines living in or out of the family, without the legal separation or divorce of the parents, is not uncommon in the traditional Chinese family. In many instances, this situation is compensated for by increased maternal dominance over child-rearing and decision-making in the family. This type of family situation apparently has considerable impact on the child's personality development. Father-child relations of both sexes appeared to be more disturbed than those between mother and child. The fathers were usually described as authoritative, bossy, demanding, and egocentric with little concern or responsibility for family affairs. The other type of father was reported to be quiet, weak, and indecisive, with low status and little influence on the decision-making at home. In both instances, the children were distant from the father; they were afraid of him in the former instance and frustrated by him in the latter. In the families with weak fathers, the mothers were reported to be domineering, capable, and devoted, and the children were much closer to them.

A typical case was seen in a very intelligent student who became paranoid soon after obtaining a Ph.D. degree from Stanford University. During the long period of treatment in this department, he was overly hostile and antagonistic toward his father and, later, toward his mother. While he was living with the parents, he was always overtly disturbed with many persecutory delusions and regressed behavior. He finally had to leave home after several hospitalizations. Only after he lived away from home did his overt psychiatric disturbances gradually subside, and he was later able to teach at a small college on a part-time basis. His father is a distinguished figure in the nation and was once a minister. During early childhood, the father was away from home for many years, first for study abroad and later because of his official duties. During this period the children were under the care of their old-fashioned, self-educated, devoted mother. They lived with the paternal grandfather who was an absolute authority figure in the family. As the eldest son, the patient was expected by his foreign-educated and Western-minded father to excel, but the father spent little time with the children because of his job and energetic social activities. The patient recalled strong feelings of inferiority, a sense of getting lost, uneasiness in the company of his father, and a tendency to avoid his father during high school days. The expectations of the highly successful, modern-minded father appeared to be a great psychological threat and burden to the patient who was raised in a traditional, old-fashioned family situation. Though he succeeded academically in the United States, he had a strong antagonism to the Western culture which his father so greatly admired.

OUTCOME OF TREATMENT

The prognosis of treatments was generally encouraging. Ten cases showed considerable improvement with fairly satisfactory social adjustments in their professions, which included college teaching, research, and government employment, while under psychotherapy and regular medication. In another 20 cases, mild to moderate improvement was obtained, though several cases relapsed later mainly because of inability to maintain treatment. Only 4 cases remained unchanged. Poor prognosis or relapse of the symptoms was significantly related to marked premorbid personality disorders and disturbed psychological relations in the family. In those cases with a favorable outcome after treatment, the return to the home country itself seemed to release psychological tension considerably, and in some cases, it served to provide an opportunity for reality-testing. With the therapist's assistance, these cases seemed to quickly strengthen ego-functions to correct their reality-distortion. It is my belief that psychotic students who break down abroad, especially paranoid cases, can be treated with much better prognosis in the home country than in foreign countries. Those persecutory delusions toward the school, immigration authorities, or the hospital staff causing the patients' compulsory hospitalization or the prospect of a forced return home generally disappeared quickly upon return to Taiwan. In one male case, delusions of being possessed by three American ghosts, including vivid somatic hallucinations of his limbs being shrunk and his blood being sucked, disappeared soon after his return to Taiwan. Sometimes the contents of delusions or hallucinations changed after the return home. A male case had visual hallucinations of being Buddha, instead of Jesus Christ as he had had in the United States, as soon as he arrived in Japan enroute to Taiwan. These changes may be understood in light of the psychodynamics in the development of delusions or hallucinations and the changes brought about by returning home.

During the course of treatment, it was observed in some cases that subsidence of paranoid psychosis was followed by depression as patients became aware of the psychological difficulties that were significant in causing their psychotic breakdown. Depressions usually diminished as patients became able to cope with their emotional difficulties through the therapist's support. Depression occurred occasionally, however, when they were faced with some problems or difficulties with job, marriage, schooling, or going abroad again, with which they were unable to cope and which had provoked the previous psychological difficulties. A male who was sent home for treatment from the United States because of a series of delusions and hallucinations of a predominantly persecutory nature committed suicide by taking a large dose of barbiturates soon after his discharge from the hospital where he had shown marked improvement after two months of hospitalization. It was found that the depression was precipitated by his receiving a letter from his American girlfriend who wished to visit him in Taiwan and who suggested the possibility of marrying him. They had once considered marriage while he was studying in the United States. He thought he did not deserve to marry her. Furthermore, marriage and subsequent departure to the United States would entail his leaving his aging mother alone in Taiwan which he felt he should not do. Also, his future in the United States would have been quite uncertain. During the long course of psychotherapy afterwards, he became depressed from time to time when he took on a new job or when he was assigned to a new project which required independent responsibility. He was overwhelmed by feelings of insecurity and getting lost. Uncertainty about his ego identity and strong ambivalent feelings of hostility and guilt toward his mother (the only member of the family who lived with him and for whom he felt responsibility) were expressed during psychotherapy. The father had died in his early childhood, and as the youngest of his siblings, he had been brought up by his illiterate, old-fashioned mother with the financial assistance of the two older brothers who lived in Japan and Malaysia. He was the only one in the family who received a college education, and the two older brothers had high expectations for his studies in the United States. While a student in Taiwan he had never had time to examine himself, his ability to study abroad, his professional career, and his future life in general. It was during graduate study in the United States that he underwent the emotional turmoil of identity crisis which resulted in a loss of confidence and in his feeling of getting lost.

Paranoia and depression are the two mental disorders which tend to be dichotomized on the basis of the entirely different psychological mechanisms in operation. Intensive family study by a psychiatrist and an anthropologist in Boston showed some significantly different patterns of intrafamily communication between parents and children and different mechanisms of ego development and control. In the families of depressed patients, the children were forced to try by themselves to attain patterns of behavior through positive "ought" channels and were taught to be responsible for their own actions and to anticipate the needs of others. In the families of paranoids, children were forced into acceptable patterns of behavior through negative "ought not" blocking procedures and were trained to be the passive recipients of action by people in authority (Hitson and Funkenstein, 1959–60). This study also found that Burmese family culture was very similar to the paranoid family culture in Boston, and the high homicide rates in Burma were interpreted on this basis. My clinical experience in Taiwan supports Yap's findings (Yap, 1967) in Hong Kong that depressive disorders among Chinese are by no means as rare as Westerners think and that the Western nosological category is also valid in the symptomatology of depression. It can be further speculated from this study that these two disorders may occur in the same person at different stages, depending on the changes of psychological mechanisms in different social environments. Denial and projection mechanisms are more frequently used as defenses against anxiety in a foreign culture where the subject is psychologically isolated and where the outside world is regarded as potentially dangerous. In the home culture, where the outside world is no longer dangerous, these mechanisms are no longer as necessary and may be replaced by another mechanism which leads to depression. Case analyses in the present study indicate that depression and other psychiatric conditions, such as psychosomatic disorders, occur in the same person along with paranoid symptoms at different stages in a long process of adjustment difficulties. The patient's uncertainty about himself and his relation with others in a strange cultural environment is responsible for the feelings of general helplessness. He may try to find an absolute solution, either through an obsessive preoccupation with self which leads to psychosomatic symptoms or through a preoccupation with the outside world which leads to paranoid patterns of behavior. The preoccupation with self also leads to intense self-awareness which includes the inferiority feelings and self-condemnation which may fluctuate with a paranoid projection.

General Discussion

A question may arise as to whether paranoid manifestations are more prevalent among Chinese students studying abroad than among other foreign students. There are no studies yet available to answer this question. Considerably more depressive symptoms and suicidal attempts among Japanese students who broke down during study in the United States have been reported (Shimazaki and Takahashi, 1967). However, when the case histories, though few in number, were carefully read, it was noted that paranoid features were so apparent that paranoid psychoses might have been the diagnosis. The psychiatric diagnosis in these cases appeared to be entirely the subjective judgment of the investigators, depending on their orientation in evaluation of symptoms. Intensive epidemiological study of the mental disorders in communities and the hospital statistics in Taiwan seem to indicate that paranoid symptoms are not more prevalent than other mental disorders among the Chinese in general, but they appear to be related to the factors of migration (Lin et al., 1969). Without going too far in regard to the prevalence rates of paranoid manifestations in Chinese students studying abroad, this discussion intends to highlight some social, cultural, and environmental factors which are thought to be relevant to explanations of their paranoid symptoms.

MIGRATION FACTORS

Psychiatric disorders have been found to be prevalent among migrating or displaced populations, and paranoid manifestations have been reported to be common symptoms (Pedersen, 1949; Tyhurst, 1957, 1951). The stress of culture shift and changes in social environment result in a confusion of value orientations, difficulty in communication, psychological isolation, and increased uncertainty concerning the self and its relation to others. These are considered to be the main psychological problems which lead to excessive denial and projection in the migrant patients. These psychological mechanisms may be partly applicable in explanation of paranoid formation among the Chinese students studying abroad.

The native country of a migrant and the country to which he migrates seem to be more important that the simple fact of his migration. The shift in culture and the relative degree of technological development ought to be considered here, among other factors. It can be assumed that the migration to a country with a basically similar culture, for example, from England to the United States, is easier than the move into a greatly different culture, from Asia to Europe or the United States, for instance. The greater the culture distance, the greater are the difficulties in adaptation and psychological adjustment. The relative degree of technological development seems to affect the psychological adjustment. Migration from technologically less developed, or so-called underdeveloped, countries to a developed country may render psychological adjustment more difficult than migration in the opposite direction. The migrants from non-Western developing countries to a highly developed Western country may be regarded as deprived, while the migrants who move in the opposite direction may be regarded as privileged. In the former case, migrants are more subject to conformity to the new culture, while in the latter case, the culture of the host countries may be, more or less, aspiring to conform to the migrants' culture. The psychological hazards in these two groups of migrants also differ. It is my contention that paranoid disorders are relatively common psychiatric disturbances among the foreign students from non-Western technologically less developed or developing countries who migrate to study in developed Western countries although the contents of delusions, precipitating factors, and the accessory symptoms may differ according to the migrants' original culture. Strong paranoid elements among psychotic foreign students from non-Western developing countries have been reported (Zunin and Rubin, 1967) which seems to support this speculation. Studies of the mental health problems of the privileged group of migrants will be significant in testing this theory.

CULTURAL FACTORS IN CHINESE BEHAVIOR

Besides the factors cited above, other characteristics of the Chinese culture appear to be relevant in the explanation of paranoid symptoms in Chinese students studying abroad. In child-rearing and in interpersonal relations, the Chinese traditionally have been situation oriented, as Hsu (1963) points out, instead of individual oriented. Filial piety and respect for elders and their beliefs are the central code of discipline in the family. Keeping harmony within the environment is also emphasized. The psychological foundation of Chinese society focuses on mutual interdependence among the members of the family and extended family group. Thus, psychological security rests largely with the family and primary kinship group. These characteristics of the Chinese may result in the following behavior patterns which appear to be relevant in an explanation of development of paranoid symptoms in our students.

1) Chinese tend to feel basically insecure outside of the family or primary kinship group, especially in foreign countries, and this may explain the strong tendency of cohesiveness among the Chinese students in the United States. Lack of emotional communication and intimacy with American and other foreign students, psychological isolation from them, and a strong tendency to maintain their own subculture in spite of their relatively successful academic adjustment are characteristics of Chinese students at a large American university reported by Alexander et al. (1969).

2) The world outside of the family or clan group is regarded as being potentially undependable and even dangerous. This is naturally more exaggerated in a different sociocultural environment.

3) Emphasis on keeping harmonious interpersonal relations makes the individual always conscious of others and sensitive to them. The generalized restraints on thought or behavior are rooted in the external social context in which the individual finds himself. The primary sources of regulating behavior in the new society appear to be the real or fantasied presence of others who have the power to shame the student. In the social environment where the outside world is regarded as potentially dangerous, the individual may tend to project his anxiety to his outside world.

4) Face-value has been known to be much emphasized, and suppression is thought to be the dominant psychological mechanism in controlling one's behavior in Chinese culture (Hsu, 1949, Hu, 1949). In a shame culture, one may tend to project his fault to others when the experienced shame is too great to be tolerated and face is lost. The phrase "long term shame turned into fury" is frequently used by newspapers in explanation of violence or homicidal acts; it seems to express this psychological mechanism.

CONTEMPORARY SOCIAL CONDITIONS

Taiwan, because of the political situation, is under strict security control. One must be extremely cautious about his behavior as well as that of others so that one will not be cheated by enemies. This attitude may account for the prevailing defensive and distrustful behavior among Taiwanese. This is reflected in the many strict regulations and formalities in government, banks, and other public organizations. Stated in the extreme, one may need to be more or less paranoid about others and one's surroundings in present-day Taiwan; this was illustrated in the results of a questionnaire study of a large group of students at a major urban university in Taiwan. More than half of the students, 54.8 percent, responded positively to the question, "Do you feel that the outside world is full of traps so you must be very cautious to be free from plots that somebody may have against you?"; 21 percent agreed with the statement, "Somebody was deliberately making trouble for you so you hate them very much"; and nearly one-fifth of the students felt that people were often criticizing them. Unless patterns of paranoid behavior are sharply deviant, they are not regarded as unusual, and may even be considered common, in present-day Chinese society. This attitude may account for lower prevalence rates of paranoid patients at home than one would expect.

PSYCHOSOCIAL IMPLICATIONS OF GOING ABROAD FOR STUDY

To study abroad for academic degrees or advanced training, especially in developed Western countries, has, for the past few decades, been the curse pursued by young Chinese intellectuals. Successful study abroad means not only obtaining knowledge or a degree, but also improved opportunities for financial security and a better life.

In a society where filial piety and conformity to elders are much emphasized, the parents' needs or wishes may play an important part in the decision-making of students. There is, consequently, some possibility that the motivation for going abroad to study is the neurotic compensation of the students themselves or of the parents or both and that the students' ability and psychological readiness have not been taken into account. The psychological pressure on these students is great. Failure in study not only means losing face for the student but for the parents and the family name as well. Therefore, the students must study hard, since they are responsible for themselves, their parents, and the family name. Chinese students seldom feel compelled to write to their parents, even during times of emotional or mental stress in the foreign country. They may even exaggerate their achievements and enjoyment of life a bit in order to reassure their parents who expect so much of them. The fear of failure in academic achievement and in losing face is so great that even the threat of failure, real or imaginary, may lead to mental breakdown.

Summary

Paranoid manifestations appeared to be prevalent among the psychotic symptoms of Chinese students who broke down during their life abroad. A variety of factors, such as marriage and sex problems, personality problems, family background, and parent-child relations were shown to be significant in causing paranoid breakdowns in these students. The migration situation as well as certain characteristics of tradtional Chinese culture and behavior were also relevant not to mention the contemporary situation.

The high rates of previous psychotic breakdowns and personality problems in this series of samples deserve our particular attention. Since studying abroad has become increasingly popular among Chinese students, more systematic studies on the adjustments and maladjustments of these students in foreign countries, preferably with international collaboration, are urgently needed. Psychiatric interviews, even one, with students going abroad before their departure will not only reliably detect any previous mental problems but also fairly well predict the risk of future mental problems. This kind of effort would also enable the students to obtain more insight into their own behavior and sensitivities, and it would prevent needless hardship and suffering.

NOTE

1.   Mainlanders refers to those persons who migrated to Taiwan after World War II or whose fathers came after that date. Taiwanese refers to those persons who were born or settled in Taiwan before World War II or whose fathers were residents before that date. These two groups of Chinese, though ethnically the same, seem to differ in way of life, value orientation, and attitude toward their children's study abroad.

REFERENCES

Alexander, A. A., K. H. Tseng, M. H. Kelin, and M. H. Miller. 1969. Foreign students in a big university—subculture within a subculture. Unpublished paper. Mimeographed.
Hitson, H. M., and D. H. Funkenstein. 1959/60. Family patterns and paranoidal personality structure in Boston and Burma. International Journal of Social Psychiatry 5:182–90.
Hsu, F. L. K. 1949. Suppression versus repression, a limited psychological interpretation of four cultures. Psychiatry 12:223–42.
———. 1963. Clan, caste, and club. New York, D. Van Nostrand.
Hu, H. C. 1949. The Chinese concepts of "face." *In* Personal character and cultural milieu. D. G. Haring, ed. Syracuse, Syracuse University Press.
Lin, T., et al. 1969. Mental disorders in Taiwan, fifteen years later; a preliminary report. *In* Mental health research in Asia and the Pacific. W. Caudill and T. Lin, eds. Honolulu, East-West Center Press.
Pedersen, S. 1949. Psychopathological reactions to extreme social displacement (refugee neuroses). Psychoanalytic Review 36:344–54.
Rin, H., K. C. Wu, and C. L. Lin. 1962. A study of delusions and hallucinations

manifested by the Chinese paranoid psychotics. Journal of Formosan Medical Association 61:46–57.

Rin, H., C. C. Hsu, and S. L. Liu. 1958. The characteristics of paranoid reactions in present-day Taiwan. Memorandum, Faculty of Medicine, National Taiwan University 5:1–15.

Shimazaki, T., and R. Takahashi. 1967. Psychiatric problems of students sent abroad for study—a study on mental disturbances, especially schizophrenia and depression during studying abroad. Clinical Psychiatry 9:564–71. [In Japanese]

Tyhurst, J. S. 1957. Paranoid patterns. *In* Explorations in social psychiatry. A. H. Leighton, J. S. Clausen, and R. N. Wilson, eds. New York, Basic Books.

Tyhurst, L. 1951. Displacement and migration: a study in social psychiatry. American Journal of Psychiatry 107:561–68.

Yap, P. M. 1967. Phenomenology of effective disorders in Chinese and other cultures. *In* Transcultural Psychiatry. A. V. S. de Reuck and R. Porter, eds. Boston, Little, Brown.

Zunin, L. M., and R. T. Rubin. 1967. Paranoid psychotic reactions in foreign students from non-Western countries. American College Health Association Journal 15:220–26.

22. Mental Illness among Western Expatriates in a Plural Society: An Exploratory Study

POW MENG YAP, M.D., F.R.C.P.E.

Division of Psychiatry
Hong Kong Psychiatric Center
Hong Kong

IN THIS PAPER we wish to ascertain what kinds of mental illness affect expatriate Westerners sojourning in Hong Kong, how these differ in both cause and presentation from illnesses among local Chinese, and to what extent the mental breakdown is attributable to the circumstances of expatriation.

Although a British Colony, Hong Kong is an industrial city-state. It lies just within the tropics but has a cold winter season. According to the 1966 By-Census, its population is nearly three and three-quarter million, of whom, if we consider the habitual language spoken, 98 percent would be Chinese and 1 percent Westerners. The great majority of the latter are Britons or of British origin, such as Australians, and they are virtually all sojourners either in business or in the Overseas Civil Service. Increasing prosperity is shared by both Chinese and expatriates. Although upper-class Chinese, who are usually bilingual, mix easily though superficially with Westerners, on the whole there remains considerable social distance between the two groups. The society is plural in that, although within one political unit, the two groups speak different languages by preference, have diverse social habits, customs, and traditions and look, in some cases, to different social institutions to accommodate their hopes and fears. There is no common identification with the locality for the majority, even of the Chinese, and shared ideals for the future are conspicuously absent. Two separate educational systems exist, and in law, certain provisions concerning marriage and succession are dissimilar for the two groups. Thus, while they have a common geographical background, technology, and economy, the two differ in a number of their social institutions, their family and class organizations, and also in some areas of their value systems. In important respects, Florence Kluckhohn's (1961) distinction between traditional Chinese and Western value orientations are valid.

Our material will not demonstrate any exotically picturesque aetiological factors or symptoms because of Hong Kong's urban, indeed metropolitan, milieu and the high standard of living enjoyed by the Western sojourners in general. But precisely because of this, particular patients will deserve study, especially where intimate social-psychological causes responsible for breakdown are concerned. Such information has potential value for the many from advanced lands sent abroad to give aid and for those in the routine foreign service.

Rationale of the Study

Whether or not expatriation precipitates breakdown is a question to be answered by epidemiologists comparing specific rates of incidence in the expatriated population and in the home population. The practical difficulties are doubtless formidable. Case-finding methods must be standardized, but the very differences in geographical and social setting would so influence procedures as inevitably to bias the results. Moreover, it is known that even within a small country like England or Wales, there are marked regional differences in the rates of psychiatric illnesses (Logan and Cushion, 1958), so that comparison of the expatriate rate with the overall rate for the home country as a whole may be quite misleading. There is finally the question of timing the exercises in the two respective countries, and here theoretical questions arise.

Bare comparison of rates cannot mean much unless we observe patients for a period of time before as well as after their emigration abroad. An increased rate overseas could mean inability to adjust to new stresses, but it could also be the result of abnormal persons trying to escape from difficulties at home.

Although a retrospective study has inherent difficulties, the anamnesis could tell us what factors might have brought about the breakdown, and we could examine how such factors are contingent upon expatriation. But even then we still cannot be certain that such expatriation experiences are specifically pathogenic; many expatriates may meet them with complete equanimity and not be brought to our notice. Comparison with a normal control group of expatriates would be important. Prospective cohort studies of persons who are examined before they leave home would be the ideal method, but here again the task is formidable.

The present research is not epidemiologically oriented. Importance is given to case studies of broadly representative samples with the aim of identifying any causally significant stresses that may be due to expatriation. We seek to understand (see Jaspers, 1968) how abnormal mental states arose in our patients because of the difficulties they experienced as expatriates. We also try to discover how such difficulties might be related to other possible aetiological factors such as previous personality, earlier life experience, and family history.

Method

Between the end of 1965 and the middle of 1968, the case histories of 100 consecutive Western expatriates who had attended or were attending the Hong Kong Psychiatric Center were analyzed. In some cases, supplementary information was also obtained. Seven patients were excluded from the samples either because of Eurasian origin or because of a non-Western, as well as non-Chinese, cultural background. Similarly, 100 consecutive Chinese patients attending the same clinic within the same period were studied, after two had been excluded for the same kind of reasons. All the patients were personally seen by the author. My consultant outpatient clinic was government-sponsored, bilingual, and in good standing with both the profession and the public. The fact that fees were charged might indicate that the patients in each group were of roughly comparable socioeconomic level. None of the patients were first referred upon discharge from a mental hospital, although several gave a history of earlier inpatient treatment. It is of interest to note that, during the same period, 55 Western patients were admitted directly to the mental hospital in Hong Kong, and one patient was sent from our clinic.[1] Although this is not an epidemiological study, some remarks concerning the relation of our two samples to their respective base populations are in order. This information might be borne in mind when considering the meaning of the age, sex, and other characteristics presented by our samples.[2] While the composition of our two samples may in some respects be biased, this should neither wholly invalidate our conclusions nor altogether pervert our understanding of relevant aspects of the subject.

Results

Most of the patients in our expatriate sample came from the United Kingdom and countries of the Commonwealth as can be seen from Table 1. Those born in Asia, including Hong Kong, were educated in Britain.

Age and sex. The age and sex distribution of the samples can be seen in Table 2. The age distribution for expatriates and for Chinese is broadly comparable except that there were fewer children and youth among

Table 1:   Origins of Expatriate Patients

Country of origin	N
United Kingdom	59
Australia, Eire	11
Canada, U.S.A.	7
S. Africa	1
Hong Kong	9
Other European countries	10
Other Asian countries	3
Total	100

Table 2:   Expatriates and Chinese, by Age and Sex

Age	Expatriates			Chinese		
	M	F	Total	M	F	Total
0– 9	5	1	6	1	—	1
10–19	2	2	4	4	2	6
20–29	6	11	17	11	15	26
30–39	20	22	42	19	17	36
40–49	8	12	20	8	10	18
50–59	1	4	5	2	5	7
60–over	2	4	6	4	2	6
Total	44	56	100	49	51	100

Table 3: Expatriates and Chinese, by Occupational Status*

Occupation	Expatriates	Chinese
Senior professions	40	19
Business managers and assistants	8	26
Junior professions	12	13
Administrative workers	11	5
Uniformed services	16	3
Technicians	3	6
Office workers	8	19
University students	2	9
Total	100	100

* In the case of housewives and children, by occupational status of head of family.

Table 4: Expatriates and Chinese, by Educational Level

Education	Expatriates	Chinese
Unschooled	4	3
Primary	8	9
Secondary	60	56
Postsecondary	28	32
Total	100	100

the former (the relatively large number of expatriate boys under five not-withstanding [3]). This is in keeping with the small number of school- and college-age persons in the expatriate population. We may conclude, therefore, that the factor of age probably did not bias our samples in any meaningful way and that these samples may properly form the basis for certain generalizations about the population groups they represent.

Socioeconomic status and occupation. These are important variables influencing the manifestation of mental illness. Unfortunately, there is no official data concerning the distribution of occupation or education, in the two groups among the general population, but it may be taken for granted that in Hong Kong expatriates as a whole enjoy a higher socioeconomic status. A glance at Table 3 reveals that expatriates in our sample are drawn from a higher economic status than Chinese. This reflects the situation in the general community in spite of a degree of selection introduced by the procedure of referral to our clinic.

Among expatriates there are more senior professionals, administrative workers and members of the uniformed services; whereas among Chinese there are more businessmen, office workers, and university students. This is in line with the fact that a greater proportion of the expatriate sample is made up of senior civil servants and their dependents than in the case of the Chinese—58 percent compared with 34 percent. The proportion of expatriate civil servants is significantly in excess, for the Staff List of the Hong Kong Government (1967) names 1,133 Western expatriates as against 1,024 Chinese senior civil servants.

It may be seen in Table 4 that, curiously, the distribution of educational levels in the two sample groups is similar. However, the three illiterate Chinese were elderly or middle-aged women, whereas the four unschooled expatriates were four young children. Also, a considerable number of the Chinese secondary and postsecondary patients never completed their courses.

CLINICAL FEATURES

Diagnosis. Table 5 shows that at least 78 percent of the expatriates exhibited disorders that are largely reactive, i.e., all those listed except the last three. (The reactive basis of schizophrenia remains, of course, a matter for debate.) In contrast, the figure for the Chinese is significantly lower, only 60 percent. It is understandable that expatriates showed less schizophrenia and organic syndromes, since they experienced some process of screening before going abroad. It is very likely that those ill with chronic brain disease or schizophrenia were returned home.

Noteworthy is the larger number of females over males in all kinds of depression, especially—among expatriates—reactive and neurotic depression. On the other hand, significantly more alcoholic disorders were found among expatriate males compared with females; but among Chinese men, as compared with women, significantly more anxiety neurosis existed.

Sexual deviation was found only among expatriates. Furthermore, there were five cases of behavior disorder in children among expatriates and only one among Chinese children.

It is probable that the increased incidence of children's behavior disorders among expatriates is largely due to their willingness to submit to psychiatric examination which is a reflection of their ability to accept their condition more readily than Chinese children. However, this cannot be the only explanation in the case of sexual disorders; the latter deserve closer examination.

Sexual disorder. Table 6a shows the occurrence in our two samples of symptoms which are unrelated as such to the number of cases labeled as sexual deviates in Table 5. This manner of analysis offers a better picture of the clinical problems presented, inasmuch as many examples of sexual pathology are polymorphous. The three homosexual males and one homosexual female comprise the four cases of sexual deviation in the expatriates mentioned in Table 5. The three hyposexual patients include two impotent males who were not included in Table 5 among deviates. Among the Chinese, not only is sexual deviation absent, but there are only two men with masturbatory worries and two with a fear of sexual exhaustion due to what they believed to be excessive coitus. One of these four also had a fear of penis shrinkage (Yap, 1964).

Table 6b further confirms the impression that complaints of sexual

Table 5: Diagnosis, by Race and Sex

Diagnosis	Expatriates			Chinese		
	M	F	Total	M	F	Total
Anxiety neurosis	8	9	17	13	2	15
Obsessional-compulsive neurosis	—	1	1	2	1	3
Hysterical neurosis	1	1	2	—	1	1
Sexual deviation	3	1	4	—	—	—
Alcoholic disorder	7	3	10	2	—	2
Personality disorder	2	—	2	2	—	2
Situational stress	3*	3	6	4*	2	6
Behavior disorder in children	4	1	5	1	—	1
Depression, neurotic and reactive	7	24	31	11	19	30
Depression, endogenous, mixed, and other	3	8	11	4†	13	17
Schizophrenia	3	1	4	7	9	16
Organic syndromes	3	4	7	3	4	7
Total	44	56	100	49	51	100

* Includes 1 patient originally classed under "no psychiatric diagnosis."
† Includes 2 postfebrile hypomanics.

Table 6a: Symptoms of Sexual Disorder, by Race and Sex*

Disorder	Expatriates			Chinese		
	M	F	Total	M	F	Total
Homosexuality	3	1	4	—	—	—
Hyposexuality (includes impotence)	3	—	3	—	—	—
Hypersexuality	1	—	1	2	—	2
Masturbatory excess	1	1†	2	2	—	2
Masochism (by flagellation)	1	—	1	—	—	—
Total	9	2	11	4	0	4

* Symptoms shown not related to number of cases.
† In a girl of 6.

Table 6b: Sexual Disorder in Spouse Contributing to Patient's Illness, by Race and Sex of Spouse

Disorder	Expatriates			Chinese		
	Husband	Wife	Total	Husband	Wife	Total
Homosexuality	1	—	1	—	—	—
Hyposexuality (includes impotence)	1	—	1	—	—	—
Hypersexuality	—	—	—	2	—	2
Masturbatory excess	—	—	—	—	—	—
Masochism (by flagellation)	1	—	1	—	—	—
Total	3	0	3	2	0	2

disorder are rare among Chinese. If complaints are encountered, they tend to be confined to anxiety over sexual exhaustion. Chinese are disinclined to seek psychiatric help for sexual disorders, save when these are related to certain overvalued ideas regarding sexual excess, but it is still possible, from what one sees and hears, that there is a genuine infrequency of such disorders among them. The fact that in the course of this study two instances of flagellation were encountered in expatriates is striking; this practice among the Chinese is probably rare. Also noteworthy is the fact that whereas three European women complained of lack of sexual satisfaction by their husbands for various reasons, not one Chinese woman did so; on the contrary, two of the latter revealed that they could not tolerate the inordinate demands made by their husbands. In this particular respect, differences in cultural norms and expectations, as well as conception of the sick-role, certainly must be considered. Normality in sexual functioning is ill-defined and largely culture-specific, but our patients, by coming to the clinic, have ipso facto defined themselves as abnormal.

It would seem that sexually functioning Westerners cover a wider range than among Chinese and meet with greater vicissitudes. This is related possibly to greater sexual freedom in Western culture, an important aspect of Western individualism. The latter often finds expression in a constant search for new experiences, as Hsu (1962) has observed. Furthermore, in the urbanized pattern of Western society, coarse physical labor is much reduced and beauty culture is widespread; sexual attractiveness is a main factor of the ideology of mass marketing, and, at the same time, opportunities for intimate social contacts between the sexes are numerous. Yet, it is obvious that sexual freedom can generate its own anxieties.

Alcoholic disorders. Alcoholic intemperance has long been linked with the expatriate east of Suez. There is some factual basis for this as can be seen in the special procedure that existed in Hong Kong under the old Mental Hospital Ordinance (rescinded in 1960) concerning the admission of patients suffering from delirium. Alcoholism has never been common among Chinese, in contrast to narcotic dependence. Table 7 shows clearly this distinction; the difference between ten expatriate and two Chinese patients is statistically significant; this takes into account only those with a major problem of alcoholism. The preponderance of this condition among expatriates is even more striking if we note that there were two expatriate female patients whose breakdowns were associated with alcoholism in their husbands. The actual diagnoses among the seventeen expatriates with both major and secondary problems of alcoholism were: chronic alcoholism, eight cases; anxiety with alcoholism, five; depression with alcoholism, two; inadequate personality with alcoholism, one; and delirium, one.

It is hard to know whether the proportion of alcoholic expatriate patients found in this sample is high or low compared with the rate in their homeland. All of our patients began drinking before leaving their home country. In any case, it is difficult to say at what point heavy social drinking becomes alcoholic addiction. Seven out of the seventeen expatriates had a predisposed personality (mostly anxious or obsessional); four had had previous breakdowns before coming to Hong Kong; and two had a family history of mental illness in first-degree relatives (i.e., parents, siblings, children).

Occupational maladjustment. The findings relating to this topic (Table 8) represent an important approach to our understanding of the patients' behavior as well as the stresses under which they labor. There is no difference in numbers between expatriates and Chinese. In both groups, all the patients were diagnosed cases of anxiety or depression except for one Chinese schizophrenic. Nine out of the eleven expatriates with a major problem of maladjustment had a predisposed personality; most of them were shy, nervous, and perfectionistic. The others included one man of inadequate personality with hysterical tendencies and one man of basically low intelligence. Among the Chinese, too, as many as ten out of the fifteen cases were predisposed by personality; nine of these were obsessional, worrying, and impatient and one felt inferior and was unduly sensitive. In regard to previous breakdown and a family history of mental illness in first-degree relatives, there was no difference in the two groups (two expatriates compared with three Chinese).

There were more expatriates who expressed their difficulties in terms of inadequate emoluments and unsatisfactory quartering rather than in terms of marked occupational pressure. None of the Chinese did so, and their stresses were more directly related to their work as such. They complained of excessive work and responsibility, and, in some cases, of business reverses leading to financial insecurity. These differences must be seen in the light of the fact that, as we have noted, there were more senior civil servants and fewer businessmen in the expatriate sample.

The expatriate group, which included two missionaries, one nightclub artist and one prostitute, had a wider range of occupations than the Chinese. The fact that these four patients figured in the samples may be an indication that these occupations are especially vulnerable in expatriate circumstances, since their numbers in the general expatriate population must be very small; certainly, analysis of the case histories bears this out, although it is true that the two missionaries also had anxious personalities.

Marital conflict. Another area in which we can study with profit the question of adjustment is that of marital relations, in the broader sense of the term. There is no overall difference between the two groups except that Chinese females appeared significantly more vulnerable to such conflict, and, also, they did not report it as a secondary problem. This could be understood in terms of the prevailing pattern of male dominance among Chinese.

The diagnoses among expatriates (primary cases) were: depression, four patients; anxiety with alcoholism, four; chronic alcoholism, one; and confusional state from self-poisoning, one. There was little difference in

Table 7: Alcoholic Disorder, by Race and Sex

Degree of Alcoholic Disorder	Expatriates			Chinese		
	M	F	Total	M	F	Total
Major problem	7	3	10	2	—	2
Secondary problem	3	4	7	1	1	2
Total	10	7	17	3	1	4

Table 8: Occupational Maladjustment, by Race and Sex

Degree of Occupational Maladjustment	Expatriates			Chinese		
	M	F	Total	M	F	Total
Major problem	7	4	11	12	3	15
Secondary problem	—	2	2	1	1	2
Total	7	6	13	13	4	17

Table 9: Marital Conflict, by Race and Sex

Degree of Marital Conflict	Expatriates			Chinese		
	M	F	Total	M	F	Total
Major problem	6	4	10	3	9	12
Secondary problem	2	1	3	—	—	—
Total	8	5	13	3	9	12

the frequency of personality predisposition among the Chinese—five expatriates and three Chinese. In regard to previous breakdowns and family history of mental illness in first-degree relatives, there was again little difference in numbers between expatriates and Chinese (four patients compared with two, and one compared with one, respectively).

As part of the major problem, marriage across racial boundaries was found in six expatriates, and all of these except one were male. In Chinese there were three instances of this, and two of the three were female. Furthermore, mixed marriage as a secondary problem was also encountered in two other· expatriate men, so that eight out of thirteen expatriates gave evidence of conflict in this respect. Taken together with the great preponderance of males concerned, this indicates that the marriage of Western colonial sojourners with local women is a potent cause of disharmony and mental breakdown. It is commonly observed that, in such unions, there is frequently a large difference in social class between the partners so that the normal principle of assortative mating does not apply. While it is true that in our overall material there were three examples of harmonious mixed marriage (two to Chinese women and one to a Creole girl) in which race difference played no part in the illness, all three women were in fact well-educated and Westernized to a varying extent. Of the six expatriate patients in whom intermarriage was a major problem, four were additionally alcoholic. Of all cases mentioned in Table 9, five expatriates were alcoholic compared with one Chinese.

Information as to extramarital relations was difficult to elicit from our patients, but it is interesting that among the Chinese this condition appeared to take a more traditionally sanctioned pattern in that there were six patients involved with either concubines or, less formally, with dance hostesses. (The latter represent a social institution originating in East Asia some forty years ago.) The comparative anonymity of life abroad may sometimes loosen conventional restraints, so that disturbances in marital relations, perhaps with sexual dysfunction, are an additional hazard. Leon (1963) has also noticed this in a study of the psychiatric problems facing North American wives expatriated to Colombia.

It is apparent that marital discord is commonly associated not only with mixed marriage but also with alcoholism in men and attempted suicide in women. Among expatriates, out of six cases of recent and three of earlier suicidal attempts, four occurred in the group with marital conflicts. Similarly with the Chinese, out of nine recent cases and one earlier attempt, five were in this group. As other studies of attempted suicide found (Yap, 1958; World Health Organization, 1968), women outnumber men (expatriates, six female and three male; Chinese, six female and four male).

Physical illness or death in patient or close relative. Mental breakdown was precipitated by physical illness in the patient or a close relative in the cases of four expatriates and twelve Chinese, a difference that is statistically significant. Close relative here covers first-degree relatives and parents-in-law whether or not they were living in Hong Kong. Illness includes deafness (one Chinese case) and sterility (one Chinese case), but it does not include examples of acute or chronic brain syndrome. The difference could reflect preselection for physical health and fewer physical illnesses in expatriates as well as intimacy of family ties and relatively large family size in the Chinese. It would appear that realistic fears and traumatic experiences associated with bodily illnesses are more important as precipitating causes of illness for Chinese than for expatriate patients.

The Stresses of Expatriation

Special difficulties. Table 10 shows that there were seventeen patients in whom major stress arose from adversities resulting from their expatriation. Of these, ten were of a pure kind, without other and secondary difficulties of a general nature unrelated to sojourn abroad. It is a striking fact that all but two of the seventeen patients were female, and one of the two males was a boy only 9 years old, newly arrived and exhibiting behavior disorder. This sex difference is significant statistically. The female patients were all in their late twenties or thirties, with the exception of one, aged 46. Ten of the females were married, and five had never married.

The diagnoses in the seventeen cases were: depression, thirteen; anxiety, two; chronic alcoholism, one; and behavior disorder, one. The fifteen anxious and depressive patients included three alcoholics, of whom one was also sexually maladjusted because of diminished libido. Another one of the fifteen had become impotent a few weeks after arrival in Hong Kong. Personality predisposition was noted in eleven patients. This proportion of 65 percent is significantly different from that of 42 percent for the occurrence of predisposed personalities in the sample as a whole. Previous psychiatric illness before coming to Hong Kong had occurred in seven patients. A positive psychiatric history in first-degree relatives, however, was found in only two patients. We may thus conclude with some assurance that the female sex, personality predisposition, and a history of previous breakdown are characteristics commonly associated with persons vulnerable to expatriation stress.

What are the pressures that may bring about such breakdown? And are they in some way peculiar to the expatriate situation in Hong Kong? How much causal significance may be ascribed to them? A study of the clinical histories of the pure cases (Appendix I) convinces us that the factors listed in Table 11 generally in order of decreasing frequency are causal factors or situations of relevance. They are causal not because they are sufficient to bring about illness by themselves but because they are, severally together, necessary for the illness to have occurred at all, granted that personality predisposition is also present.

It will not be denied that sometimes the factors or situations presented in Table 11 may be more the result than the cause of disorder (especially in the case of items 2, 4, 6, 7, and 9), but with psychogenic

Table 10:   Expatriates with History Showing
             Special Expatriation Stresses, by
             Age and Sex

Age	M	F	Total
0–19	1	—	1
20–39	1	14	15
40–59	—	1	1
60–over	—	—	—
Total	2	15	17

Table 11:   Special Factors in Expatriation Stress*

1) Overcrowding, noise, inadequate hygiene, unpleasant summer
2) Few friends or clubs, too much gossip
3) Separation from relatives, homesickness; trouble with children at school
4) Immoderate leisure leading to boredom
5) Class snobbishness
6) Difficulty in housekeeping and/or with servants
7) Housing not up to expectation
8) Difficult occupation, e.g., artist, missionary
9) Inability to mix with, or antipathy to, Chinese; political disturbances

* Arranged roughly in order of decreasing frequency.

illnesses it is erroneous to think in terms of unilinear causality. Subjective attitudes should not be discounted: as Montaigne put it, "He who fears he will suffer, already suffers because of his fear." And if certain harmful and antagonistic postures and attitudes developed from the illness itself, they could hardly have been nurtured on other than expatriate soil.

The ethos of the colonial sojourner bears some distinct features that may be underscored here. Persons of different social origins come to live and work in close contact with one another, their sense of community heightened by the consciousness of belonging to a tiny, though privileged, minority far from home. A preoccupation with racial prestige and its manifestation in social status soon develops. Overtaking the Joneses involves acquiring servants; this is nowadays a difficulty even for Chinese employers. With servants may come unaccustomed idleness and, in turn, restlessness and boredom. While social relations with English-speaking Chinese are excellent on the whole, the illusion of high-society life, sweetened with boats and beaches ("everyday being like a holiday," as I have been told by a nurse), may induce a few to yield to unhealthy racist sentiments which, as we have seen, are often tinged with social class prejudice. Leisured wives may try to engage in social work sponsored by voluntary societies but may be hurt by the subtle class distinction, more strict perhaps than even in southern England. In these cases, a sense of bitterness and frustration is engendered. Growing dissatisfaction may prompt those who cannot keep up with the pace to wish they were in the native country, and this may lead to a conflict with the husband and a dislike of his job. It is true that some wives, having secured servants, will busy themselves in full- or part-time employment, but working wives often create pressures for their husbands and themselves.

Escape from homeland. We have seen that in the majority of cases where there was a breakdown from the stresses of expatriation, personality predisposition, as well as a history of previous illness, was found. There is some evidence that as far as mental hospital admissions in Singapore were concerned, Western colonial expatriates had a higher rate in comparison with local non-Western groups and the home population (Murphy, 1959, 1961). There has been noticeably little research on this general topic.

In our entire sample, there were only two patients with continued illness who came to Hong Kong because they wanted, or had been advised, to seek a change. One was a male obsessional-compulsive teacher and the other a male doctor whose schizophrenic symptoms were under control with heavy medication. It is, therefore, not plausible to say that an increased incidence of illness among expatriates is attributable to their escape from home being due to the social complications caused by such apparent illness. Probably such illnesses would prevent rather than encourage departure abroad.

It could well be otherwise with faults of personality, whether or not they have previously erupted into episodes of clinically definable illness. In our sample, there were patients whose histories showed clearly that they had moved abroad to evade distress, frustration, or embarrassment at home, and these troubles were often linked understandably to personality weaknesses (Appendix II). Table 12 shows that there was a total of ten such patients; if only adults in our sample were counted the proportion of these would be ten out of eighty-eight.

The diagnoses were: anxiety state, four patients; alcoholism, two; inadequate personality, one; situational stress reaction, one; obsessional state, one; and schizophrenia, one. As many as eight patients showed personality predisposition. This proportion of 80 percent is significantly higher than in the sample as a whole where the proportion is 42 percent. As far as previous breakdowns are concerned, it has already been mentioned that one schizophrenic and one severely obsessional patient carried their illnesses out with them; as for the four patients with anxiety state and the two with alcoholism, the question may be raised as to whether they were not ill before they left their homeland. Thus, only two patients out of ten had not experienced any illness, or near breakdown, previously.

The high incidence of previous illness as well as the evidence of nonresilient personality in this group would suggest that those who "escape" are susceptible persons. Very likely they would in due course have broken down, or relapsed into illness, even without expatriation stress. It should be noted that of the seventeen cases classified under expatriation stress, only one was an escapee (case 6, Appendix II). Thus, only one out of ten escapees succumbed to special expatriation stresses as against those of a pedestrian and universally human variety.

Flight abroad therefore does not always, or necessarily, prevent

Table 12:   Expatriates with History Showing Theme of Escape

Reason for Escape	M	F	Total	Remarks
Illness	2	—	2	One schizophrenic, one obsessional.
Extramarital affair	1	1	2	Male patient with older wife had to run away from lover. Female patient left to preserve her marriage and family; affair became too serious.
Inadequate at work	3	—	3	Two pensioners (one of them alcoholic). One inadequate fire services officer.
Marital conflict	1	—	1	Alcoholic lawyer with unfaithful wife.
Aimless, anxious	1	—	1	Bored, nervous engineer; "could not stand England."
Flight from family	—	1	1	"Bohemian" girl, hating middle-class family.
Total	8	2	10	

vulnerable persons from having a breakdown, as is seen in our cases. To what extent it can help to achieve this end, we do not know, for such persons would not come our way. It is undoubtedly possible that some who go abroad may be able to make a better and more constructive adjustment than they would at home; an example would be the Briton, married to a continental European woman, who finds the British way of life disagreeable.

Conclusion

The association of personality predisposition with earlier illness, as well as final breakdown, is of interest in our cases. It is possible to view all this as one continuous psychopathological process occurring in a patient under repeated but independent stresses of no particular specificity, with cumulative effects (Langner, 1961; Langner and Michael, 1963). Because of characteristic stresses which burden the expatriate colonial sojourner and also, the tendency for some susceptible persons troubled at home to seek relief abroad where they in due course succumb to different pressures, it is possible that the incidence of mental illness among colonial expatriates may be higher than in the home population. We need properly designed epidemiological research, ideally along the lines of a cohort (or panel) study, to test this surmise.

In the meantime, a clinical study like ours is necessary to help identify some of the relevant aetiological factors as a step toward the planning of large-scale investigation. It is all too easy in pursuing epidemiological interests to fall into an ecological fallacy, that is, to ignore the attitudes and feelings of our subjects in concentrating only on external sociological and demographic facts. A clinical study serves to correct our perspective and, also, to enhance our understanding of the meaning of epidemiological data. Furthermore, it is particularly germane to research on the psychiatric implications of social change (Kantor, 1965), a singular and much neglected instance of which is colonial expatriation.

Appendix I: Cases Showing Direct Expatriation Stress *

1)   C.B. F, 27. Reactive depression. A trained commercial artist married to a civil engineer. Born in England. Father was a teacher. By personality inclined to be anxious. Only European female in her office in Hong Kong. Found expatriates unfriendly, odd: "You never know whether they'll say good morning to you or not." Missed her natural cultural amenities. Husband did not entirely share her interests. Also worried about ill treatment of mother by father back at home; unhappy because she could not intervene. No children. Elder sister treated for anxiety state.

---

* All initials used to designate patients are fictitious.

2)   B.R. F, 28. Mixed depressive state. Born in England of an engineer;
        married to subinspector. Previous attacks of depression and one
        attempt at suicide before coming to Hong Kong. High-strung per-
        sonality. Mother in England also treated for depression, had leg
        amputated just before patient's present illness. She had opposed
        patient's expatriation and wanted her to return. Homesick, never
        liked Hong Kong, although had been living there several years.
        Complained bitterly of lack of diversion and boredom. Difficulty in
        making friends; friends ceased to visit her when she appeared ill.
        Hated husband's career, wanted him to retire prematurely or resign.

3)   D.B. F, 31. Hysteria (psychogenic somnolence). Born in South
        Africa of company director. Rather attention-seeking by personality.
        Worked as secretary-stenographer in civil service. Lived alone. No
        male friends, but desired marriage. Hardly ever went out. Unhappy
        with "atmosphere" in her department (special branch), pressed for
        transfer. Determined not to go back to Hong Kong after her next
        home leave, confessed general unhappiness in Hong Kong, especially
        from loneliness and boredom.

4)   E.D. F, 28. Reactive depression with psychosomatic symptoms;
        treated for sprue. Single. Born and bred in England. Father was an
        author. Previous suicidal attempt. Qualified as dietician, joined
        Hong Kong Government. Found summer heat trying, thought work
        excessive in hospital, could not converse with her patients. Illness
        started two months after arrival. Intellectual interests, only a few
        friends. Found Hong Kong people too "status-conscious": "I hate
        them inquiring into my family background. I have nothing to be
        ashamed of." Wished to go home immediately.

5)   A.B. M, 9. Behavior disorder. British-born son of university lecturer,
        newly arrived from Australia. No one of his age in multistoried
        block of flats, but two older children around. Adventurous,
        wandered into Australian bush once before. Now felt rather
        cramped, found school system difficult. Frightened by 1967 riots,
        trembled visibly in street. Developed tantrums, threatened to run
        away, and succeeded in getting lost.

6)   A.F. F, 30. Neurotic depression. Born in Singapore, brought up in
        Scotland. Father was senior civil servant in Hong Kong. Worked as
        secretary in different places, finally with Hong Kong Government.
        Timid, immature and uneasy by personality. Lived with parents in
        Hong Kong until they left, then remained alone. Had always been
        with parents in a united family. Disclaimed interest in men, denied
        desire to get married, and was socially isolated. Was all right when
        home for a few weeks, relapsed again on return to Hong Kong.

7)   E.T. F, 46. Reactive depression. English-born. Father was an elec-
        trician. Worked as secretary. Married to government accountant.
        Pleasant personality. Was in Africa 18 years and liked open spaces.

Three months after arrival in Hong Kong became ill. Disappointed with place, especially first few weeks in hotel. Felt enclosed, too crowded, everything on top of her. Humidity unpleasant, no close friends, could not manage servants. Also upset by daughter's divorce and son's failure in examinations; both away in England, worried about them.

8)   E.H. F, 26. Alcoholic toxic psychosis. Born in Ireland. Father was an engineer. Had been to Borneo and Aden with husband, a school teacher in Overseas Civil Service. Fairly heavy social drinker before going to Hong Kong. On arrival lived first in hotel, engaged an *amah* to help look after three young children. Did not like new acquaintances in Hong Kong: "too artificial"; American men tried to make advances to her: "Hong Kong is a man's paradise." Could not stand noise and pace of life. Drinking increased, became paranoid and hallucinated.

9)   J.H. F, 36. Reactive depression. Born in England. Father was a bus conductor. Receptionist before marriage to government engineer. Went to Africa, Australia, and arrived in Hong Kong in 1967. Worked briefly as confidential assistant. Previous personality pleasant. Mother of two children; husband became interested in local women. Patient had dreams of other women mocking her, fought them off. Bored, no clubs she could join. Husband would not take her out, had no friends of her own. Wanted to go back to Australia, after less than one year in Hong Kong.

10)   E.L. F, 37. Neurotic depression. A perfectionistic-worrier, born in England. Father was a shopkeeper. Was confidential assistant. Married an engineer who was posted to remote island, and had only one "European" neighbor to keep her company. Could not get interested in the locals. Husband was likely to be in charge of water-works there for 12 years, and in due course they might be only expatriate family there: son away in England. Fear of traveling on ferry made her isolation worse.

Appendix II: Cases Showing Theme of Escape *

1)   J.B. F, 36. Situational stress reaction. Tense and tearful. English-born, daughter of a company director, whom she detested because he was mercenary, "sadistic," and cold: "Worse thing my mother ever did was to marry him." A feminine, muddled, and rather immature person, expressing herself with mock-Bohemian vehemence: "My father has settled some money on me to escape death duties, but I wish I could earn enough to say 'f--k you' to him; I hate myself for being so English, they are so hypocritical, so dishonest with

---

* All initials used to designate patients are fictitious.

themselves." Had tried to get away from family by taking jobs in Austria for room and board only and secretarial work in Malaysia, Singapore: "It is easier to get jobs out here." In Hong Kong, lonely, started affair with a married Englishman, wanted his baby badly: "I am prepared to be his concubine."

2) K.H. M, 44. Alcoholism, inadequate personality. Father was lawyer. War pensioner from Australia (diagnosed hysteria with personality defect). Now a free-lance journalist, married to Chinese teacher. Had not been able to hold jobs and make ends meet in homeland, so went to Hong Kong to live in a country cottage. With low cost of living and help of wife could manage. No children.

3) H.R. M, 35. Alcoholism. Born in Burma, schooled in Britain. A lawyer in the civil service. Father was a merchant-banker. Irritable and jealous, with long history of heavy drinking. Abandoned by mother at the age of 5. While in Canada, alcoholic wife had two affairs with married men; the second caused lover's wife to become mentally ill. After this thought marriage irreparable, came to Hong Kong, where however he could find no satisfaction in his work. Wife, after having been relinquished by lover, came back to him with his three children, but left again shortly thereafter.

4) W.A. M, 53. Inadequate personality, below average intelligence. Referred by Australian authorities. Born in Australia. Father was a farmer. Superannuated postal clerk, married thrice; first two wives left him. Lived in water-front shack near Sydney, moved around a great deal, had visited Hong Kong two years previously. Jobless when seen, living on superannuation. Mild affective symptoms. "Normal life would be too much, but in Hong Kong, where I am living, there is nothing to upset me." Planned to go to the Seychelles where cost of living would be lower.

5) R.H. F, 38. Reactive depression. Musician, born and trained in England. Father a school teacher, committed suicide. Serious-minded, emotional. When she learned of father's suicide four years previously, cried and stayed in bed for several days. Married a man of quite different interests and outlook, then had a violent affair with another. Told husband; and in order to preserve family, with the two children, they decided to leave for Hong Kong, where she lost libido completely, developed menstrual irregularity, and remained downcast.

6) H.E. M, 39. Anxiety state. Father, a metal worker. An English Fire Services Officer of weak and nervous personality, not very intelligent, and married to an ambitious, overbearing woman who dominated him: "She is a social climber, she pushed me up." Had quarreled with wife over another woman, was for a time neurasthenic. Wife decided they could do better abroad, and they came out. Found Hong Kong unpleasant, complained of being housed in

poor area, too much noise and dirt, next to ordinary Chinese people. Uneasy over meeting Chinese, wanted to have European companion with him whenever he stepped out. Could not work. Both patient and wife very much on defensive, resenting diagnosis of illness: "A lot of it is just Hong Kong."

7) S.B. M, 36. Anxiety state. An English engineer in the civil service, the son of another. Inclined to worry. Married to a woman ten years older than he. Had serious affair with a married woman in Kuwait, and when back in United Kingdom continued intimacy with her. Wife ambivalent about divorce; he felt he could not abandon daughter he loved, saw several doctors, marriage counselors, solicitors, but could not arrive at a solution to problem. Then they decided to go to Hong Kong to get away from it all. Continued to have chronic arguments with wife. Disliked his work.

8) M.P. M, 43. Anxiety with psychosomatic symptoms. A P.W.D. engineer. Born and brought up in London. Father was property owner. High-strung, inhibited, stammered. Badly teased in school. First marriage failed because wife left him and in-laws were hostile. Could not stand living in England, went to Africa, Malaya on contract jobs. Married again. Salary insufficient, insecure, feared parenthood and practiced contraception for several years. Drank heavily. Back in England had cricothyroid spasm, belching, tension. Went to Hong Kong on permanent job, in consideration of imminent old age, but remained chronically irritable.

9) H.F. M, 31. Schizophrenia. Single, born in England. A doctor; father, a lawyer. Previous schizoid personality. First attack four years previously. On recovery became ship surgeon, then went into general practice. Had second attack, after which went to Zambia as G.P. Returned home, continued general practice, then ill again three months before going to Hong Kong, having been accepted to a post in charity hospital. When first seen, symptoms well controlled by heavy medication. Felt he was losing sense of humility, getting "inflated sense of status," "taking advantage of others' deference for him." Uncomfortable with people, no friends. Work unsatisfactory, returned home after five months.

10) J.B. M, 33. Obsessional-compulsive neurosis. A single school teacher, born in England. Father was a journalist. Both parents were nervous, father drank heavily. Obsessional personality trait, argumentative. Previous spells of debility, only once saw doctor. Marriage in Canada failed, wife left him. Although a university graduate, drifted from job to job, last one was deck-chair attendant. Went to Hong Kong to escape unhappiness and frustration, but could not teach properly there. Exhausted, compulsion to speak backwards, etc., sent home after fourteen months.

NOTES

1.   The diagnoses were: manic-depressive illness, 20; schizophrenia, 20; psycho-organic syndromes, 5; alcoholic disorders, 5; neurosis and personality disorders, 3; drug dependence, 1; no psychiatric diagnosis, 1.
2.   From Tables 28 and 30 of the 1966 Hong Kong By-Census (Commissioner for Census and Statistics 1968) it can be computed that, as regards age distribution, those we must take as Western expatriates, i.e., people classified as "speaking English habitually," differ from Chinese in that there are fewer young people of school and university age among the former. In regard to sex, expatriates resemble Chinese in that males outnumber females at all age groups excepting the minority over 55. For the total number of all ages, among expatriates men form 49 percent of their total population, and among Chinese, the proportion is only slightly higher—51 percent. When these data are compared with the sex difference in each one of our two samples (expatriates 44 percent male and Chinese 49 percent male), the difference for expatriates is statistically significant. (In this study the level of $P = .05$ is taken as the level of statistical significance.)
3.   This unusual number was probably due to referral by a child guidance clinic to our center during a period when its principal psychologist was away; usually this clinic saw a large number of European children.

REFERENCES

Hong Kong Government, Commissioner of Census and Statistics. 1968. Report of the by-census, 1966.
Hsu, F. L. K. 1962. Psychological anthropology. Homewood, Illinois, Dorsey Press.
Jaspers, K. 1968. The phenomenological approach in psychopathology. British Journal of Psychiatry 114:1313–23.
Kantor, M. B. 1965. Mobility and mental health. Springfield, Illinois, Charles C Thomas.
Kluckhohn, F., and F. L. Strodtbeck. 1961. Variations in value orientations. Evanston, Row, Peterson Co.
Langner, T. S. 1961. Environmental stress and mental health. *In* Comparative epidemiology of the mental disorders. P. H. Hoch and J. Zubin, eds. New York, Grune and Stratton.
Langner, T. S., and S. T. Michael. 1963. Life stress and mental health. New York, The Free Press of Glencoe.
Leon, C. A. 1963. Adaptive problems of a group of North American housewives in Latin America. Acta Psiquiatrica y Psicologica Argentina 9:114–21.
Logan, W. P. D., and A. A. Cushion. 1958. Morbidity studies from general practice, vol. I (General). London, H.M.S.O.
Murphy, H. B. M. 1959. Culture, society and mental disease in South East Asia. M.D. thesis, University of Edinburgh.
———. 1961. Social change and mental health. *In* Causes of mental disorders: a review of epidemiological knowledge. New York, Milbank Memorial Fund.

World Health Organization. 1968. Prevention of suicide. Geneva.

Yap, P. M. 1958. Suicide in Hong Kong, with special reference to attempted suicide. Oxford, Oxford University Press.

————. 1965. Koro, a culture-bound depersonalization syndrome. British Journal of Psychiatry 111:43–50.

23.   Psychiatric Concomitants of Fusion in Plural Societies

H. B. M. MURPHY, M.D.

Department of Psychiatry
McGill University
Montreal, Canada

THE INFLUENCE of rapid social change on mental health has been a constant subject of discussion for a hundred and fifty years or more and is still not properly understood. For a long time, the effect was believed to be harmful; but this is not necessarily so (Murphy, 1961), although the types of change favoring and disadvantaging mental health have until quite recently been difficult to distinguish (Murphy, 1965, 5–29). Part of our difficulty has lain in the crudeness of the measures of health and of change which were customarily used, and part has been due to the absence of a suitable typology. Traditional approaches to a typology of change have nearly always been sociological and have focused on the broad setting—speed and content of the change—whereas mental health considerations demand more attention to individual experience. In the past five years, however, our knowledge of the subject has expanded considerably, so that a more appropriate typology is now available. In this paper, I propose to explore one such typology and to apply it to data collected many years ago in Singapore, hopefully demonstrating its potential relevance to understanding the psychiatric significance of much of the change going on in Asia at the present time.

     The typology to be explored is one focusing on the subjective sense of personal involvement rather than on objective measures and is thus more in harmony with the psychiatrist's concern with intrapsychic conflicts than most view of change employed in the past. There are four main categories of change proposed, namely: A) self-motivated change toward a known or imagined model; B) self-motivated change toward an unknown model; C) unmotivated change away from a highly valued state; D) unmotivated change away from an indifferently valued state.

These are ideal types, unlikely to be found in pure form, and it may be necessary in the future to distinguish several subtypes. Type A has been considerably studied in recent years (see brief review below), and some of the theory which applies to it might apply to type C as well. Type B, however, has been almost wholly ignored, and it will be the main subject of the present paper.

Type A change is the most familiar to us, since it is exemplified by acculturating European immigrants to the U.S. and by the earlier westernization of non-Western peoples. Such people strove toward an ideal represented by a known person or group either of their own culture or of another, and although rejection of some of the model's characteristics might have existed, enough were usually retained for the goal to be clear. When the relation of such change to mental health was formerly investigated, the focus was customarily on single, relatively objective concepts such as externally induced stress or social selection, and results were unclear. Work done in the past ten years, however, has chosen for its target the interaction between two or more variables of a more subjective character, employing hypotheses quite closely related to Festinger's theory of cognitive dissonance, and this has been more fruitful. Combining the findings of such contrasting studies as Kleiner and Parker's analyses of Philadelphia mental hospitalizations (Kleiner and Parker, 1965, 78–85), Chance's investigation, using the Cornell Medical Index, of a small Eskimo community (Chance, Rin, and Chu, 1966), the "disparagement syndrome" data from the Stirling County study (Cleveland and Longaker, 1957, 167–200), and perhaps Rosenberg's childhood data in a situation of "contextual dissonance" (Rosenberg, 1962), one gets the firm impression that the best mental health is found in persons whose goals are in accord with their perceived means of reaching these, while considerably poorer mental health is shown by persons who experience a dissonance between what they think should be their position in the world and what they think actually is, or can eventually be, their position in it. Such measures of dissonance correlate better with the Philadelphian and Alaskan mental health ratings than do such matters as status consistency, orientation toward change, or access to means of change. To some extent, it .may be possible that the dissonance is the result rather than the cause of unhealthy mental conditions, for a marked discrepancy between goal and means suggests weak reality-testing; but the rule appears to apply even when goals are quite modest, and in other situations the theory offers a potential explanation for apparent paradoxes.[1]

However, while the concept of dissonance between goals and means or between expectations and perceived reality would appear useful for explaining the mental health of those moving purposefully toward a known or clearly imagined target (type A change), and while it might also be applicable to those who feel themselves being pulled away from their ideal (type C change), it should not theoretically apply to type B situations and might also not apply to type D. The theory of cognitive dissonance requires that two or more pieces of knowledge are sufficiently defined for their incompatibility to be manifest, and this is not likely to be the case if one's goal is unknown and has been imagined only in part or if personal judgments and decision-making are absent. Accordingly, this theory would predict that the correlation between dissonance and mental health would be strongest where there was a close correspondence between the chosen ideal and a known model but would steadily weaken insofar as the chosen model, and all others, were felt to be defective and inadequate. This expectation appears borne out by Rin's findings from his Taiwan survey (Chance, Rin, and Chu, 1966) and by some of the data from Grave's Tri-ethnic community study (Graves, 1967).

Rin, while working with Chance and me in Montreal, had attempted to replicate Chance's findings with his Taiwan survey data. He found that the mental health ratings showed the expected trend when subjects born in mainland China were considered, but not when he worked with those born in Taiwan. That difference could have been accidental, but a more plausible reason is that the mainlanders lacked the support of their traditional milieu and saw promise in change to an American model, while the Taiwanese were still supported by their traditions and preferred a form of change that would achieve an as yet undefined compromise between the American model and these traditions. Similarly, the Tri-ethnic study data on alcoholism and deviance (Graves, 1967) yielded a clear correlation between mental health and access to modernization when only those members of the minority groups most strongly oriented to the major culture were considered, but no such correlation existed when those who were not so oriented were analyzed.

In these last instances, I would suggest that the type of change being followed is predominantly type B (though in some of the Tri-ethnic subjects, there may be no change to speak of), and the dissonance concept fails to indicate how such change is related to mental health. The question now is: can we discover how Type B change relates to mental health, if it relates at all. Populations in which type B change is taking place must be common, but they are not so easy to distinguish from, or to contrast with, contiguous populations in which change is not taking place. Moreover, in many instances of type B change, there is a complicating element of upward social mobility for which allowance has to be made. However, one situation which offers an appropriate contrast with little vertical mobility is that exemplified in a number of African societies recently by the development of an indigenous church with Christian and non-Christian elements. Another is the movement toward fusion or synthesis which can occur in plural societies when these are put under external pressure before any one of the participant cultures has been permitted to attain absolute dominance.

A Plural Society

Plural societies occur wherever two or more peoples of substantially different cultures live in close proximity but with little interaction, and where each people possesses the essentials of a complete society with its own distinct institutions, leadership, proletariat, and economic base. Fusion is initiated when, by force of circumstance, such peoples must cooperate more closely in order to avoid being dominated by their neighbors or in order to form a nation state. It is irrelevant to the present paper whether plural societies can form naturally or are only the result of constraint, for example, under colonial domination.[2] In the short run, it is irrelevant, also, whether they can remain viable without one of the cultures becoming wholly dominant. What is relevant is that many such societies exist at the present time, that most are attemping to arrive at a fusion or, at least, better accommodation between the disparate peoples within them, and that the attempts at fusion imply a change toward a hybrid culture whose vague character can be inferred but whose precise lineaments are unknown. In most such situations in the present-day, postcolonial era, the individuals actively striving toward fusion are few and relatively easy to identify among the masses who retain a traditional orientation or look to existing foreign models as their ideals. However, the former are not so few as to be only the self-selected, and since the movement is not likely to result in either an increase or a decrease in social status, the psychiatric aspects of vertical mobility can conveniently be disregarded.

Singapore, with its distinct populations of Chinese, Malay, Indian, and European origin, was not the first location to which the term "plural society" was applied, but it could well have been (Freedman, 1960), and in the 1950's, it had good reasons to start seeking a greater unity among its peoples than had been necessary hitherto. As a predominantly Chinese city surrounded by Malay neighbors, Singapore did not desire affiliation with mainland China or Taiwan and was dependent on its functions as a warehouse and a naval base after the colonial power moved out. Its only chance of survival seemed to lie in the establishment of its right to be considered a legitimate political entity, distinct from the various nations that had contributed to its population. Before and after independence, therefore, there was governmental pressure to reduce cultural barriers, although without any real attempt at describing the sort of synthesis being sought. Thus, the public looked spontaneously toward the same goal. At many social levels, people attempted to establish contact with their neighbors of other cultures, to understand why each did ordinary things in different ways, and, perhaps, to see whether some habits might be exchanged. Even more important than this deliberate reaching-out was a readiness to accept and to socialize with members of other cultures on a relatively equal basis, if employment, housing, schooling, or other factors (often manipulated by the government) made assimilation beneficial. Meanwhile, elaborate social surveys in 1947 and 1955 had augmented a relatively good decennial census, and these combined with good mental hospital records to permit the calculation of first admission rates for a wide variety of groups within the population. It is possible to ascribe to several groups, of different ethnic origins, a fairly distinct orientation toward change.

Among the Chinese, a major division had been created by the existence of two school systems—one in the mother tongues and the other in English. Most of those educated in Chinese followed traditional career ideals for which suitable models existed, so that if they sought change, it was usually of type A. Most of those educated in English aimed at taking over the known roles of the now disappearing Europeans, so that type A change also predominated, although the same does not necessarily apply for the English-educated women.

Among the Malays, a majority were tradition-oriented with little inclination toward change, except possibly in the direction of greater dominance of Malay culture and the Mohammedan religion. Distinct from that majority, however, was a highly visible group of traders who were attempting to compete with the Chinese and Indians in the general market and who, I think, had as an ideal a compromise with tradition, for which they had no clear model, rather than a return to tradition or an imitation of European ways. Hence, this minority is one example of people pursuing a type B change.

The majority of Indians, like the majority of Malays, were not really oriented to cultural change but merely aimed at gaining material wealth and security along traditional lines and dreamt of returning to India after having experienced no change other than becoming richer. However, there also was a minority of Malays who regarded Singapore as their home and who saw their chances of continuing success there as doubtful, unless the Chinese majority ceased to think of itself as Chinese and became instead Singaporean. Consequently, this minority also had as an ideal a merging of cultures such as would permit its minority status to be forgotten without absorption of its identity by the Chinese life style.

Finally, there were the Eurasians and Europeans, each divided roughly into those who regretted the imminent loss of their former colonial privileges and those who saw it necessary to strive for a modern democratic state in which both the old colonial privileges and the old cultural barriers would be removed. Among the Eurasians, it was difficult to differentiate the holders of these attitudes demographically. Among the Europeans, however, there was a fairly clear age split—the older members derived from the prewar colonial period, and the younger ones had been sent out by the postwar Labor government to assist the territory in gaining its independence.

Although ethnic grouping is the most relevant population subdivision for our needs, it is useful to view the population in terms of geography or neighborhood. For the purposes of studying the relation of cultural isolation (in Faris's [1934] original sense) and social interaction to mental hospitalization rates, I identified, with the aid of the city planning department (actually, the research branch of the Singapore Improvement Trust), six sectors which had fairly distinct characteristics in respect to ethnic composition and type of neighborhood interaction. One of these was a Western style suburb of small modern bungalows with no outward manifestations of Asian influence, although the population was almost wholly Asian. My assumption is that the people who chose to live there were pursuing type A change with Europeans as their model. Another was a semisuburban locality with new, government-owned, high-rise apartments and a mixed population, and conditions conspired to make it highly desirable for the different cultural groups to understand one another. Since there was much interaction between groups beyond that imposed by the organizational structure at the same time that there was no evidence that European styles of life were the ideal, I regard this as a strong example of type B change. A third central sector exemplified the traditional Chinese orientation, and two further sectors appeared to experience cultural mixing without shared goals. In theory, therefore, a comparison of their mental hospitalization patterns should enable us to see whether the different types of change have different psychiatric concomitants, and in particular, whether there is anything distinctive about the type B example.

Patterns of Mental Hospitalization

During the 1950's, first admissions to mental hospitals in Singapore were running at about the same rate as in Western countries. There were no psychiatric facilities outside of the mental hospital, and a rough check for unhospitalized psychoses revealed that although they could be found through the public health nurses, the patients had nearly all been to a hospital at least once, because families avoided recourse to Western medicine only after it had been used and found unsuccessful. Moreover, parallel studies of suicide (Murphy, 1954), juvenile delinquency (Murphy, 1963), psychosomatic illness (Murphy, 1959, thesis), and student mental health (Murphy, 1959, 164–222) yielded results similar to many found in the analysis of hospitalizations. Therefore, I feel that the first admission data represent a fair, even if not wholly accurate, measure of community mental health.

Starting with the data for the different ethnic groups, the first results of interest concern the English-educated Chinese. They should have had lower hospitalization rates than the Chinese-educated, since they belonged on the average to a higher social class and since among the Singapore Chinese, class-specific admission rates declined as status rose (Murphy, 1959, thesis). As Figure 1 shows, however, the expectation is disproved. Among males, the rate for this group is higher than that for those educated in Chinese, at nearly

Figure 1: Comparative Rates of Mental Hospitalization
in the Singapore Chinese by Age, Sex, and
Education

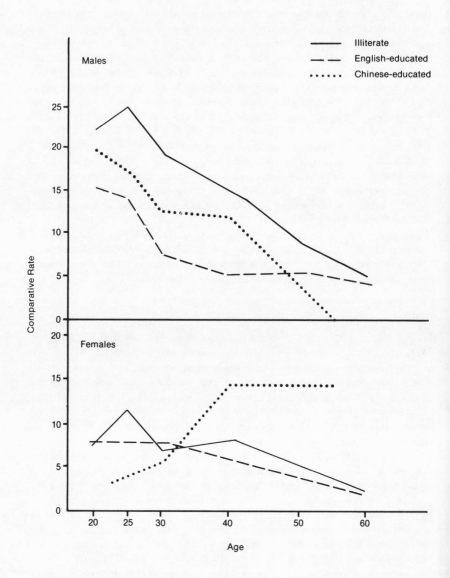

all ages; among the females it is lower than those for the other groups in early adult life but then climbs higher than not only the Chinese-educated group's rate but the illiterate group's as well.

By themselves, these figures tell us little beyond the fact that the group undertaking the greater change had higher hospitalization rates. In the case of the males, however, it was possible to arrive at rough estimates of incidence for different occupational strata within each of the two educational categories, and that makes the picture more interesting. For the higher occupational strata in which Europeans formerly predominated, the English-educated had hospitalization rates substantially below those of the Chinese-educated. For other occupational strata, however, the hospitalization rates for the English-educated were considerably above those for the Chinese-educated. In other words, mental health is better where change was initiated and was not attempted. Where it was initiated and the goal not reached, however, mental health suffers, despite some rise in social status—an illustration of the results of type A change.

For Chinese women, the story is different, since there is no evidence that the high mental hospitalization rate among the older English-educated derives disproportionately from those who have failed to reach the social class of European predecessors nor any evidence that the life of the prewar Singapore European woman had been the Chinese ideal. Most Singapore Chinese girls, in pursuing an English education, must have been attracted by the greater freedom which the younger European females enjoyed and perhaps by the chance of marrying someone of high status, but it is very doubtful that they had a clear image of what they wanted their lives to be like when they were older. Chinese culture rewards the later years of life better than British culture does, at least within the family, and in Singapore, the Chinese career women, who has, in Western style, retained her independence beyond the normal Chinese age for marriage, may find it difficult to marry thereafter. A disproportionate number of the English-educated female patients were unmarried beyond the age of thirty, a state which they are unlikely to have intended, but regardless of that, it seems likely that this group embarked on a change toward an inadequately defined goal and found the result disappointing. In any event, we must conclude that this type B change has been accompanied by signs of worsened mental health.

The same conclusion applies to the second example of type B change —namely, that of the Malay trading community. As Table 1 shows, the rate of mental hospitalization is higher for this group, despite their superior economic status, than for almost every other occupational category. Interpretation here is complicated by the fact that Malay occupation-specific rates of mental hospitalization did not follow the expected pattern, and it can be argued that the high incidence among traders was merely an expression of the tendency of rates to rise as responsibility and demand for effort increased in these people. However, other features of Table 1 can also be interpreted as reflecting the intensity of change to which different strata are exposed, and whether one considers the change as type B or type C, greater change does appear to be accompanied by more mental illness. Among the females whose lives were little affected by such change, on the other hand, there is, as far as can be judged, no rise of incidence in the higher classes.

Turning now to the Europeans, the picture is more complex. Taking all subgroups together, Singapore mental hospitalization rates for Europeans were above those for Asians despite the former group's higher social status. The rates for Europeans were also, above the corresponding rates in Britain at this time, even though seamen were excluded from consideration and some patients avoided local hospitalization by repatriating themselves. However, for those over 45 years old, the rates were relatively low, and below that age, they varied greatly with background and sex. Of the males, a disproportionate number of the psychoses occurred in those who did not belong to the dominant British group, and in the native British males, the rate was relatively low, especially if one considers the psychoses only (Table 2). Among females, however, there were very few mental hospitalizations of those of non-British origin but a marked excess of cases among the British, with schizophrenia being a frequent diagnosis.

Viewed in terms of experience with social change, each of these groups is different. The non-British can hardly be classified, since although their move to Singapore undoubtedly exposed them to change, some individuals sought that change, others regretted it; some had a clear goal in view, and others moved aimlessly. The older British can be classed on the average as having experienced a type C or type D process, since a majority had been prewar colonials who viewed the recent political changes with regret or indifference. Consequently, their relatively low hospitalization rates may tentatively be interpreted as indicating that passivity in the face of change is less stressful than participation. Among the younger British, however, there were many who saw it as their function to assist in the break-up of the colonial system. They had come to Asia not with the idea of economic exploitation or paternalistic suzerainty but to act as equals to Singaporeans in a move toward national independence. Since the form of the society they were seeking to create was unknown, this must be called, for the majority of the young, involvement in type B change. In this change, both men and women were involved, since the wives recognized their task to work towards a new joint society with the Asian wives while their husbands attempted to create something new alongside the Asians in their occupations. The local women, however, had a high rate of mental hospitalization while the men had a relatively low one. How can this difference be explained, given the fact that in the non-British and in the older generation there was no excess of female admissions?

The most plausible answer relates to the relative structuring of the man's task and that of his wife. In most work settings, there already existed a set of shared expectations about how people of different cultures could cooperate, and every day there were short-term tasks whose solutions offered

Table 1: Comparative Malay First Admission Rates at Singapore Hospital 1950–54, by Occupational Group

Occupation	Rates	Occupation	Rates
Manager, tradesman	85.7	Shop assistant	50.0
Professional	66.7	Domestic	25.0
Office worker	41.2	Trishaw operator	85.7
Police-, post-, fireman	48.0	Hawker	33.3
Artisan	110.0*	Laborer	74.2
Driver	35.4	Messenger, watchman	18.2
Services	28.0	Fisherman, farmer	41.5

* Rate questionable for internal reasons

Table 2: European Mental Hospitalizations in Singapore, 1950–54*

Group	Psychoses M	F	Other Admissions M	F	Total M	F
†Chinese	11.5	8.7	2.4	1.4	13.9	10.1
‡Europeans	5.6	10.2	8.6	6.8	14.2	17.0
‡British	12	18	13	13	25	31
‡Other Europeans	9	2	3	2	12	4

* Note: The British origin comprised approximately two-thirds of the European population aged 15+, the proportion being slightly higher for males than for females. Hospitalizations from shipboard and of sailors in transit through Singapore are excluded.
† Rates per 10,000 aged 15–44
‡ Number of cases, all ages

Table 3: Comparative Rates of Schizophrenia and the Affective Psychoses in Different Social Milieux in Singapore, 1950–54

Urban Sectors	N	Schizo-phrenia	Affective Psychoses	Organic Psychoses	Total Admissions	Ratio
New style sector	100	39.0	10.5	17.3	75.0	3.71
Western style suburb	38	23.3	18.0	30.3	78.4	1.30
Old style suburb	241	22.1	17.5	15.4	62.0	1.26
Central cohesive area	831	25.5	17.4	23.0	78.8	1.47
Central mixed area	607	28.5	25.0	31.2	102.3	1.14
Transitional area	127	31.1	27.7	30.3	109.1	1.12

* Ratio of schizophrenics to those with affective psychoses

opportunities for exploring cooperation more deeply. The men, therefore, possessed landmarks and short-term goals to assist them during their efforts at achieving change. In their households, the wives also had such tasks and landmarks, but the contact was only with subordinates, and in their main efforts towards cultural change, their effort at contacting their Asian neighbors, the short-term tasks and the landmarks were missing. Common problems could offer points of contact, but there was not the necessity of achieving common, short-term solutions, and when they made assumptions about common viewpoints, these often proved illusory. In reaching out towards the other cultures and in seeking a common future culture which Singapore Chinese and British families would share, therefore, the women had a much more difficult and intangible task than the men had. To say that the sex difference in mental hospitalization rates found in Singapore's British population in the five years of my survey is wholly attributable to the difference in their means of approaching social change would be unjustifiable, for other factors may have been at work, and some of the difference may have been accidental. But similarities between this picture and others which arise under conditions ·of what seems to be type B change suggest that a connection exists.

Among the Indian and Eurasian sections of Singapore's population, it is difficult to distinguish groups having clearly different orientations to change, and many other factors can be detected as affecting their mental hospitalization rates. We can, therefore, pass on to the second group of data which concerns the different urban sectors.

Table 3 presents the essential data for the six sectors chosen for special study, with the one in which, I believe, type B change has occurred placed first and the one most likely to contain people with type A orientation second. The rest are intended to represent various degrees of ethnic mixture and residential locality without an orientation to sociocultural change. In interpreting the rates which Table 3 presents, consideration must be given to the social class structure in each locality. The Western style and old style suburbs were predominantly middle class, the two central areas were predominantly lower class, and the remaining two sectors, new style and transitional, were mixed. Given these facts, one sees that the Western style sector representing type A change manifested more mental illness than one would expect (though the difference is not statistically significant), if one assumes the old style sector to be representative. The new style sector, standing for type B change, had a healthier rate of hospitalization, if one takes into account the difference in average social class, and it is definitely healthier than the transitional sector of approximately equivalent socio-economic range. However, in the new style sector, what is striking is not so much its low overall admission rate as the high ratio of schizophrenia to affective disorder that pertains here, a ratio almost three times as high as that arising from the other sectors. Because of the method of deriving these sector rates (each case had to be spotted on a large map), the sex of the patients was not ascertainable. This is unfortunate since one might suspect that the excess of schizophrenia in the new style would rest mainly in the women, and, thus, it would repeat the findings in the two other main instances of type B change—the younger British group and the English-educated Chinese females. However, even without this information, it is instructive to note that in the type B situation, schizophrenia remained quite high in respect to other forms of mental illness. Such a finding might have been anticipated if the sector were inhabited mainly by young unmarried individuals; but the contrary was the case, since it was virtually impossible to find accommodations in this sector unless one were married and had children. Probably, then, the finding is in some way linked to the changing situation in which these people found themselves.

Discussion

The purpose of this paper was to explore the utility in mental health research of a new typology of social change with emphasis on cultural change in Asia. The data used happened to be at hand and, therefore, were not particularly suited to the purpose in mind, but they have yielded some pointers.

For type A change, i.e., motivated change toward a well-defined goal, a single general illustration presented itself, though we are able to approach it from two distinct viewpoints. The shift from Asian to Western modes of living, which is assumed to be represented by the English-educated Chinese males and by the Western style suburb, was accompanied by somewhat higher levels of mental hospitalization than were occurring in comparable populations that had not made this shift. However, upon closer examination this higher-than-expected level is seen to be derived disproportionately from that sector of the changing population that failed to attain its goal when the change was embarked on. Of course, failure to attain any goal is stressful, and mental illness can induce some failure as well as follow it. However, all the Singapore Chinese had the goal of improving the economic security of their families, whereas the Malays did not, and many failed; yet, among the Chinese-educated there was no sharp difference in rates from different socioeconomic strata which can be inferred to occur among the English-educated. Accordingly, the findings here did harmonize with the theory of type A change proposed earlier, although they did not illustrate it as well as some other more directly pertinent studies have done.

For type B change, i.e., motivated change towards an imprecise goal, four illustrations have been offered with different results according to circumstance. In the Malay traders and the English-educated Chinese female sections of the population, mental hospitalization rates were definitely higher than were expected. In the new style sector, they were lower than expected, but with an unusually high ratio of schizophrenia to affective disturbance. In the younger British generation, the rates were somewhat lower than expected for the males but much higher than expected for the females, and schizophrenia was again in excess among the latter. On the average, the groups that embarked on type B change had markedly poorer rates of mental hospitalization than one would have expected on the basis of their cultural background and mean socio-economic status. There were two instances where this general tendency is abandoned. We cannot say that these exceptions arise from having attained or having come close to the intended goal, since none of these groups could at that time be said to be within sight of its ideal. If mental health during type B change is to be protected, however, it is important to know how these exceptions differ from the rule: how the young British males maintained a more markedly improved level of mental health than their wives, and how the new style sector maintained low rates of mental hospitalization for conditions other than schizophrenia.

The answer seems to be that in each case the long-range goal could be pursued through, or at least parallel to, a series of short-range goals, each of which was represented by a fairly concrete need best pursued through cooperation. The Europeans in their workplaces shared daily problems with their Asian colleagues, and each cooperative tackling of a specific problem could be seen both as a task in itself and as a step in the process of improved culture contact. The inhabitants of the new style sector, packed together in high-rise apartments and forced to deal with unfamiliar regulations, administrative procedures, and service breakdowns, found that their shared experiences were of greater immediate relevance than their separate cultural backgrounds, and they pursued friendships with each other while solving local difficulties. In the other less happy instances of type B change, these conditions were lacking. The Malay traders had short-term goals, but they pursued them not in cooperation but in competition with their Chinese and Indian neighbors who saw no personal benefits in the Malay traders' learning to please the non-Malay customer. (It would have been different if the Malays had apprenticed themselves to some Chinese or Indian businessmen, but they tended to keep themselves apart.) The European wives had the potential cooperation of their Asian neighbors, but not the short-term, practical goals on which this cooperation could be exercised. The English-educated Chinese women probably had neither the cooperation nor the short-term goals, for the compromise which they desired probably had been too poorly defined from the start for a series of shared and circumscribed changes to be possible.

Therefore, it appears that, under conditions of type B change, mental health is best served if the individual can advance along a series of short steps, each with its own limited and attainable goal, and share his experience with others having similar long-rang goals. Conversely, mental health seems most likely to be endangered during such change if the individual must pursue his journey alone and cannot break it into modest stages with fairly concrete targets. This statement may echo Durkheim's remarks concerning anomic suicide, since the vagueness of the goal in type B change may be such that, in his words, "the limits between the possible and the impossible are unknown." Although Durkheim stressed the value of socially defined norms, he did not mention the advantages of a shared confrontation with the anomic situation. Possibly he would have said that if the confrontation were shared, it became itself a norm. I have seen catastrophic anomie, or abandonment of norms, occur in war-time situations without apparent damage to mental health, and, in most instances, the whole community's sharing in the abandonment was probably the key protective factor. Furthermore, Durkheim did not concern himself with different types of mental distress or breakdown. The foregoing results have suggested that, when conditions are suitable, the general mental health of the population may actually be raised during type B change, except for the schizophrenia-prone sector.

As I have argued elsewhere (Murphy, 1968, 74–92), I believe that schizophrenia is evoked in suitably predisposed persons when they are confronted with a continuing demand for action or for decisions under conditions of confused, contradictory, or inadequate information. If a goal is inadequately defined, the pre-schizophrenic is confused; then, if there is group pressure on him to participate in a move towards that goal, the situation becomes dangerous for him. If conditions are such that exploration of unorthodox answers is permitted or encouraged, and there is an expectation that one will be able to come out with a socially acceptable solution, the situation is healthier for the schizophrenia-prone than if he is trapped in a rigid cultural tradition which does not face up to its own consistencies. But in most situations of type B change, the schizophrenia-prone person is in danger, and we should, therefore, not be surprised if the rate for this form of illness is high.

Almost no examples for types C and D change have been presented, although the older European generation in Singapore may be thought to represent one or the other. It is highly unlikely that type C, i.e., change away from a highly valued state, can occur without damage to mental health. The exile and the reversionary individual are not prototypes of superior mental health. That the ex-colonial administrator should regret the passing of his glory, however, does not mean he is experiencing type C change; he may, with another part of his mind, accept the idea of change or he may, as was true for many, find a niche where he can continue his former role until retirement. The latter can be relatively unstressful. Regarding type D change, i.e., unmotivated change away from an indifferently valued state, it seems likely that what little influence the experience of change would have on mental health is greatly outweighed by the question of whether the state arrived at was more or was less rewarding than the state which had been left. However, this may be an oversimplification.

It is hoped these considerations will be of relevance when it comes to estimating the probable impact on mental health of anticipated social change, but it must be realized that the experience of change itself is only one of the factors which will determine the outcome. Largely excluded from this discussion have been the questions of the acceptance of change and the question of whether the resultant state is more or less rewarding than the original one. Ambivalence toward change is likely to involve some mental distress, particularly if there is an inner conflict between two equally powerful needs. The immigrant, undecided whether to stay in the new land or to return home, is in such a state, and he not infrequently develops paranoid defenses against the demands of one side or the other, defenses which need not, however, be of much prognostic significance once the choice is made. Conversely, after the change has been accepted, the rewards available in the new state may result in an improvement in mental health which outweighs any adverse effects induced by the process of change. It is toward an understanding of this process, and not with reference to any appreciation of the end result, that this paper has been addressed.

NOTES

1.   For instance, one such paradox is that in Canada the mental hospitalization rate of immigrants from certain European countries is higher for the better educated than for the lesser educated, although one normally expects the former to have the lower rates. The paradox begins to resolve itself, however, if one considers what the different educational classes experienced in Europe and what they would expect in Canada, for then one realizes that it is relatively easy to find in the new country the greater material prosperity which the lesser educated customarily seeks; but it is quite hard to find something that will improve on the bourgeois comforts and sociability to which the better educated immigrant from these lands had been accustomed.

2.   For detailed discussion see the opposing views of Furnivall (1948) and Wertheim (1965).

REFERENCES

Chance, H. A., H. Rin, and H. Chu. 1966. Modernization, value identification and mental health: a cross-cultural study. Anthropologica VIII 2:197–216.

Cleveland, E. J., and W. D. Longaker. 1957. Neurotic patterns in the family. *In* Explorations in Social Psychiatry. A. Leighton, J. Clausen, and R. N. Wilson, eds. New York, Basic Books.

Faris, R. E. L. 1934. Cultural isolation and the schizophrenic personality. American Journal of Sociology 40:155–64.

Freedman, M. 1960. Growth of a plural society in Malaya. Pacific Affairs 33:158–68.

Furnivall, J. S. 1948. Colonial policy and practice: a comparative study of Burma and Netherlands India. Cambridge, Cambridge University Press.

Graves, T. D. 1967. Acculturation, access, and alcohol in a Tri-ethnic community. American Anthropologist 69:306–21.

Kleiner, R. J., and S. Parker. 1965. Goal striving and psychosomatic symptoms in a migrant and non-migrant population. *In* Mobility and Mental Health. M. Kantor, ed. Springfield, Illinois, Charles C Thomas.

Murphy, H. B. M. 1954. The mental health of Singapore, part I: suicide. Medical Journal of Malaya 9:1–45.

———. 1959. Cultural factors in the mental health of Malayan students. *In* The Student and Mental Health: An International View. D. Funkenstein, ed. London, World Federation for Mental Health.

———. 1959. Culture, society and mental disorder in South East Asia. M.D. thesis, Edinburgh University.

———. 1961. Social change and mental health. Milbank Memorial Fund Quarterly 39:385–445.

———. 1963. Juvenile delinquency in Singapore. Journal of Social Psychology 61:201–31.

———. 1965. Migration and the major mental disorders: a reappraisal. *In* Mobility and Mental Health. M. Kantor, ed. Springfield, Illinois, Charles C Thomas.

———. 1968. Sociocultural factors in schizophrenia: a compromise theory. *In* Social Psychiatry. J. Zubin and F. A. Freyhan, eds. New York, Grune and Stratton.

Rosenberg, M. 1962. The dissonant religious context and emotional disturbance. American Journal of Sociology 68:1–10.

Wertheim, W. F. 1965. East-West parallels: sociological approaches to modern Asia. Chicago.

EPISTEMIC PROBLEMS

24.   Pathologies of Epistemology

GREGORY BATESON, Ph.D.

Biological Relations Division
Oceanic Institute
Waimanalo, Oahu, Hawaii

FIRST, I would like you to join me in a little experiment. Let me ask you for a show of hands. How many of you will agree that you see me? I see a number of hands—so I guess insanity loves company. Of course, you don't "really" see me. What you "see" is a bunch of pieces of information about me, which you synthesize into a picture image of me. You make that image. It's that simple.

The proposition, "I see you" or "you see me," is a proposition which contains within it what I am calling "epistemology." It contains within it assumptions about how we get information, what sort of stuff information is, and so forth. When you say you "see" me and put up your hand in an innocent way, you are, in fact, agreeing to certain propositions about the nature of knowing and the nature of the universe in which we live and how we know about it.

I shall argue that many of these propositions happen to be false, even though we all share them. In the case of such epistemological propositions, error is not easily detected and is not very quickly punished. You and I are able to get along in the world and fly to Hawaii and read papers on psychiatry and find our places around these tables and in general function reasonably like human beings in spite of very deep error. The erroneous premises, in fact, work.

On the other hand, the premises work only up to a certain limit and, at some stage or under certain circumstances, if you are carrying serious epistemological errors, you will find that they do not work any more. At this point, you discover to your horror that it is exceedingly difficult to get rid of the error; that it's sticky. It is as if you had touched honey. As with honey, the falsification gets around; and each thing you try to wipe it off on gets sticky, and your hands still remain sticky.

Long ago, I knew intellectually, and you, no doubt, all knew intellectually, that you do not see me, but I did not really encounter this truth until I went through the Adalbert Ames experiments and encountered circumstances under which my epistemological error led to errors of action.

Let me describe a typical Ames experiment with a pack of Lucky Strike cigarettes and a book of matches. The Lucky Strikes are placed about three feet from the subject of experiment supported on a spike above the table and the matches are on a similar spike six feet from the subject. Ames had the subject look at the table and say how big the objects are and where they are. The subject will agree that they are where they are and that they are as big as they are, and there is no apparent epistemological error. Ames then says, "I want you to lean down and look through this plank here." The plank stands vertically at the end of the table. It is just a piece of wood with a round hole in it, and you look through the hole. Now, of course, you have lost use of one eye, and you have been brought down so that you no longer have a crow's eye view. But you still see the Lucky Strikes where they are and of the size which they are. Ames then says, "Why don't you get a parallax effect by sliding the plank?" You slide the plank sideways, and, suddenly, your image changes. You see a little tiny book of matches about half the size of the original and placed three feet from you, while the pack of Lucky Strikes appears to be twice its original size and is now six feet away.

The effect is accomplished very simply. When you slid the plank, you, in fact, operated a lever under the table which you had not seen. The lever reversed the parallax effect; that is, the lever caused the thing which was closer to you to travel with you and that which was far from you to get left behind.

Your mind has been trained or genotypically determined—and there is much evidence in favor of training—to do the mathematics necessary to use parallax to create an image in depth. It performs this feat without your volition and without your consciousness. You cannot control it.

I want to use this example as a paradigm of the sort of error that I intend to talk about. The case is simple; it has experimental backing; it illustrates the intangible nature of epistemological error and the difficulty of changing epistemological habit.

In my everyday thinking, I see you, even though I know intellectually that I don't. Since about 1943 when I saw the experiment, I have worked to practice living in the world of truth instead of the world of epistemological fantasy; but I don't think I've succeeded. Insanity, after all, takes either psychotherapy to change it or some very great new experience. Just one experience which ends in the laboratory is insufficient.

This morning I raised a question which nobody was willing to treat seriously, perhaps because my tone of voice encouraged them to smile. The question was whether there are true ideologies. We find that different peoples of the world have different ideologies, different epistemologies, different ideas of the relationship between man and nature, different ideas about the nature of man himself, the nature of his knowledge, his feelings, and his will. But if there were a truth about these matters, then either only those social groups which think according to that truth could reasonably be stable or, if no culture in the world thinks according to that truth, there would be no stable culture.

Notice again that we face the question of how long it takes to come up against trouble. Epistemological error is often reinforced and, therefore, self-validating. You can get along all right in spite of the fact that you entertain, at rather deep levels of the mind, premises which are simply false.

I think perhaps the most interesting—though still incomplete— scientific discovery of the twentieth century is the discovery of the nature of mind. Let me outline some of the ideas which have contributed to this discovery. Emmanuel Kant in the *Critique of Judgment* states that the primary act of aesthetic judgment is selection of a fact. There are, in a sense, no facts in nature; or if you like, there are an infinite number of potential facts in nature, out of which the judgment selects a few which become truly facts by that act of selection. Now, put beside that idea of Kant, Jung's insight in *Seven Sermons to the Dead,* a strange document in which he points out that there are two worlds of explanation or worlds of understanding, the *pleroma* and the *creatura*. In the *pleroma,* there are only forces and impacts. In the *creatura,* there is difference. In other words, the *pleroma* is the world of the hard sciences, while the *creatura* is the world of communication and organization. A difference cannot be localized. There is a difference between the color of a desk and the color of a pad. But that difference is not in the pad, it is not in the desk, and I cannot pinch it between them. The difference is not in the space between them. In a word, a difference is an idea. The world of *creatura* is that world of explanation in which effects are brought about by ideas, essentially by differences.

If, now, we put Kant's insight together with that of Jung, we create a philosophy which asserts that there is an infinite number of differences in this piece of chalk but that only a few of these differences make a difference. This is the epistemological base for information theory. The unit of information is difference. In fact, the unit of psychological input is difference.

The whole energy structure of the *pleroma*—the forces and impacts of the hard sciences—have flown out the window so far as explanation within *creatura* is concerned. After all, zero differs from one, and zero, therefore, can be a cause which is not admissible in hard science. The letter which you did not write can precipitate an angry reply, because zero can be one half of the necessary bit of information. Even sameness can be a cause, because sameness differs from difference.

These strange relations obtain because we organisms (and many of the machines that we make) happen to be able to store energy. We happen to have the necessary circuit structure so that our energy expenditure can be an inverse function of energy input. If you kick a stone, it moves with energy which it got from your kick. If you kick a dog, it moves with the energy which it got from its metabolism. An amoeba will, for a considerable period of time, move more when it is hungry. Its energy expenditure is an inverse function of energy input.

These strange creatural effects (which do not occur in the *pleroma*) depend also upon circuit structure, and a circuit is a closed pathway (or network of pathways) along which differences (or transforms of differences) are transmitted.

Suddenly, in the last twenty years, these notions have come together to give us a broad conception of the world in which we live—a new way of thinking about what a mind is. Let me list what seem to me to be those essential minimal characteristics of a system which I will accept as characteristics of mind. (1) The system shall operate with and upon differences. (2) The system shall consist of closed loops or networks of pathways along which differences and transforms of differences shall be transmitted. (What is transmitted on a neuron is not an impulse, it is news of a difference.) (3) Many events within the system shall be energized by the respondent part rather than by impact from the triggering part. (4) The system shall show self-correctiveness in the direction of homeostasis and in the direction of runaway or both. Self-correctiveness implies trial-and-error.

Now, these minimal characteristics of mind are generated whenever and wherever the appropriate circuit structure of causal loops exists. Mind is a necessary, an inevitable, function of the appropriate complexity wherever that complexity occurs.

But that complexity occurs in a great many other places besides the inside of my head and yours. We'll come later to the question of whether a man or a computer has a mind. For the moment, let me say that a redwood forest or a coral reef with its aggregate of organisms interlocking in their relationships has the necessary general structure. The energy for the responses of every organism is supplied from its metabolism, and the total system acts self-correctively in various ways. A human society is like this with closed loops of causation. Every human organization both shows the self-corrective characteristic and has the potentiality for runaway.

Now, let us consider for a moment the question of whether a computer thinks. I would state that it does not. What thinks and engages in trial and error is the man plus the computer plus the environment. And the lines between man, computer, and environment are purely artificial, fictitious lines. They are lines across the pathways along which information or difference is transmitted. They are not boundaries of the thinking system. What thinks is the total system which engages in trial and error, that is, man plus environment.

But if you accept self-correctiveness as the criterion of thought or mental process, then obviously there is thought going on inside the man to maintain various internal variables at the autonomic level. And similarly the computer, if it controls its internal temperature, is doing some simple thinking within itself.

Now, we begin to see some of the epistemological fallacies of Occidental civilization. In accordance with the general climate of thinking in mid-nineteenth-century England, Darwin proposed a theory of natural selection and evolution in which the unit of survival was either the family line or the species or sub-species or something of the sort. But today it is quite obvious that this is not the unit of survival in the real biological world. The unit of survival is organism plus environment. We are learning by bitter experience that the organism which destroys its environment destroys itself.

If, now, we correct the Darwinian unit of survival to include the environment and the interaction between organism and environment, a very strange and surprising identity emerges. The unit of evolutionary survival turns out to be identical with the unit of mind.

Formerly, we thought of a hierarchy of taxa—individual, family line, sub-species, species, etc.—as units of survival. We now see a different hierarchy of units—gene-in-organism, organism-in-environment, ecosystem, etc. Ecology, in the widest sense, turns out to be the study of the interaction and survival of ideas and programs (i.e., differences, complexes of differences, etc.) in circuits.

Let us consider now what happens when you make the epistemological error of choosing the wrong unit. You end up with the species versus the other species around it or versus the environment in which it operates. Man against nature. You end up, in fact, with Kaneohe Bay polluted, Lake Erie a slimy green mess, and "Let's build bigger atom bombs to kill off the next-door neighbors." There is an ecology of bad ideas, just as there is an ecology of weeds, and it is characteristic of the system that basic error propagates itself. It branches out like a rooted parasite through the tissues of life, and everything gets into a rather peculiar mess. When you narrow down your epistemology and act on the premise "what interests me is me, or my organization, or my species," you chop off consideration of other loops of the loop structure. You decide that you want to get rid of the by-products of human life and that Lake Erie will be a good place to put them. You forget that the eco-mental system called Lake Erie is a part of your wider eco-mental system and that if Lake Erie is driven insane, its insanity is incorporated in the larger system of your thought and experience.

You and I are so deeply acculturated to the idea of self and organization and species that it is hard to believe that man might view his relations with the environment in any other way than the way which I have rather unfairly blamed upon the nineteenth-century evolutionists. So I must say a few words about the history of all this.

Anthropologically, it would seem, from what we know of the early material, that man in society took clues from the natural world around him and applied those clues in a sort of metaphoric way to the society in which he lived. That is, he identified with or empathized the natural world around him and took that empathy as a guide for his own social organization and his own theories of his own psychology. This was what is called "totemism." In a way, it was all nonsense, but it made more sense than most of what we do today. The natural world around us really has this general systemic structure and, therefore, is an appropriate source of metaphor to enable man to understand himself in his social organization.

The next step, seemingly, was to reverse the process and for man to take clues from himself and apply these to the natural world around him. This was "animism," extending the notion of personality or mind to mountains, rivers, forests, and such things. This was not a bad idea in many ways, but the next step was to separate the notion of mind from the natural world, and then you got the notion of gods. When you separate mind from the structure in which it is immanent, such as human relations, the human society, or the eco-system, you thereby embark, I believe, on fundamental error which in the end will surely hurt you.

Struggle may be good for your soul up to the moment when it becomes easy to win the battle. When you have an effective enough technology so that you can really act upon your epistemological errors and can create havoc in the world in which you live, then the error is lethal. Epistemological error is all right, it's fine, up to the point at which you create around yourself a universe in which that error becomes immanent in monstrous changes of the universe that you have created and in which you now try to live.

We're not talking about the dear old Supreme Mind of Aristotle, St. Thomas Aquinas, and so on down through ages—the Supreme Mind which was incapable of error and incapable of insanity. We're talking about immanent mind which is only too capable of insanity, as you all professionally know. This is precisely why you're here. These circuits and balances of nature can only too easily get out of kilter, and they inevitably get out of kilter when certain basic errors of our thought become reinforced by thousands of cultural details.

I don't know how many people today really believe that there is an overall mind separate from the body, separate from the society, and separate from nature. But for those of you who would say that that is all superstition, I am prepared to wager that I can demonstrate with them in a few minutes that the habits and ways of thinking that went with those superstitions are still in their heads and still determine a large part of their thoughts. The idea that you can see me still governs your thought and action in spite of the fact you may know intellectually that it is not so. In the same way, we are most of us governed by epistemologies that we know to be wrong. Let us consider some of the implications of what I have been saying.

Let us look at how the basic notions are reinforced and expressed in all sorts of detail of how we behave. The very fact that I am monologuing to you—this is a norm of our academic subculture, but the idea that I can teach you, unilaterally, is derivative from the premise that the mind controls the body. Whenever a psychotherapist lapses into unilateral therapy, he is obeying the same premise. I, in fact, standing up in front of you, am performing a subversive act by reinforcing in your minds a piece of thinking which is really nonsense. We all do it all the time, because it's built into the detail of our behavior. Notice how I stand, while you sit.

The same thinking leads, of course, to theories of control and to theories of power. In that universe, if you do not get what you want you will blame somebody and establish either a jail or a mental hospital, according to taste, and you will pop them in it, if you can identify them. If you cannot identify them, you will say, "it's the system." This is roughly where our kids are nowadays in blaming the establishment, but you know the establishments aren't to blame. They are part of the same error, too.

Then, of course, there is the question of weapons. If you believe in that unilateral world, and you think that the other people believe in that world (and you're probably right; they do), then, of course, the thing is to get weapons, hit them hard, and control them.

They say that power corrupts, but this, I suspect, is nonsense. What is true is that the idea of power corrupts. Power corrupts most rapidly those who believe in it, and it is they who will want it most. Obviously, our democratic system tends to give power to those who hunger for it and gives every opportunity to those who don't want power to avoid getting it. This is not a very satisfactory arrangement, if power corrupts those who believe in it and want it.

Perhaps there is no such thing as unilateral power. After all, the man in power depends on receiving information all the time from outside. He responds to that information just as much as he causes things to happen. It is not possible for Goebbels to control the public opinion of Germany, because, in order to do so, he must have spies or legmen or public opinion polls to tell him what the Germans are thinking. He must then trim what he says to this information, and then again find out how they are responding. It is an interaction, and not a lineal situation.

But the myth of power is, of course, a very powerful myth and probably most people in this world more or less believe in it. It is a myth which, if everybody believes in it, becomes to that extent self-validating. But it is still epistemological lunacy and leads inevitably to various sorts of disaster.

Last, there is the question of urgency. It is clear, now, to many people that there are many catastrophic dangers which have grown out of the Occidental errors of epistemology. These range from insecticides, to pollution, to atomic fallout, to the possibility of melting the Antarctic ice cap. Above all, our fantastic compulsion to save individual lives has created the possibility of world famine in the immediate future.

Perhaps, we have an even chance of getting through the next twenty years with no disaster more serious than the mere destruction of a nation or group of nations.

I believe that this massive aggregation of threats to man and his ecological systems arises out of errors in our habits of thought at deep and partly unconscious levels.

As therapists, clearly we have a duty. First, we must achieve clarity in ourselves and then look for every sign of clarity in others, implement it, and reinforce them in whatever is sane in them.

There are patches of sanity still surviving in the world. Much of Oriental philosophy is more sane than anything the West has produced, and some of the inarticulate efforts of our own young people are more sane than the conventions of the establishment.

ACKNOWLEDGMENT

Prepared under Career Development Award (K2–21, 931) of the National Institute of Mental Health. This paper is Contribution No. 64 of the Oceanic Institute, Hawaii.

25. Group Perceptions and Group Relations

JEROME D. FRANK, M.D.

Department of Psychiatry and Behavioral Sciences
Johns Hopkins University
Baltimore, Maryland

STUDENTS OF CULTURE have long concerned themselves with how members of different groups and societies perceive themselves and each other, and they have amply documented the universality of ethnocentrism—that is, the overvaluation of one's own group and the derogation of members of other groups. Ethnocentrism has been a potent source of violent group conflict throughout the ages. Today, many forces converge to increase occasions for such conflict, and the means available to the combatants for inflicting damage on each other have become vastly more lethal than ever before. This combination creates an actual danger to survival for the first time in history.

The speed and unevenness of change in conditions of life has heightened tensions between nations, ethnic groups, social classes, and generations. These tensions have been aggravated by enormous increases in the volume of electronic communication, other forms of mass communication, and in mass transportation. These increases in volume have caused groups to impinge on each other, symbolically or physically, before they are psychologically ready. Finally, the rapidity of change has weakened the social controls, political structures, and value systems that, in the past, held conflicts resulting from intergroup tensions within bounds.

Not only have occasions for conflict multiplied, but warring groups have biological, chemical, and nuclear weapons at their disposal whose lethal power defies imagination. One depot of nerve gas is estimated to contain sufficient lethal doses for thirty times the world's population. Botulinus toxin, fatal in doses of millionths of a gram, has been stockpiled by the gallon, and as everyone knows, the destructive potential of nuclear weapons is limitless. Hence, human survival depends not only on overcoming the propensity to resort to violence to settle group conflicts, but also on learning to replace ethnocentrism with mutual appreciation between members of different groups. The purpose of this presentation is to stimulate your thinking about the second aim by reviewing a few of the psychosocial determinants of group hostility and amity.

The main theme I wish to develop is that group members' perceptions of themselves and of members of other groups depend primarily on the relation between the groups. To be sure, individual characteristics of group members make a difference. It appears, for example, that ethnocentrism characterizes persons who reveal themselves to be authoritarian on certain psychological tests (Frank, 1967, 121–24). However, by and large, the relations between the groups are the overriding determinant of their mutual images. This has been neatly illustrated by the findings of repeated surveys of Americans concerning their characterizations of people of other countries. In 1942 and again in 1966, respondents were asked to choose from a list of adjectives those that best described the people of Russia, Germany, and Japan. In 1942 the first five adjectives chosen to characterize both Germans and Japanese, our enemies, included warlike, treacherous, and cruel, none of which appeared among the first five describing the Russians, our allies. In 1966, all three had disappeared from American characterizations of the Germans and Japanese who had become allies. But now the Russians, no longer allies, although more rivals than enemies, were described as warlike and treacherous. Data were reported for the mainland Chinese in 1966, and predictably, they were seen as warlike, treacherous, and sly (The Gallup Poll, 1966). The adjectives applied to the Japanese and Germans as wartime enemies no doubt accurately described their behavior, as they do for all nations at war including the United States. It is noteworthy that Americans did not apply these adjectives to the Russians when they were allies. The Germans undoubtedly saw the Russians, their enemies, as warlike and treacherous. Americans now use these terms for the Russians and the Chinese, although there is no direct evidence that they apply. The Russians have been talking and acting with great restraint, and Chinese bellicosity is restricted to words; neither nation has shown any particular signs of treachery, unless one so views the Russian invasion of Czechoslovakia, but the same may be said of the United States' invasion of the Dominican Republic.

Groups become enemies when each perceives its goal as obtainable only at the other's expense. I should like to consider now some of the effects of this type of group relation on inter-group perception when the groups are classed as superior and inferior ones in the same society, and when they are roughly equal, as often occurs on the international scene. The superior-inferior relation occurs among classes or castes within societies, among subject peoples and their conquerors, and in a sense, between the under-developed and industrialized nations, although the limitation of face-to-face contact here may alter the situation significantly. Of course, groups in a superior and subordinate position are not automatically in conflict. Enmity arises only when the superior oppresses the subordinate one by preventing it from achieving its aspirations. My examples of how this situation affects inter-group perception come entirely from Negro-white relations in the United States, since these are the only ones with which I am familiar.

With respect to the whites, until recently the two outstanding features were relative blindness to the resentment, distrust, and general hostility felt by the Negroes, and the attribution of personal characteristics that the whites, themselves, wished to disown. The blindness of the whites was exposed when Negroes suddenly found the courage to speak up and tell it like it is. One example, brought to light in interracial group meetings at the Johns Hopkins Hospital, may suffice. White wives of physicians who work as volunteers in the clinics are unaware that they are deeply resented, by both Negro patients and Negro hospital employees, because the Negroes sense the patronizing attitude underneath their courtesy. As evidence of the whites' underlying contempt, Negroes seized on the fact that they questioned Negro adolescent girls about their sex practices and tried to convince them to use contraceptives in the hearing of other patients and the staff. The attitude implied by this behavior is that all Negro girls are promiscuous and have no shame or reticence about their sexual behavior.

It is easy to see why the whites have been blind. First of all, it is much more comfortable not to know how the oppressed group really feels, especially since there is no need to do so. Until recently the power relation between whites and Negroes was so unequal that regardless of how the Negro felt, he had to submit and pretend to be content. Apparently members of subordinate groups through the ages have developed sly ways of expressing their real feelings which are understood by each other but which the superior group does not catch. Negro spirituals are said to be full of such allusions, as in the line "everybody talk about heaven ain't a-going there." Similarly, the famous "Go down Moses" apparently became a way of signaling under-ground railroad routes for spiriting slaves out of the South.

The whites see themselves, by and large, as generally benevolent and well disposed toward the Negro. They point out frequently, and they exaggerate, how much they have done for Negroes, and they fail to recognize that the offer of aid on one's own terms is humiliating to the recipient and, therefore, characteristically elicits resentment rather than gratitude. Whites also ignore the amount of violence they have inflicted on Negroes, because this is mainly done by agents of the law under the guise of preserving law and order. Thus, when Negroes display their resentment openly, the whites overact because it challenges their image of themselves as benevolent and suggests that the Negro, besides all his other evil traits, is ungrateful. The recent urban riots in the United States caused a great outcry against Negro violence. In actuality, the violence of Negroes against whites was almost entirely directed against property and was infinitesimal compared with the three centuries of violence of whites against Negroes which was directed at their persons.

One function of the attribution to the members of the oppressed group of the characteristics that the superior person wants to disown in himself is, of course, to justify his oppressive behavior, but it has disquieting consequences. One consequence is the arousal of a latent fear of what the oppressed might do should they gain power, since they are seen as violent, sexually aggressive, and generally bestial. As a result, the superior group characteristically overreacts savagely to any overt expression of hostility or even to strivings to break out of their place by members of the oppressed group.

In turning to the perceptions of the subordinate group, my experience is confined to the American Negro, and even this is very sketchy. The Negro is peculiar in that he has been cut off from his own culture for several generations and has been totally dependent on the white group for his welfare. To what extent observations about him would apply, for example, to lower and upper caste Hindus or to the attitudes of Indians or Chinese toward the whites when the latter controlled their nations, I would have to leave to others to determine. In any case, the perception that the Negro has of the white man is rapidly changing and varies sharply among Negroes. Negroes share many of the values and attitudes of the whites, especially since they have no culture of their own on which to fall back. This leads to the well-known phenomenon of self-hatred, in which the prestige in the Negro community went to those who looked and acted most like whites, and they, in turn, tried to divorce themselves from Negroes who came closest to the negative stereotype that the whites had of them. This phenomenon has, of course, been observed with many minority groups. On the other hand, the Negro fears and resents the white man, and although he often has good reason for these feelings, they lead him sometimes to interpret behavior which is merely thoughtless as based on evil intent. Much of what Negroes now attribute to racism is a product of heedlessness rather than maliciousness. In a harassed out-patient department of a teaching hospital, for example, the personnel, regardless of their racial attitudes, are likely to be short-tempered with everyone, regardless of their race. Negro patients tend to interpret this attitude toward them as a sign of racism even when it is not.

The most striking feature of mutual images of antagonistic groups that are not also mutually dependent, such as enemy nations, is that they are, to a large extent, mirror images of each other as has been pointed out by many observers. This point may be illustrated by the findings of a quantitative study that compared Russian and American views of themselves and each other as revealed by statements in some of their mass media and elite publications. Each nation's media portray the other as aggressive and treacherous. Thus, 63 percent of the American and 88 percent of the Soviet items, attribute war to one state's aggressiveness, and virtually 100 percent of those in both countries describe the other's national goal as domination or expansion and its military doctrine as including a pre-emptive or preventive strike.

Each nation sees its own motives for offering foreign aid as altruistic, but the other's as in the service of expansion, and both nation's media are in virtually unanimous agreement that the other offers foreign aid not to help the recipients but to strengthen its own position and weaken the opponent's (Angell, Dunham, and Singer, 1964).

The enemy image creates and is reinforced by what has been called the double standard of political morality; that is, the same behavior is seen as in the service of good motives if performed by our side and bad if performed by an enemy. This is well illustrated by a study conducted in 1965 in which a large number of college freshmen were presented with 50 statements concerning belligerent and conciliatory actions that had been taken by both the United States and Russia. Half the students attributed the acts to the United States; the other half attributed the acts to the Soviet Union. As might be expected, an action was scored more favorably when attributed to the United States than when attributed to Russia. To cite two examples, on a 6-point scale, the average score for "The U.S. (Russia) has established rocket bases close to the borders of Russia (the U.S.)" was 4.7 for the United States version and 0.5 for the Russian version. "The U.S. (Russia) has stated that it was compelled to resume nuclear testing by the action of Russia (the U.S.)" was scored 4.2 in the United States form and 1.0 in the Russian form (Oskamp, 1965).

As Konrad Lorenz has persuasively maintained, humans are the only predators that lack inhibitions against killing their own kind (Lorenz, 1966). There are undoubtedly many reasons for this characteristic which today threatens race suicide, but important among them is that feature of the enemy image termed dehumanization. Enemies feel free to slaughter each other without restraint because, in some sense, they regard each other as no longer being members of the human race. This is facilitated by the development of methods of mass killing at a distance which reduce the enemy to faceless numbers. Enemies have slaughtered each other in face-to-face combat since time immemorial, so other sources of dehumanization must be involved. An especially powerful one is the adherence of the enemy to an antipathetical ideology, especially one which claims exclusive possession of the truth and, therefore, views other ideologies as intolerable threats.

Ideological components of conflict remove constraints on violence for two reasons. In contrast to fights over tangible goods like land or resources which end when the aim is achieved, ideological struggles have no natural end. A fight over property stops when one side has firmly secured it, but an idea ceases to be a danger only with the death of the last survivor who holds it, and even then it may crop up again. Hence, religious wars tend to be especially bitter, stopping only when both sides are exhausted with the survivors still clinging to their beliefs. Furthermore, ideologies, by giving meaning to existence, are often more important sources of psychological security than possessions. For many humans, the loss of their ideology may be worse than biological death so they prefer to die. The enemy who holds an antipathetical ideology is no longer a human but the embodiment of a hated abstraction, such as Communism, Imperialism, Islam, and the like. As a believer in false gods, he partakes of the demonic and so must be destroyed. Once enemies are at war, they further dehumanize each other by perceiving each other as bestial on the grounds that they commit atrocities. Whether or not a method of killing is viewed as an atrocity depends on whether it is considered legitimate, not on the amount of pain or suffering it inflicts. Who can say whether it hurts more to be disemboweled or to be roasted to death by napalm? Yet in war, each side continually invokes the atrocities of the other to arouse martial spirit and increase mutual hatred.

In short, the propensity of humans to form unfavorable images of members of groups other than their own is enhanced when the groups are in competition. These mutual negative images easily progress to the creation of the stereotype of the enemy. Since this stereotype includes the perception of the enemy as a demon or beast rather than a fellow human, it weakens whatever restraints humans may have against killing their own kind. Today, this represents a serious threat to the survival of our species. To overcome this danger permanently requires the creation of new international military, political, and legal institutions for handling international conflicts, analogous to those that preserve the peace within societies. The devising of such institutions is beyond our area of competence, but as students of human behavior we can contribute to the development of a sense of community among the world's peoples on which the viability of such institutions must depend.

The goal of achieving the brotherhood of man is probably as old as humanity itself, but until our generation, it was hopelessly Utopian. Today, for the first time, startling advances in mass communication, transportation, and in science and technology have brought it within the range of possibility by creating new, powerful means for combating enthnocentrism. Technical advances are, of course, only tools, and their effects depend on how they are used. International telecommunications and travel may well exacerbate tensions if they cause groups that are in a competitive posture to impinge on each other. Some of the unrest in the world today is undoubtedly caused by the transistor radio and television which, for the first time, have made the poor of many nations directly aware of the discrepancy between their standard of living and that of the rich, thereby intensifying their resentments. Similarly, mass media fanned urban riots in the United States and intensified racial antagonisms, because the whites were shocked by seeing the Negroes' behavior, and the Negroes were stimulated to emulate those who were already rioting. But in the long run, international mass communication media will promote international understanding simply by supplying an increasing volume of information. Given free access to information about another group, normal curiosity will impel people to try to learn more, and the more they learn, the harder it will be to maintain mutual hatred based on partial or distorted views. Experiences of each other at work and play rather than only as participants in formal or staged activities, such as political rallies or military parades, help especially to substitute favorable for unfavorable stereotypes.

One sign that a genuine group exists is the emergence of public opinion, that is, opinions held in common by many of a group's members. There are growing signs that mass media are developing a world public opinion which already may be exerting constraints on the actions of national leaders. The Soviet Union's greater restraint in its invasion of Czechoslovakia, as compared to its actions in Hungary a decade ago, strongly suggests that the outraged opinion of other nations, and of Communist parties in these nations, exerted a constraining effect. As a recent report of a Congressional subcommittee on international organizations and movements says, "Few things are undertaken in today's world without regard for the opinions of mankind." (Congressional Subcommittee on International Organization and Movements, 1968).

The facilitation of international person exchanges through mass travel can also cause more harm than good if improperly managed. When persons with different cultural backgrounds meet, opportunities for misunderstandings, embarrassment, and humiliation are legion. Social scientists are gradually delineating the conditions that maximize the chances that these contacts will lead to increased rather than decreased mutual understanding and respect. Studies of student exchanges, for example, have suggested that to produce more than fleeting changes in attitude, visits should be long and should include as numerous and varied experiences as possible with people in the host country and should be rewarding for both host and guests. Visitors want to be treated as individuals rather than as members of a category, and this can be done very effectively by involving them in some ongoing enterprise. Some studies have revealed change in attitudes six months after the visitors have returned home, suggesting that well managed, extensive, and massive visiting programs could help to promote world-mindedness and break down negative international stereotypes (Frank, 1967, 238–45).

Since the way members of each group perceive each other, however, depends primarily on relations between them, main hope must be placed on extensive exploitation of the new opportunities for international scientific cooperation. Of these, the most spectacular is, of course, the exploration of outer space. Although primarily competitive, it represents a kind of middle ground in that a gain for either Russia or the United States is potentially a gain for the other as well. This is in sharp contrast to the Middle East, Vietnam, and other areas of competition in which a success for one nation is a defeat for the other. Evidence that the exploration of space is in some sense a joint enterprise is that both nations mourn when a spaceman of either nation is lost, and they can sincerely congratulate each other on new space triumphs which would be inconceivable, for example, in the case of the construction of an improved missile. The space exploits of Russians and Americans, furthermore, inspire mutual respect for such characteristics as courage, adventurousness, and other virtues that do not necessarily imply militancy or hostility, thereby helping to counteract unfavorable aspects of their images of each other. Actually, the space race is a venture of all humanity. The cosmonauts and astronauts capture the imagination of all peoples, and all humanity derives a sense of success from their achievements.

Potentially the most powerful means, however, of increasing the sense of world community lies in collaborative efforts by nations to achieve goals that all seek but none can achieve alone; that is, goals that can be attained only by cooperation. The effectiveness of such goals in breaking down mutual hostility was elegantly demonstrated by an experiment conducted in a boys' camp some years ago. In this experiment, boys who were initially strangers to each other were formed into two groups. Then, the groups were made enemies through athletic competitions. In time, they became like two hostile nations. The members of each group chose their friends only from their group, looked down on members of the other, and the two groups fought at every opportunity. Simply bringing the two groups together did nothing to reduce their mutual antagonism. However, when the camp director arranged matters so that both groups had to cooperate, mutual hostility rapidly diminished. For example, he secretly arranged for the camp water supply to be interrupted, and the whole camp had to get out and repair it. The truck carrying food for an overnight hike unaccountably ran into a ditch and stalled, and all the boys had to get on the tow rope to pull it out. It took a series of such events to break down the hostility between the groups, but friendly relations were eventually completely restored (Sherif, Harvey, White, Hood, and Sherif, 1961).

I would hestitate to generalize from eleven-year-old boys to nations in conflict were it not for certain obvious parallels. In a sense, the nations of the world today are in the same predicament as the boys in the camp. They will have to cooperate in order to survive so, at first glance, survival would seem to be the superordinate goal that would counteract international enmities. Unfortunately, however, under some circumstances, survival takes a backseat to the urge to destroy the enemy. Moreover, the long-term measures required for national survival, such as general disarmament, appear to increase the short-term risks of destruction by an enemy, so mobilizing the urge to survive works both ways. Modern science, however, has created many opportunities for cooperative activities among nations to attain goals that all of them want, but none can achieve alone. We know from the experience of one continuing, cooperative, international scientific project in the Antarctic that grew out of the International Geophysical Year that such activities foster habits and attitudes of cooperation which gradually become embodied in institutions. Scientists have devised dozens of such projects which can be activated as soon as the world's leaders are willing. One set, which cannot be launched too soon, lies in international measures to control the accelerating pollution of the biosphere which may prove to be a greater threat to the continuance of our species than war.

To conclude, if the passengers on our small overcrowded spaceship are not to destroy each other, they must learn to understand each other's point of view and to accept and live with their differences while searching for and exploiting shared beliefs and goals. As educators and researchers, we can promote these aims by continuing to study and analyze the effects of group perceptions and misconceptions on political decisions and the forces that combat ethnocentrism and promote a sense of community among the peoples of the world. We have the additional responsibility of striving to bring our findings to the attention of political leaders who, in the last analysis, are the only ones who can put them into practice. Time is very short and social scientists are not very influential, but we have made some headway, so there is reason to hope that our efforts, joined with those of lawyers, political scientists, and members of many other disciplines, may yet suffice to tip the balance toward survival.

REFERENCES

Angell, R. C., V. S. Dunham, and J. D. Singer. 1964. Social values and foreign policy attitudes of Soviet and American elites. Journal of Conflict Resolution 8:329–491.

Frank, J. D. 1967. Sanity and survival: psychological aspects of war and peace. New York, Random House.

Gallup Poll. "Image" of Red powers. *In* The Santa Barbara News-Press, June 26, 1966.

Lorenz, K. 1966. On aggression. New York, Harcourt, Brace & World.

Oskamp, S. 1965. Attitudes toward U.S. and Russian actions: a double standard. Psychological Reports 16:43–46.

Sherif, M. et al. 1961. Intergroup conflict and cooperation: the robbers' cave experiment. Norman, University of Oklahoma Book Exchange.

United States Congress, Subcommittee on International Organization and Movements. 1968. The future of United States public diplomacy: report no. 6 on winning the Cold War: the U.S. ideological offensive, p. 3R.

26. On Reason and Sanity: Political Dimensions of Psychiatric Thought

THOMAS J. SCHEFF, Ph.D.

Department of Sociology
University of California, Santa Barbara
Santa Barbara, California

ABOUT SEVENTY-FIVE YEARS AGO, a psychologist named Stratton conducted a series of excellent studies of the individual's perceptual world (Stratton, 1897). His procedure was unusual but simple; he designed a pair of prismatic spectacles which inverted his field of vision. He wore these glasses during all his waking hours for several periods of many weeks. One of his finds, as might be expected, was that the experience, at least initially, was almost totally disorienting. The inversion of up and down destroyed his customary world so that even the most trivial kind of activity, such as tying his shoelaces, was well nigh impossible.

It can be argued that the individual's experience is mediated by a whole series of absolute dimensions which give him a sense of continuity, mastery, and agency in his endeavors. Some of the dimensions are physical such as up and down, left and right, the geographic sense of location in space, the temporal or historic sense of location in time (with respect to a calendar, say). Some of these axes are not physical but social and/or psychological. In a racist society, for example, the axis of racial separation is probably one such absolute dimension. Any perturbation along this axis is perceived by the members of the society as a cataclysmic dislocation with the concommitant feelings of vertigo, nausea, and paralysis. The worth and value of a white man, his sense of self-esteem, for example, is constantly witnessed and affirmed by his sense of the inferiority of the black. The racial axis allows him constantly and continuously to locate himself, not in physical time and space but in social time and in moral space.

In an experiment somewhat analogous to Stratton's, a white man, Griffin, changed the color of his skin and became a Negro (Griffin, 1960). Like Stratton, he experienced almost total disorientation. An interesting difference between the two studies, however, was that Griffin's experience proved to be irreversible. He was thrown out of orbit, so to speak. When Stratton took off the glasses, he returned to his customary place in his society, an ordinary man among men. But Griffin's experiment so perturbed his position in the society that he found himself unable to return to his customary place.

In modern mass societies, there are probably many other important absolute axes such as nationality and ideology. In the United States, particularly, the capitalist-communist axis and the closely related axis of patriotism which separates Americans from aliens probably operate in a way similar to the racial axis discussed above. All three of these axes are similar psychologically in that they identify an ingroup, the white American free enterprise population, at the expense of outgroups, the blacks, the communists, and the aliens.

There is another more subtle axis of contemporary experience which, because it is more pervasive, is even more important than those already mentioned. This is the axis of reason and unreason, rationality and irrationality, or, most relevant to our discussion here, the closely related axis of sanity and insanity which, in its most contemporary guise, is the axis of mental health and mental illness. In this paper, I wish to make two points. First, the dimension of mental health and mental illness is not an absolute fact of nature like the physical directions of up and down but a moral axis like the social separation of whites and blacks. Secondly, the confusion of the absolute and social bases of the distinction between sanity and insanity has political consequences. I will first discuss the cultural arbitrariness of contemporary concepts of sanity and insanity.

Although most researchers in the area of mental illness speak with assurance about diagnostic entities such as schizophrenia, the scientific basis for these classifications remains obscure at best. For the major mental illness classifications, none of the components of the medical model have been demonstrated: cause, lesion, uniform and invariate symptoms, course, and treatment of choice (Scheff, 1966). Studies of the reliability of psychiatric diagnosis show the levels to be abysmally low. Even at the theoretical level, there is little consensus about the nature of these diseases. The two most flagrant examples are the concepts of schizophrenia and sociopathy.

In the areas of positive mental health, the confusion is even more apparent. In a recent review of concepts of mental health, Jahoda found six competing concepts: (1) mastery of the environment, (2) self-actualization,

(3) self-esteem, (4) integration of self, (5) autonomy, and (6) adequacy of perception of reality (Jahoda, 1958).

The prospect of choosing between these six different criteria, as advanced by different experts, is disquieting enough. When one notes that some of the criteria may be contradictory (for example, mastery of the environment as against self-actualization and perception of reality as against autonomy) and that none have been operationally defined or investigated, one begins to perceive the state of chaos which characterizes the concept from a scientific point of view. It would appear that mental health is not a physical fact, but a value choice about what kind of men we should be and what kinds of values should be encouraged in our society. Whether one selects a notion like aggressive mastery of the environment, traditionally a Western ideal, or the more inward turning goal like self-actualization, more akin to traditional ideals in the Orient, is not dictated by the natural order of stably reoccurring regularities in nature but by human choice.

Just as mental health may be seen as a value choice as to how men should behave, so the symptoms of mental illness can be seen as value choices of how men should not behave. Thought and behavior that are taken to be correct in each culture are so taken for granted that the assumptions of propriety are largely invisible to its members. If one goes to the local cafeteria and butts in at the head of the line, there would be a reaction from those standing in line. If the intruder asked what the trouble was, he would be told, "First come, first served," or some such explanation. Suppose however, he continued in line and decided not to carry his own tray for his food but placed his food on the tray of the stranger behind him. He might be told that in this cafeteria, one carries one's own tray. More likely, the others in the line would feel that everybody knows that and would eye him with suspicion and alarm. Continuing the example, suppose that after sitting down with the stranger, the intruder notices some food on the other's plate that looks particularly tempting. He reaches across the table and spears some of the food with his fork. This action, although it is no more than the violation of custom, would probably place the offender beyond the pale. There are literally myriads of customs associated with each culture that go without saying to the point that violations leave the conforming members of the society baffled. His society has not prepared him for violations; they exist outside his vocabulary of motives. In speaking even simple sentences, there are thousands of understandings about proper grammar, syntax, pitch, loudness, rhythm, gesture, etc., that are part of any living language. The most elementary conversation is embedded in a whole network of under-standings about comportment. For example, there is a conversational distance, neither too far nor too close. When one speaks, one looks in certain directions: at the hearer's eyes or mouth but not at his ear or forehead. Breaking so simple a custom results in the most violent kind of reaction. If one looks at another's ear, for example, during the conversation, the other will try to save the situation by moving his eyes into your line of vision. If you persist in looking at his ear, you can get him to move around in a full circle. The result of shifting one's line of vision from the eyes to an ear, merely an angle of a few degrees, is enormous: the transaction is completely disrupted.

Although the reaction to the violation of customs such as the ones discussed here is violent and complete, it must be remembered that these customs are largely conventions in a particular culture and, as such, are, for the most part, arbitrary and subject to change and transformation. They are not absolute, sacred, or immutable.

Let us now turn to the so-called mental illnesses such as schizophrenia. There are two major issues here. The first deals with the question of the existence of a behavioral system, an entity that is referred to as schizophrenia. As indicated above, the scientific basis for this label is somewhat cloudy, i.e., there has been no demonstration beyond a reasonable doubt that there is a pattern of behavior which has a known cause, a lesion, uniform and invariate symptoms, a course, and a treatment of choice. The second point is independent, to some degree, of the first. Even if it were granted that there were such a system, would it necessarily follow that the energies of reasonable men be directed toward finding, analyzing, and changing such behavior? According to the concept of schizophrenia held by some psychiatrists, the attributes of schizophrenia are withdrawal, flatness of affect, thought disorder, language aberrations, and hallucinations or delusions. The schizophrenic is pictured, therefore, as a passive, inward-dwelling, remote person who lacks interpersonal and other competences that other members of the society see as necessary to maintain or improve one's status in society.

Although these symptoms are stated in such a way as to suggest that they are in some way deviations from absolute and immutable standards, this is not necessarily the case. Withdrawal may be considered to be a violation of customary expectations about the degree of social and interpersonal distance that are held in the society, flatness of affect, a violation of expectations about expressive gestures. The language aberrations can obviously be seen as transgressions, not against the rules of nature but of language which are, of course, arbitrary. What about thought disorder, and hallucinations and delusions? It has already been suggested that there are culturally derived rules about propriety. Similarly, it is suggested there are culture-bound rules about thought and about reality. To illustrate rules about reality, consider the effort Western parents go through to convince their children that dreams and nightmares are not real but that disease germs are real. The child has seen and experienced nightmares and has never seen germs. After some struggle, the parents convince him. But in some traditional societies, the scheme is reversed; the dreams are real, and the germs are not.

Not only are the expectations which lead to the absolute rejection of schizophrenic symptoms arbitrary, but it may be argued that the evaluation of conventional sanity as desirable and mental disease, e.g., schizophrenia, as undesirable should be reversed. According to the conventional picture of schizophrenics, they would not have the competence or the motivation to napalm civilians, defoliate forests and rice crops and to push the button that would destroy much of the world that we know. These activities are carried out by persons sane by conventional definition and encouraged, or at least not discouraged, by the great majority of the sane people in the society.

Perhaps my point can be illustrated by the recent episode concerning the mental status of Richard Nixon. There was a flurry of public interest when a columnist disclosed that Nixon had consulted a psychiatrist at one point in his career. Unfortunately, the conventional definitions of sanity and insanity that are used today give Nixon, Johnson, Humphrey, and John Kennedy a clean bill of health. These definitions, rather, are used to mobilize society to want to change the behavior of schizophrenics and other relatively inoffensive persons.

I am not suggesting that the President of the United States is insane but that the contemporary vision of reason and sanity is arbitrary and distorted and, further, that the distortion is given support and substance by the inadvertant assistance of practitioners and researchers in the field of mental health. To the extent that these workers argue and act as if mental illness is largely a technical, scientific issue rather than an area that is almost completely governed by moral values, they are functioning as accomplices in the current moral status quo. It is always tempting for the scientist to take the easiest way, to treat his job as exclusively concerned with means rather than ends. This bureaucratization of science demeans the scientist to a mere technician and induces him to avoid his responsibilities as an intellectual and citizen.

> To become worthy of his power the scientist will need to develop enough wisdom and humane understanding to recognize that the acquisition of knowledge is intricately interwoven with the pursuit of goals. It has often been pointed out that the nineteenth century slogan, "Survival of the fittest," begged the question because it did not state what fitness was for. Likewise it is not possible to plan man's future without deciding beforehand what he should be fitted for, in other words, what human destiny ought to be—a decision loaded with ethical values. What is new is not necessarily good, and all changes, even those apparently the most desirable, are always fraught with unpredictable consequences. The scientist must beware of having to admit, like Captain Ahab in Melville's *Moby Dick,* "All my means are sane; my motives and objects mad." (Dubois, 1959).

I am not suggesting that psychiatrists and other workers in the field of mental illness are more at fault than the rest of the society. As it becomes increasingly clear that the United States is committed to overt imperial dominion in Asia and covert counterrevolutionary terror in the rest of the world, virtually all of the segments of American society fall into place either by acts of commission or omission (Houghton, 1968). What Conor Cruise O'Brien has called the "counterrevolutionary subordination" of science and scholarship has been proceeding apace for the last twenty years. Many social scientists are directly involved in planning brutal and inhuman procedures to be used by the military, for example, the "population influence and control" programs in Vietnam. Other scholars, though not directly involved, approve and assent to the steps taken. Still others, and this includes most of the brightest scholars, conduct their work in such a way that objective scholarship is suborned to the interests of American power (Chomsky, 1969).

What I am suggesting is that researchers in the field of mental illness, to the extent that they follow contemporary social definitions of sanity and insanity, reason and unreason, without question or investigation, are helping to further confound the moral issues by giving laymen the impression, however subtly or unintentionally, that there is absolute scientific justification for the prevailing American world view. It is our responsibility as scholars and students of human behavior to make the hidden moral values in psychiatry and mental health visible so that they can be made the subject of research and open public discussion. Only in this way will we have borne witness as scientists and scholars by contributing our knowledge of human affairs to the area of politics. With patience and ingenuity, it should be possible to make the invisible visible. We have the example of Stratton and Griffin before us. Goffman, in *Asylums,* has suggested one avenue for exploration. The enterprise I have in mind is not a small one: to explore and help recreate current concepts, first, of sanity and, more broadly, of reason and rationality.

REFERENCES

Chomsky, N. 1969. American power and the new mandarins. New York, Pantheon.
Dubois, R. 1959. Mirage of health: utopias, progress, and biological change. New York, Harper.
Goffman, E. 1961. Asylums. Garden City, N.Y., Doubleday & Company.
Griffin, J. H. 1960. Black like me. New York, Signet.
Houghton, N. D., ed. 1968. Struggle against history: U.S. foreign policy in an age of revolution. New York, Simon and Schuster.
Jahoda, M. 1958. Current concepts of positive mental health. New York, Basic Books.
Scheff, T. J. 1966. Being mentally ill. Chicago, Aldine Publishing Co.

Stratton, G. M. 1897. Some preliminary experiments on vision without inversion of the retinal image. Psychological Review 3:611–17.
———. 1897. Vision without inversion of the retinal image. Psychological Review 4:463–81.

27. Reflections of a Tender-Minded Radical

ALEXANDER H. LEIGHTON, M.D.

Department of Behavioral Sciences
Harvard School of Public Health
Boston, Massachusetts

MY SENSE of gratitude for the opportunity to attend this meeting, great at the start, has grown enormously during the course of the week. It could hardly be otherwise given the quality and significance of papers and discussion, and yet there has been a disadvantage for me: the corresponding increase in my anxiety at having to fill this terminal spot. I have organized my presentation by headings which may not be self-evidently logical, but, on the other hand, they may serve to highlight some of the areas stressed during this conference.

Overviews of Mankind—Moral Issues and Mind Stretching

I should like to begin with a word of full appreciation to Drs. Frank, Bateson, and Scheff for the wide horizons and compelling ideas they have put before us. Several of the people here from Asian cultures expressed pleasure in seeing that Americans were capable of something more than science and pragmatism. Dr. Lapuz murmured that perhaps the American conscience is stirring.

Such remarks rest on the view that an abiding contrast between Asian and American cultures is the presence of deep moral and philosophical concern in the former and its comparative absence in the latter. This is possibly a true generalization, but the points of exception should not be overlooked. Surely there is much common ground for East and West in the ideas of such men as Thomas Paine, Jefferson, Lincoln, Herman Melville, and Henry David Thoreau. Was not Thoreau, in fact, an influence on Gandhi—especially with regard to his ideas of civil disobedience?

Certainly, we all have to agree that values and moral issues are root matters in human behavior and that the function of science, when not heuristic, is to provide ways and means toward fulfillment. This is diagrammatically clear in medicine. Health and illness are value concepts which are not primarily scientific. People are opposed to being ill; scientific medicine's task is to clarify the nature of illness and discover methods of treatment and prevention.

The same relation to science holds when we replace the words "health" and "illness" with "happiness" and "suffering"—a matter that has been much to the fore in our discussions here. We have been especially concerned with the individual's right and freedom to find happiness how and as he chooses.

Now in this regard, an obvious but easily overlooked fact is that man is a social animal, and it readily happens that individual A's pursuit of happiness interferes with that of B and even C and D. In consequence, we have the social regulation of behavior which man has always imposed on himself and to which he has always objected. Much of history consists of struggle and vacillation between too much freedom and too little. For, if the members of a social system reach too great a degree of individual liberty, social chaos sets in, bringing about deterioration in the functional prerequisites of a society which in turn leads to formidable constraints on opportunity and open choice. The alternatives for the individual then become few and stark. The pursuit of freedom, therefore, is a relative matter, a question of the best possible within a set of contingencies.

If we look at justice instead of liberty, the inevitability of constraint is much less in evidence. No human being can ever be completely free, but there is nothing in the nature of things to prevent every man and every woman having equal access to justice. A task for the behavioral sciences, therefore, might well be to find how this can be effected, to discover means for giving everyone a fair share of choice and opportunity and for dealing reasonably with those who try to preempt someone else's margin of freedom.

The matter is urgent because of the rapidity with which the values of justice drop from sight in struggles for the reform of social systems. They become quickly overrun with battles for position and revenge. Bleeding hearts and wounds from knives in the back become hard to distinguish. As in the crusades of the Middle Ages, the fervor of ideals and rhetoric are high but so, too, is greed and the lust for attention, and the long range good is a matter of doubt.

The deterioration of values pertaining to justice during the process of social and cultural change is, if I may repeat, well worth serious scrutiny by the behavioral sciences. It is inherent in such problems as better treatment of the mentally ill, the elimination of poverty, and the eradication of discrimination based on skin color or religion. A critical matter is that despite the fact that virtually all social struggles begin with the aim of correcting injustice, they seem to carry the seeds of their own destruction. They rouse passions that seek shortcuts, and as these passions mount, the just perspective fades into a war among Titans, all equally unjust. If Hamlet will forgive, I would like to say that passion makes bigots of us all. This is surely one of the lessons to be learned from the French Revolution, the Civil War, the Congo, Nigeria and our campuses.

Scientific inquiry does not, of course, have to wait on such massive occurrences. It can start with more commonplace phenomena as, for example, the fact that prejudice and stereotypic thinking are able to grow to cancerous proportions in relatively small movements that have as their aim the correcting of these very barriers to justice. Such an approach would put emphasis on looking at the sentiments and behavior of the weak as well as the strong, the underdog as well as the top dog, those against as well as those for the system, those under 30 as well as those over.

These remarks draw inspiration from Gregory Bateson's impeachment of simplistic explanations. It is very easy to treat a part as the whole, especially when that part fits with one's feelings and the rest does not. It is easy to think that because a proposition has some truth in it, it is necessarily all true or that because a negation is in part correct, the totality is, therefore, contaminated and false. Occam's razor was corrective to the rococo elaborations of scholasticism, but it can be a knife that kills understanding of relations in living things. Life is complex at all its levels of integration from molecular to social, and the task of the behavioral sciences is to comprehend, not caricature.

The fact that we in the behavioral sciences are divided into disciplines presents us with some difficulties and some illustrations of points made above. Any explanation from the viewpoint of one discipline is bound to be incomplete and lacking in sophisticated complexity. It is also apt to be prejudiced and stereotypic and to have a high potential for arousing emotions. During the last twenty years, the Stirling County Study (A. H. Leighton, 1959; Hughes, 1960; D. C. Leighton, 1963) of psychiatric disorder and sociocultural environment has had, as project members, people from East, West, and Africa, and their religions have included Protestant, Catholic, Jewish, Buddhist, Moslem, and atheist. These ethnic and religious divisions have never provided any serious threat to the morale and working ability of the study. On the other hand, the divisions constituted by disciplines—psychiatry, psychology, sociology, anthropology, and statistics—these have been continually explosive, calling for unremitting effort to prevent disruption.

Surely, we can do better than to train students so that they go forth with discipline-centric banners streaming and stereotypic views of everyone else's field. When I was a physiologist, I never heard anything good about psychology. In medical school, I learned that social science was like "Holy Roman Empire," a name for something that never existed. In psychiatry, I discovered that many people held to a closed system of ideas that purported to explain the real meaning of all human motivation. Later, I found that some anthropologists worship at an exclusive shrine named "cultural" and that there are sociologists who appear to use role theory as a line with which to measure depth in all the seas.

Let me take the currently popular attacks on "the medical model" as a case in point (Brown and Long, 1968). What is called in question is the applying of a monocausal explanatory model based on infectious diseases to processes that do not have these kinds of components and relations. So far, so good, but one soon leaves the issue behind and comes on the exchange of polemics over entrenched positions. The fact that medicine has other explanatory models that it employs much more extensively nowadays is ignored by many people. The possibility that some of these might aid in understanding and training research workers regarding the interplay of social, psychological, and organic factors in the genesis of psychiatric disorders does not get a fair examination. With so many other valuable fish in the waters of the world, it is surely wasteful to spend time on red herrings.

Intradisciplinary stereotypes have other disadvantages. For example, by isolating a given discipline from knowledge available in other fields, such stereotypes foster extreme positions as I illustrated a moment ago with reference to psychiatry. A parallel is now looming up in regard to sick-role theory as applied to psychiatric disorders. Some of what I hear from protagonists of this viewpoint borders on magical thinking. The reasoning appears to go like this: step one is the recognition that there is the phenomenon of the sick role; step two asserts that in psychological disorders that role is paramount in determining the disorder; step three indicates that role definition and role labeling are part of the social system; step four proposes to abolish psychiatric disorder by altering the social system so as to abolish the sick roles.

Somewhere in this chain, the as yet unanswered question of the degree and way in which role definition determines illness-behavior disappears. With this goes the possibility of inquiring into how much variation there may be with different kinds of disorder patterns—senility, mental retardation, neuroses, psychophysiological disorder, schizophrenia, etc. Acuity of thinking retreats when the use of words becomes vague; it is as if the entire illness phenomenon were driven out into the role as into a surrounding shell, and when this is snatched away, behold: the illness is gone. One is reminded of an Eskimo Shaman brushing illness from the patient onto a dog and then destroying the dog.

It is highly probable, indeed virtually certain, that there is important truth in sick-role theory, but we need to give our attention to finding out how much truth, under what circumstances it is found, and whether the relation to chronicity is greater than to etiology. When bad generalizations in psychiatry are countered by overclaims from sociology, it is unlikely that the advance of knowledge is being favored.

Cultural relativity is another example that has come up a number of times in the course of our deliberations. The concept is, of course, derived from anthropology, and the aspect for attention here is the observation that a value or practice highly approved in one culture may be roundly condemned in another. Everyone can think of examples. From this the inference is made that contrary to European religious and humanistic traditions, there are no absolute values but rather all matters of choice are relative. The notion has spread far beyond anthropology and has been further elaborated to say that all values are a matter of personal choice. In this guise, cultural relativity is used to batter down standards, especially those of the middle class, and, also, to justify individual conduct, however idiosyncratic and at variance with the societal prerequisites for the survival of people. In the mental health field, this takes the form of claiming the right of individuals to have delusions and hallucinations, commit suicide or, like Diogenes, live in a kennel and adopt the habits of dogs. (This, as you well recall, is the origin of the word cynic.)

In saying all this, I am not arguing for or against the merits of any particular set of values but rather wish to point out that this use of cultural relativity constitutes an amputee and leaves out the rest of the anthropological original, namely, the answer to the question—relative to what?

The reply has to be in terms of another anthropological concept: each culture is a totality, a system upon which a given population is dependent for survival and the meeting of individual needs. The minimal statement about cultural relativity, therefore, is that each cultural pattern (including values) has functional significance relative to the total cultural system of which it is a part. It is the total context that explains why polygyny, cattle-stealing, or being an entrepreneur is acceptable here and unacceptable there. Anthropological observations do not encourage the view that it is feasible for individuals to make an eclectic compilation of values from around the world according to fancy or, contrariwise, to reject all values. The more plausible inference is that while cultural systems may vary from one to another—have different ground plans—no group of people can survive that does not have such a system, and there cannot be a cultural system without a component consisting in a network of values which serve to maintain and interrelate behaviors.

Cultural relativity, therefore, does not mean that values are a matter of free choice, but, on the contrary, that values are functionally relative to whole cultures and that this is a pragmatic relation, one that is often essential for human survival. Change is, of course, also functional, and the above remarks are not in defense of status quo but rather protest against willy nilly.

The nature of pathology is another topic with which we have dealt in the course of our deliberations. Because of different underlying assumptions, the discussants have sometimes appeared to be trying to reach each other by traveling in trains which approach but go by on different tracks. One of these tracks is concerned with an anatomical model; pathology is a lesion constituting a structural and visible block to proper functioning. As is obvious to everyone, this model in such a form is of use in psychiatric disorders only in cases of brain damage. By adding one word, however, and removing another, the model has been widely employed. The modified form runs something like this: pathology is an invisible lesion constituting a structural block to proper functioning. As is easily seen, this has much in common with the "medical model."

There are, however, a number of other ways of looking at the matter. One such takes its origin in a man who is often called the father of pathology which is to say he is credited with founding the discipline. The name is Rudolf Virchow, and his long life spanned the greater part of the nineteenth century. Virchow was explicit in some of his writings in saying that the essential in pathology is not mangled physical matter nor is it the presence of a foreign body. Rather, he said, pathology is a process, and it differs from a normal process only in "the character of danger" it implies for the survival of the organism. "It is," he said, "a question either of the obstruction of normal physiological processes, or the stimulation of the same in unusual locations or at unusual times." Nowadays, we would be inclined to express this in relational terms or in terms of general systems and field theory.

If we follow Virchow, psychiatric disorder can be viewed in terms of patterns of behaviors that weigh against survival for the individual who manifests them. Suffering for himself, damaging effects on other people, and lack of ability on the part of the individual to control his feelings and behavior are also to be considered as elements in various syndromes. The basic frame, however, is the element of danger resulting from a particular configuration of otherwise normal processes. Such perspective makes it possible to avoid fruitless arguments about what is normal, to avoid monocausal traps, and to proceed from definitions of specified behavior to the examination of the multiple processes involved in bringing them into existence. Further, it increases one's chance of distinguishing between issues which are concerned with understanding and altering phenomena (what causes condition X, and where can one intervene to prevent it occurring?) and issues which are jurisdictional (should the psychiatrist, the sociologist, or the psychologist be in charge of the action?). The problems of gaining knowledge and the problems of management are both easier to solve when they are conceptually distinct.

In harmony with Virchow's way of looking at pathology and with much that has been said at this meeting is the dawning of a focus in behavioral sciences which seems to me an advance in thinking, one that opens many roads for the development of theory and method relevant to all our disciplines. This is the notion that the behavioral pattern is the basic unit of study. In using this term, I am referring to the fact that nature—whether we are studying individuals or societies—presents us with behavior in packages. It always comes in patterns that have functional significance. This makes enough specification possible so that reliable results can be obtained by independent observers regardless of whether the investigation is experimental or observational. In the mental health field, there is the particular advantage of escape from building etiological assumptions into diagnostic entities. Questions of cause are opened for discussion rather than prematurely answered, and they are elicited in a way that makes it possible to take into account multiple etiologies.

Dr. Gallimore touched on this matter in referring to a rat pressing a bar. This is an example of an extremely simple behavior pattern. But even here we should not begin by asking why the rat presses the bar, much less by forming a hypothesis and trying to test it. On the contrary, there are many questions to be asked first. Does he press the bar? How often? What variations seem to occur spontaneously? Eventually we are in a position to introduce experimental variations, but this is with the full recognition that bar pushing can be the final common path for processes that have many different points of origin—physiological, psychological, and social. The explanatory system built up in this way is one which does not sacrifice understanding of nature for the sake of simplicity.

In the field of psychiatric disorder, in contrast to that of the behavioral studies of animals, we have the disadvantage that tradition is sometimes against us. The sheer complexity of phenomena is a problem, too, as is often asserted, but to my mind this complaint dodges a more fundamental issue which consists in a variety of etiological dogmas that color our views whether we look as psychiatrists, psychologists, sociologists, or anthropologists. As scientists, we can handle complexity and theories, but we cannot handle dogma.

Social and Cultural Studies

Under this heading, I should like to consider the reports by Drs. Dusit, Lebra, Higa, Dipojono, Caudill, Yeh, DeVos, Kim, and Triandis. These important contributions have in common their exemplification of what was said above about behavior patterns constituting a basic unit of study. It can be seen that this holds true whether a study is focused on the individual or on the actions and reactions of groups.

Starting from this basis, it is possible to discern a number of dimensions that are relevant to the problems of mental health and mental illness. One dimension is that of cultural contrast; one can compare, for example, behavior patterns that have to do with dependency and independency of individuals as seen in different cultural groups. Another dimension is that of cultural change with the double possibility of investigating the change of patterns within a given culture and, also, comparing two or more cultures.

Thirdly, one can focus on cross-cultural comparison in terms of patterns related to certain worldwide phenomena such as population increase, technological development, migration to urban centers, and wars.

A fourth dimension is the investigation of the emergence of new cultural patterns, those arising out of the present situation of flux. Dr. Lebra's presentation might be considered an example, and there are many others that could be cited. Noteworthy is the transworld pattern of youth protest and revolt. The posture of many older people today regarding youth is like that of the king who, when told that his subjects were revolting, replied, "I know, but I love them anyway."

One of the great but as yet insufficiently exploited approaches to cultural studies is that of systematic exchange of behavioral scientists between two cultures. That is to say, Japanese scientists might study U.S. culture while a parallel team from the United States makes a related study in Japan with appropriate sharing in both teams of theory and technique. Dr. Hahn touched on this when he pointed out that the response, "I feel like a million bucks," to the question, "How are you?" can make a person from an oriental culture feel put down. From the viewpoint of occidental culture, this is not the manifest intent, but rather the expression is used to share good feelings. Nevertheless, it is possible for an occidental to see the implications this might have for an oriental, and as he reflects further, he may well conclude that there is actually an element of competition and egocentric assertiveness in the remark.

I trust that Dr. Hahn will forgive me if I report a counterpart experience that happened to me in Japan. Over and over again people would greet me by saying, "You look tired." I knew perfectly well, intellectually, that this was a polite expression intended to convey sympathy. Nevertheless, it was impossible to quell altogether a reflex resentment at having weakness pointed out. I felt "one-upped," in spite of myself.

Ralph Linton in one of his seminars many years ago mentioned what he said was a Japanese anthropologist's account of "The American Cigar Ceremony." This interesting folk ritual, the Japanese said, was most often seen among businessmen. When two businessmen meet on the street, the first move after shaking hands is for each to put a hand into his upper left vest pocket, draw forth a cigar, and present it to the other gentleman. Both gentlemen take the offered cigar. The man of lower rank proceeds to bite his, light it, carefully thrust his thumbs into the armholes of his vest, hold his head back to a prescribed angle, and exhale smoke with a prolonged "Aah." The man of superior rank puts the cigar he has received into the upper right hand pocket of his vest, takes a second cigar from his left pocket, and smokes it quietly.

In addition to cross-cultural comparisons, there are also studies to be done in which various degrees of difference between culture and no culture are compared. The end of the continuum toward no culture, where the social prerequisites of a society are seriously failing, has been labeled by my colleagues and myself as sociocultural disintegration. Other people have noted the same or similar phenomena under a variety of names; one example is Lewis's (1961) culture of poverty. A striking feature of recent decades is the evident increase in the populations which are caught up to a growing extent and degree in this malfunctional condition. One is tempted to believe at times that as Neanderthal man was succeeded by civilized man, so the civilized in turn will be succeeded by the anomic man.

It appears that the world is afflicted with a parallel to entropy, that is, a descent away from patterning toward randomness. Communities, like individuals, appear to be losing a sense of identity and to be moving toward undifferentiated mass, a nonsystem kind of state, perhaps Hobbes's "war of all against all." This trend is accompanied by massive individual suffering of which psychiatric disorder is one variety.

There are, of course, countertrends manifest; among them are revivalistic religion, political action groups, encounter forms of psychological rehabilitation, and back to nature colonies. However, their capacity to reverse the overall trend is dubious at this time.

It is fairly clear that such groups often provide comfort, identity, and modes of expression for individuals. Their capacity to stop the deterioration of the social system as a whole is less evident. In fact, a case can be made for asserting that they foster the deterioration. In the larger urban areas especially, they appear to form societal lumps which are inert or negatively charged toward each other and hence are destructive to the functioning of the total social system and the fulfilling of its prerequisites. Lump formation results in flocculation rather than synthesis and as such is a form of social pathology. New York City with its strikes and conflict among garbage collectors, police, teachers, school boards, bus drivers, subway workers, and, of course, students, faculty and administration in colleges, constitutes a kind of exemplar of flocculation.

Dr. Caudill, in talking about Japanese industrial organization, indicated that the Japanese appear to do best in a social system providing small groups with which individuals can and do identify. This proclivity could well be a human universal rather than particularly Japanese. The organization of Japanese society is thus far such that the small subgroups are orchestrated so as to be supportive for individuals and also contributive to the functioning of the whole society. It may be that flocculation has emerged in the large metropolitan areas of the West due to population growth and the disappearance of subgroups that are both meaningful to the individual and contributive to the societal whole. Flocculation can be seen as an abortive form of reconstitution—a reaction against the anomic mass and state of nonsystem, one that falls short and, in so doing, increases the failing of the social system.

The fact of widely distributed sociocultural disintegration and flocculation inevitably raises the question of why. There is, perhaps, some illumination to be had from a study conducted almost twenty years ago at Cornell (A. H. Leighton and Smith, 1955). It happened that a number of us were engaged for various reasons in studies of seven small communities at widely scattered points around the earth: namely, Burma, India, Japan, Navaho country, Nova Scotia, Peru, and Thailand. Because of the cultural contrasts, it seemed of interest to compare these communities with each other in order to see if any common features or processes could be identified. As comparative description and qualitative analysis proceeded, a number of points soon became evident.

First, it was clear that in all seven communities, more services were being provided to more individuals than had ever been the case before. By services I mean such activities as welfare, health protection, formal education, and technical training in agriculture.

Secondly, hand in hand with the first, there was loss of local autonomy and increase of central bureaucratic control. Local leadership roles which, in the past, had been determinate in virtually everything except taxes and military services were being stripped down to positions of little influence, and with this, there developed sentiments of helplessness and powerlessness. In many instances, the services of health, education, and welfare were being greatly improved by the change, but the price everywhere in our seven communities was reduction in self-determination.

The third similarity was a matter of individual rights. While actual power was diminishing at the community level, strong sentiments were growing with regard to individual rights. People were becoming less and less willing to accept fatalistic ideas of being locked forever into low-ranking and uncomfortable roles. The widening of horizons through education and communication generated comparisons of self with others and a resultant ever increasing sense of relative deprivation. Distant, often fictional, reference groups became motivational forces in discontent. More and more people were growing to believe in the possibility of making life better for themselves and in their right so to do.

That these three trends are incompatible was evident to us at the time of the original study, and we were surprised at how widespread the phenomenon was and how similar in patterning. Differences from place to place seemed primarily matters of specific cultural content, duration, and degree of intensity in feeling. I think now that we were looking at an earlier phase of that psychological chain reaction and sociological explosion which has since traveled around the world and which has left so many millions of people as isolated particles uncertain of their identity, struggling in all directions for something to believe in and for membership in a group small enough to have meaning.

Could studies in the behavioral sciences now make it possible to find ways of converting flocculation within social systems into a viable rather than a suicidal process for mankind?

The Clinical Viewpoint

Under this heading, I am thinking of the papers by Drs. Yap, Takagi, Tan, Marsella, and Chu. These exceedingly valuable studies take much of their significance from the fact that they are not statistical but rather descriptions of processes. The fact that they come from a variety of cultural settings further augments their worth when they are considered together. I put emphasis on this point because in this day when tremendous capability has been placed in our hands by quantitative techniques, it is important not to overlook other vital components in the total complex of activities through which scientific discoveries are made. In the mental health field, there is no substitute for the perceptive eye and astute brain of the able clinician.

Looking to the future, it is to be hoped that the clinicians of today and tomorrow who, like Dr. Hahn, are considering these kinds of issues will embark on trials of radically new methods for delivering services. In Europe and North America, for example, the stone castles we call mental hospitals are, by and large, as outdated as their Norman counterparts. We are able to conceive what seem to us far better community based types of treatment and prophylactic services. But the solid masses of architecture and the money bound up in them stand in the way of much we should like to do. In many parts of the United States, the stone of the hospitals is almost literally millstone about the neck of psychiatry.

Countries which are not as yet so heavily committed to these institutions can, perhaps, establish world leadership through creating alternate modes for delivering services aimed at both treatment and prevention. In saying this, I realize that there are formidable difficulties to be overcome. In many places, both professional and political leaders are so imbued with the idea of the Western hospital and its type of organization that they will regard anything else as second best, if not worse, and hence unworthy of their country. It would be all too human if they were to insist on building bigger and more impressive millstones for their psychiatry to wear, but it would be regrettable. Perhaps the mental health workers can exert a helpful influence.

It would be appropriate to ask at this point what I mean by innovations in both treatment and prevention. I cannot answer properly because I am throwing out a challenge and talking about what has not yet been conceived. The general direction, however, can be sketched.

One possibility is to break the healing and care functions down into a much larger number of role categories. Para-professionals can then be trained for these positions in less time than is presently required. If adequately carried out, it seems likely that a system of this sort could serve more people and serve them better at no greater cost. Buildings would, of course, be needed, but these could be small, of simple construction, and decentralized so as to serve local areas with intimacy and fitness.

A second trend, which can be combined with the first, is the utilization of indigenous institutions that already in some degree care for the psychiatrically disturbed. Many native healers and religious groups function this way. Why not try to develop and set standards rather than displace them?

There are, I concede, extremely strong feelings against both of these suggestions. I think I understand on what these are based, and I can respect them even though I think they are in error, just as I think the American Medical Association has been in error in many of its positions. Social and psychological processes are in motion which will prevail in their demand for more services at lower rates, and it is my belief that sooner or later drastic restructuring will arrive. Sooner rather than later will be better for people generally, and it is here that the challenge for leadership lies.

An actual example that includes the ideas sketched above can be seen in the clinic at Khartoum North in the Republic of Sudan. Established by Tigani El Mahi and developed by T. A. Baasher, it maximizes its service through the use of medical assistants and cooperates with selected religious healers. More recently a similar relationship with native healers has been developed by Collomb at the Fann Hospital in Dakar. Lambo's use of Nigerian villages as residential and therapeutic centers is, of course, well known and has existed now for over a decade. His plan includes both especially trained assistants and native healers. At our meeting here, Dr. Tan and Dr. Schmidt have told me of programs that incorporate some of the same ideas.

Professions that are neighbors to psychiatry in the health field, such as internal medicine and surgery, have, of course, also established some working models of the same general kind. The program in Fiji is one of these, and another, more recent model, was established among the Navajos by Walsh MacDermott (1960). A feature here was the development of a para-professional role called "health visitor."

Outside the field of medicine, there have also been examples of redesigning technical functions so that subspecialist roles are developed for which people with limited formal education can be quickly trained. I have been informed that the retiring vice-chancellor of the East-West Center, Baron Goto, has been outstanding in the successful development of para-technical aids in agriculture for much of the Pacific.

These examples indicate that such programs are feasible, and this encourages further endeavor. A main frontier now is evaluation. How well do these systems work? Surely, the next efforts along these lines should be designed with a view to measuring effectiveness and so rescue us from the cloudy and treacherous shores of opinion. It is here that behavioral science methods and the clinical viewpoint might join forces with great effect.

Basic to all ideas about providing services is comprehensive understanding with regard to peoples' concepts of mental health and mental illness. What is the specific content of each culture, and how do these ideas compare one with another? Except for the work of Dr. Yap and a few others, very little has been done in this field. Yet it is one that has not only the pragmatic importance indicated above, but it has great heuristic value as well. Psychiatry would greatly benefit from a series of systematic studies that took up language by language and dialect by dialect the full list of words that refer to mental health or disorder and gave for each descriptive accounts and case history examples. This is work requiring only a small budget, and it is of such a nature that with a little linguistic advice it could be undertaken by clinicians during free time and could start with cultural groups within easy reach. Annotated glossaries of this kind would vastly enhance our background knowledge as a basis for providing services and, at the same time, would give basic information necessary for understanding the interrelation of culture and psychiatric disorder.

Another suggestion for a research area that is low budget and within the reach of most clinicians has to do with the fact that psychiatric disorder appears to be different in men as compared to women. Numbers of epidemiological studies have now shown that there are not only differences in overall frequencies, but also differential rates among various patterns of symptoms, differential rates with regard to age and, finally, with regard to sociocultural stresses. The statistics, however, only point to relationships and differences. To get leads on "why," it is appropriate to return to the clinic and develop accurate descriptions of the natural history and process of disorder as seen in selected men and women. From such investigations, new light may come regarding causal factors—intrapsychic, interpersonal, and cultural. This is apposite to what Dr. Hahn said about comparative personality studies and also to Dr. Takagi's interest in unusual syndromes. It is possible that much can be learned of transcendent importance for the current and future problem of family and social stability and for population control.

Psychiatric Epidemiology

This final topic is relevant to the papers by Drs. Chu, Escudero, Murphy, and Tung, and all my personal biases incline toward underscoring its importance. We know so little about how much psychiatric disorder there is in populations and how it is distributed in relation to social and cultural factors that the field has some of the characteristics of basic sciences, such as genetics and biochemistry as applied to human behavior. There is also, however, a practical aspect and that is its use as a guide to services, the evaluation of results from giving services, and, ultimately, the development of preventive action.

Outstanding, therefore, is the task of mapping distributions in all the populations of the world. Gateways toward understanding many aspects of etiology will be opened when this task is accomplished. I believe that there is a parallel here to the importance that species description had for the development of ecology, oceanography, ethology and other fields comprehensive of the living processes on earth.

The exciting thing is that recently comparative epidemiology has come within our grasp. There is now enough experience to show that if investigators focus on behavior patterns of psychiatric relevance, high degrees of reliability are obtainable. Not all the operational criteria are, of course, sufficiently defined and standardized, but I do believe that it has been demonstrated that the way is open.

This does not mean that everything is easy. Saying that the objective is achievable is not the equivalent of saying it is free of difficulties. My contention is that trials made thus far suggest very strongly that the issues, complex though they be, are resolvable. What we have at our disposal are ways of conceptualizing psychiatric phenomena that create new possibilities for quantification, methods that gather data in accordance with these conceptualizations, and statistical and computer resources that can handle complex relations among large numbers of variables in a manner that would have been impossible a few years ago.

Because of these potentialities, I would like to suggest that the time has come to begin thinking of what might be called a standard core to be employed in surveys of psychiatric disorder prevalence in all parts of the world. The assumption underlying this notion is that various research workers in different countries will always have a prime desire to answer questions germane to their own research interests and to the culture and socioeconomic conditions of the population they are studying. This does not, however, prohibit gathering a certain limited amount of data according to prescribed techniques that would be the same from one study to another. All those participating in the use of such a standard core could then work cooperatively toward the mapping of the psychiatric phenomena and in comparative analysis.

The studies of Dr. Zubin and his British-American colleagues (Gurland et al., 1969) are an outstanding example of cross-national comparison where the subjects are hospitalized patients. They promise to clarify whether differences in the psychiatric statistics of the United States and Britain are in fact differences in labels or differences in phenomena. The work of Katz in Hawaii in comparing the behavior of patients from different cultural groups is also germane to this central idea. The current World Health Organization study of schizophrenia in various cultures is another case in point. Developed by the genius of Tsung-yi Lin, this work is concerned with establishing standard criteria and procedures in terms of which the distribution of this major pattern of disorder (or group of disorders with similar manifestations) can be assessed.

The work of our Stirling County group has been more heterogeneous, utilizing samples and covering all kinds of psychiatric disorders in the population at large without regard to whether there has been treatment. Collaborative and comparative studies have been undertaken by us with researchers in Sweden (D. C. Leighton, in press), Nigeria (A. H. Leighton, 1963), and Senegal, and this has given support to the idea that a standard core for epidemiological investigation is both highly desirable and possible and, further, that certain standard computerized techniques for analysis can be widely applied.

I should like to suggest that the time is at hand when it would be profitable to form some kind of international group interested in cooperating and collaborating in comparative studies of psychiatric epidemiology. I shall not spend time here speculating about how this might be done nor about its structure, but I do wish to lay it before each of the members of this meeting for his consideration and before our hosts at the East-West Center.

In the meantime, pending the development of a collaborative institution, there is much work that can be done by individuals without mobilizing large amounts of money. Thus, for example, some of the methodological fundamentals can be accomplished. Reference has already been made to creating lexicons of mental health and illness terms in various languages and local dialects. A further step might be the translation into one of those languages of the questionnaire items that might be candidates for a standard score. Such a task involves much more than literal translation. It comprehends translation of essential meaning and identifying parallels in different systems of thought, and it marks out the areas in which comparison is impossible as well as those in which it can be done.

In adapting its questionnaire items to the Yoruba in Nigeria and the Serrer in Senegal, the Stirling group has found the task both illuminating and absorbing. We are at present engaged in further exploration of this kind in collaboration with the Musée de l'Homme in Paris. The language and cultural groups in question are the Bassari, another tribe in Senegal, and the Ammassalik Eskimos of Greenland. Quite aside from the actual surveys, the work is of immense value in clarifying conceptual problems by texts against nature, problems which otherwise remain the topic of endless, paralyzing speculation. Such studies, though very modest in cost and manpower, can yield results as worthy of publication as the large scale surveys.

All my comments so far have dealt with the dependent variable. Because I have already taken so much time, I shall only briefly mention one point. The independent variable—social and cultural factors—is of coequal importance with the dependent variable, if we are to make progress in understanding the relations between the two. Conceptualization and method are not so well developed here as for the dependent variable, but they are not too far behind. Enough has been done to show promise of major advances as commensurate effort is applied to this other half of the total problem.

Conclusion

Even the longest river eventually reaches the sea, and so with apologies for being prolix I shall close. In doing so, I should like to return once more to the wide view of our beginning.

One way of summarizing and interpreting man's adaptation to

change is to say that ever since he has appeared on the stage of history he has been causing changes and has always been frightened by the consequent effects on human relations. To escape from his fears he is always constructing myths and institutions. But these myths and institutions are never more than partially successful, and as change continues, they become progressively less so and have to be replaced. This process of replacement is generally accomplished at enormous cost in destruction, death, and especially, suffering—incalculable suffering.

This is primitive and wasteful. Could we as behavioral scientists consider that, whatever the avenue of our approach, our central task in these times is to find ways and means for humanizing change and adaptation to change? Can we make a contribution by pointing out how the destruction and the suffering might be reduced, the cruelty of the price made less?

We spoke earlier about complexities. One of the ways in which myths and institutions fail and bring disaster with their tumbling is through being too simple for the actual complexities of man's social and psychological nature. Fear and disorientation generate polarizations and definitive targets with the result that adaptations are self-defeating. Is one of our functions to find ways to make complexity manageable? Can we keep before the eyes and minds of policy makers, politicians, and the public the realization that the notion of good guys and bad guys is a disastrous guide and that myths and institutions must be created that comprehend the actual dynamic complexities of man's psychological and social being in order for him to survive?

It was said at this meeting that the fatalism of the East, contrary to what many people think, is positive and purposeful, while the fatalism of the West tends to be nihilistic. Could we blend in the behavioral sciences the activism and pragmatism of the West with the confident and purposeful fatalism of the East?

REFERENCES

Brown, B. S., and S. E. Long. 1968. Psychology and community mental health, the medical muddle. American Psychologist 23:335–41.

Gurland, B. J., et al. 1969. Cross-national study of diagnosis of the mental disorders: some comparisons of diagnositc criteria from the first investigation. American Journal of Psychiatry. April Supplement:30–39.

Hughes, C. C., et al. 1960. People of Cove and Woodlot. New York, Basic Books, Inc.

Leighton, A. H., and R. J. Smith. 1955. A comparative study of social and cultural change. Proceedings of the American Philosophical Society 99, No. 2, April.

Leighton, A. H. 1959. My name is legion. New York, Basic Books, Inc.

Leighton, A. H., et al. 1963. Psychiatric disorder among the Yoruba. Ithaca, Cornell University Press.

Leighton, D. C., et al. 1963. The character of danger. New York, Basic Books, Inc.

———. In press. Psychiatric disorder in a Swedish and a Canadian community: an exploratory study.

Lewis, O. 1961. The children of Sanchez. New York, Random House.

McDermott, W., et al. 1960. Introducing modern medicine in a Navajo community. Science 131:197–205, 280–87.

Index